T0226488

Aortic Valve Disease

Editors

MARIE-ANNICK CLAVEL
PHILIPPE PIBAROT

CARDIOLOGY CLINICS

www.cardiology.theclinics.com

February 2020 • Volume 38 • Number 1

ELSEVIER

1600 John F. Kennedy Boulevard • Suite 1800 • Philadelphia, Pennsylvania, 19103-2899

http://www.theclinics.com

CARDIOLOGY CLINICS Volume 38, Number 1
February 2020 ISSN 0733-8651, ISBN-13: 978-0-323-71161-6

Editor: Stacy Eastman
Developmental Editor: Laura Kavanaugh

Cardiology Clinics (ISSN 0733-8651) is published quarterly by Elsevier Inc., 360 Park Avenue South, New York, NY 10010-1710. Months of issue are February, May, August, and November. Business and Editorial Offices: 1600 John F. Kennedy Blvd., Ste. 1800, Philadelphia, PA 19103-2899. Customer Service Office: 3251 Riverport Lane, Maryland Heights, MO 63043. Periodicals post-age paid at New York, NY and additional mailing offices. Subscription prices are $352.00 per year for US individuals, $706.00 per year for US institutions, $100.00 per year for US students and residents, $432.00 per year for Canadian individuals, $885.00 per year for Canadian institutions, $466.00 per year for international individuals, $885.00 per year for international institutions, $100.00 per year for Canadian students/residents and $220.00 per year for international students/residents. To receive student/resident rate, orders must be accompanied by name of affiliated institution, data of term, and the *signature* of program/residency coordinator on institution letterhead. Orders will be billed at individual rate until proof of status is received. Foreign air speed delivery is included in all *Clinics* subscription prices. All prices are subject to change without notice. **POSTMASTER:** Send address changes to *Cardiology Clinics*, Elsevier Health Sciences Division, Subscription Customer Service, 3251 Riverport Lane, Maryland Heights, MO 63043. **Customer Service: 1-800-654-2452 (U.S. and Canada); 314-447-8871 (outside U.S. and Canada). Fax: 314-447-8029. E-mail: journalscus-tomerservice-usa@elsevier.com (for print support); journalsonlinesupport-usa@elsevier.com (for online support).**

Reprints. For copies of 100 or more, of articles in this publication, please contact the Commercial Reprints Department, Elsevier Inc., 360 Park Avenue South, New York, NY 10010-1710. Tel.: 212-633-3874; Fax: 212-633-3820; E-mail: reprints@elsevier.com.

Cardiology Clinics is also published in Spanish by McGraw-Hill Interamericana Editores S. A., P.O. Box 5-237, 06500, Mexico D. F., Mexico; in Portuguese by Reichmann and Alfonso Editores Rio de Janeiro, Brazil; and in Greek by Dimitrios P. Lagos, 8 Pondon Street, GR115-28 Ilissia, Greece.

Cardiology Clinics is covered in *MEDLINE/PubMed (Index Medicus), Excerpta Medica, The Cumulative Index to Nursing and Allied Health Literature* (CINAHL).

Contributors

JOHN B. CHAMBERS, MD, FESC, FACC
Professor of Clinical Cardiology and
Consultant Cardiologist, Cardiothoracic
Center, Guy's and St Thomas' Hospitals,
London, United Kingdom

MARIE-ANNICK CLAVEL, DVM, PhD
Associate Professor at Faculté de Médecine,
Institut Universitaire de Cardiologie et de
Pneumologie de Québec (IUCPQ) - Université
Laval, Québec Heart and Lung Institute,
Québec City, Québec, Canada

NANCY CÔTÉ, PhD
Institut Universitaire de Cardiologie
et de Pneumologie de Québec (IUCPQ) -
Université Laval, Québec Heart and
Lung Institute, Québec City, Québec,
Canada

JORDI S. DAHL, MD, PhD
Department of Cardiology, Odense University
Hospital, Odense, Denmark

MARC R. DWECK, MD, PhD
British Heart Foundation Centre for
Cardiovascular Science, University of
Edinburgh, United Kingdom

ISMAIL EL-HAMAMSY, MD, PhD
Division of Cardiac Surgery, Montreal Heart
Institute, Université de Montréal, Montreal,
Québec, Canada

MIHO FUKUI, MD, PhD
Minneapolis Heart Institute Foundation,
Cardiovascular Imaging Research and Valve
Science Centers, Minneapolis, Minnesota,
USA

PHILIPPE GÉNÉREUX, MD
Division of Cardiology, Morristown
Medical Center, Morristown, New Jersey,
USA

REBECCA T. HAHN, MD
Division of Cardiology, Columbia University
Medical Center, NewYork–Presbyterian
Hospital, New York, New York, USA

ROGER HALL, MD
Department of Cardiology, Norwich Medical
School, University of East Anglia, Norwich,
United Kingdom

ANDREW W. HARRIS, MD
Fellow, Department of Medicine, Division of
Cardiology, University of Washington, Seattle,
Washington, USA

PATRIZIO LANCELLOTTI, MD, FESC, FACC
Professor, Department of Cardiology,
Heart Valve Clinic, CHU Sart Tilman, Liège,
Belgium

AMINE MAZINE, MD, MSc
Division of Cardiac Surgery, University
of Toronto, Toronto, Ontario, Canada;
Montreal Heart Institute, Montreal, Québec,
Canada

TAMIM M. NAZIF, MD
Division of Cardiology, Columbia University
Medical Center, NewYork–Presbyterian
Hospital, New York, New York, USA

VIVIAN G. NG, MD
Division of Cardiology, Columbia University
Medical Center, NewYork–Presbyterian
Hospital, New York, New York,
USA

CATHERINE M. OTTO, MD
Professor, Department of Medicine, Division of
Cardiology, University of Washington, Seattle,
Washington, USA

CÉCILE OURY, PhD
Laboratory of Cardiology, Department of
Cardiology, GIGA-Cardiovascular Sciences,
University of Liège Hospital, University of
Liège, CHU du Sart Tilman, Domaine
Universitaire du Sart Tilman, Liège,
Belgium

PALINA PIANKOVA, MSc
Centre for Clinical Epidemiology, Jewish
General Hospital, McGill University, Montreal,
Québec, Canada

PHILIPPE PIBAROT, DVM, PhD
Full Professor at Faculté de Médecine,
Université Laval, Canada Research
Chair in Valvular Heart Disease, Head of
Cardiology Research, Institut Universitaire
de Cardiologie et de Pneumologie
de Québec, Québec Heart and Lung
Institute, Québec, Canada

JOSEP RODÉS-CABAU, MD
Doctor, Institut Universitaire de Cardiologie et de Pneumologie de Québec, Québec Heart and Lung Institute, Laval University, Québec, Québec, Canada

ERWAN SALAUN, MD, PhD
Fellow, Institut Universitaire de Cardiologie et de Pneumologie de Québec, Québec Heart and Lung Institute, Laval University, Québec, Québec, Canada

JULIEN TERNACLE, MD, PhD
Institut Universitaire de Cardiologie et de Pneumologie de Québec, Québec Heart and Lung Institute, Université Laval, Québec City, Québec, Canada; Cardiology Department, Expert Valve Center, Henri Mondor Hospital, INSERM Unit U955, Team 8, Paris-Est Creteil University, Val-de-Marne, Créteil, France

CHRISTOPHE TRIBOUILLOY, MD, PhD
Department of Cardiology, Amiens University Hospital, Jules Verne University of Picardie, Amiens, France

EVANGELOS TZOLOS, MD
British Heart Foundation Centre for Cardiovascular Science, University of Edinburgh, United Kingdom

PHILIPPE UNGER, MD, PhD
Department of Cardiology, CHU Saint-Pierre, Université Libre de Bruxelles, Brussels, Belgium

KANG H. ZHENG, MD
Department of Vascular Medicine, Amsterdam UMC, University of Amsterdam, The Netherlands

Contents

Calcific aortic valve stenosis is the commonest form of heart valve disease in high-income countries and set to become a major health care burden. Currently, there are no medical therapies that have proved to slow down or halt disease progression. The only available treatment is aortic valve replacement, of which the optimal timing is unknown and to which not all patients are suited. This review discusses the pathophysiology of aortic stenosis, how noninvasive imaging techniques have improved our understanding of the underlying biology, and how these emerging insights might translate into potential novel treatments targeting oxidized lipids, fibrosis, and calcification.

Severe aortic stenosis (AS) is associated with a progressive cardiac remodeling that ultimately leads to heart failure and death if the valve is not replaced. The confirmation of AS severity is therefore crucial to adequately manage patients with AS. Transthoracic echocardiography is the first-line examination to confirm AS severity, but it may be inconclusive in discordant cases. In this setting, AS severity should be confirmed using a multimodality imaging approach. This review gives an overview of how to assess and/or confirm AS severity, especially in case of discordance.

Severe aortic stenosis (AS) causes chronic pressure overload of the left ventricle (LV), resulting in the progressive cardiac damage, which extends beyond the LV. Several previous studies have shown a relationship of the cardiac damage to AS, rather than the stenosis severity, with adverse events after aortic valve replacement (AVR) in patients with severe AS. A new staging system for AS patients has important prognostic implications for clinical outcomes after AVR. This review summarizes the importance of assessment of cardiac damage in patients with AS.

Aortic stenosis presenting as part of a multiple valve disease scenario or as mixed valve disease is frequent. These scenarios induce hemodynamic interactions that may result in diagnostic pitfalls. Echocardiography is the cornerstone technique for diagnosis of valve disorders, but other modalities may be useful. In addition to assessment of each individual lesion, the heart valve team must integrate numerous parameters into the management strategy, including global assessment of clinical and hemodynamic effects, operative risk, life expectancy, natural history of untreated valve disease, valve reparability, and/or suitability for single or multiple transcatheter valve procedures.

clinical practice, frailty can be evaluated by a tiered approach starting with a brief screening tool such as the Essential Frailty Toolset.

Procedures and Outcomes of Surgical Aortic Valve Replacement in Adults   89

Amine Mazine and Ismail El-Hamamsy

The ideal aortic valve substitute remains elusive. Bioprosthetic valves are the replacement option of choice in elderly patients undergoing aortic valve replacement (AVR). When implanted in young and middle-aged adults, both bioprosthetic and mechanical valves are associated with excess mortality compared with the age- and sex-matched general population. The Ross procedure is the only operation that can restore normal life expectancy in young and middle-aged adults undergoing AVR. In this article, the authors review the various options for surgical AVR and examine their contemporary applications and outcomes.

Planning for Success: Pre-procedural Evaluation for Transcatheter Aortic Valve Replacement   103

Vivian G. Ng, Rebecca T. Hahn, and Tamim M. Nazif

Advancements in transcatheter heart valve technology have greatly improved the ease and safety of the TAVR procedure. Nevertheless, multi-modality imaging remains vital to performing these procedures safely and effectively. Pre-procedural echocardiography and MSCT facilitate procedural planning, guide the choice of valve type and size, and allow prediction of potential complications. Furthermore, intra-procedural echocardiography can be used to provide additional real-time guidance.

Transcatheter Aortic Valve Replacement: Procedure and Outcomes   115

Erwan Salaun, Philippe Pibarot, and Josep Rodés-Cabau

Initially, transcatheter aortic valve replacement (TAVR) was only used in patients with severe symptomatic aortic stenosis and prohibitive risk for surgical aortic valve replacement. Subsequently, TAVR was extended to patients with high and intermediate surgical risk. Recently, the results of randomized trials in low-surgical-risk patients showed superiority or noninferiority of TAVR versus surgical aortic valve replacement in this population. Procedural outcomes have been improved. Long-term durability of transcatheter heart valves remains to be confirmed. This article presents the evolution and current status of TAVR, with respect to the different types of devices and procedures as well as its outcomes.

Sex Differences in the Pathophysiology, Diagnosis, and Management of Aortic Stenosis   129

Nancy Côté and Marie-Annick Clavel

For years, calcific aortic stenosis (AS) was considered to be similar in men and women, and the underrepresentation of women in research studies prevented any alternate conclusions. With new sex-specific studies and data, the landscape of AS is evolving and recently important sex-disparities were revealed. These sex-specific discrepancies are of utmost importance to stratify and personalize treatment according to sex. It is important and urgent to elucidate the sex-related differences and similarities in the pathophysiology of AS to develop and validate sex-

CARDIOLOGY CLINICS

SERIES OF RELATED INTEREST

Cardiac Electrophysiology Clinics
Heart Failure Clinics
Interventional Cardiology Clinics

THE CLINICS ARE AVAILABLE ONLINE!
Access your subscription at:
www.theclinics.com

Preface
A Decade of Revolutions in Calcific Aortic Stenosis

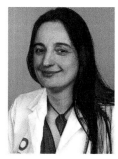 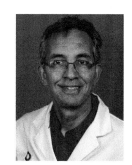

Marie-Annick Clavel, DVM, PhD   Philippe Pibarot, DVM, PhD

Editors

Calcific aortic stenosis (AS) is the most frequent valvular heart disease in high-income countries and the third most frequent cardiovascular disease after hypertension and coronary artery disease. The prevalence of aortic sclerosis (ie, the preclinical stage of AS) is estimated at 25% in the general population older than 65 years and close to 50% in those older than 80 years.[1] The prevalence of AS is less than 1% in the population less than 60 years old,[2] but increases exponentially to more than 10% in elderly people older than 75 years.[3,4] The prevalence of this disease is expected to triple by 2050 due to population aging. If left untreated, AS is inevitably fatal, and there are currently no pharmacotherapies that can halt or delay its progression. The only available option for the treatment of severe AS is thus aortic valve replacement (AVR) by a prosthetic valve using open heart surgery or transcatheter valve implantation. AS is directly responsible for approximately 20,000 deaths and 150,000 AVR procedures per year in North America.

Despite important discoveries and major progress in the understanding and management of AS during the past 10 to 15 years, some important unmet clinical needs persist with regards to the prevention, diagnosis, and treatment of AS. The advent of unbiased approaches, genetics, and epigenomics led to the identification of new promising therapeutic targets that will need to be tested in randomized trials. Multimodality imaging, including aortic valve calcium scoring by multidetector computed tomography and quantitation of myocardial fibrosis by cardiac magnetic resonance imaging, has been recently developed and validated and may be useful to enhance (i) grading of AS severity; (ii) staging of associated cardiac damage; and (iii) decision making for timing and type of AVR. Transcatheter AVR has emerged as an alternative to surgical AVR in patients with intermediate- or high-surgical risk and will likely be extended to the low-risk patients in the near future.

This issue of *Cardiology Clinics* presents a state-of-the art overview of the different aspects of AS, including pathophysiology, diagnosis, and treatment.

Marie-Annick Clavel, DVM, PhD
Associate Professor at Faculté de Médecine
Université Laval
Institut Universitaire de Cardiologie et de
Pneumologie de Québec
2725 Chemin Sainte Foy #A-2047
Québec, G1V4G5, Canada

Philippe Pibarot, DVM, PhD
Full Professor at Faculté de Médecine
Université Laval
Canada Research Chair in Valvular Heart Disease
Head of Cardiology Research
Institut Universitaire de Cardiologie et de
Pneumologie de Québec
Québec Heart and Lung Institute
2725 Chemin Sainte Foy #A-2039
Québec, G1V4G5, Canada

E-mail addresses:
Marie-annick.clavel@criucpq.ulaval.ca
(M.-A. Clavel)
Philippe.Pibarot@med.ulaval.ca (P. Pibarot)

cardiology.theclinics.com

REFERENCES

1. Coffey S, Cox B, Williams MJ. The prevalence, incidence, progression, and risks of aortic valve sclerosis: a systematic review and meta-analysis. J Am Coll Cardiol 2014;63:2852–61.
2. Eveborn GW, Schirmer H, Heggelund G, et al. The evolving epidemiology of valvular aortic stenosis. the Tromso study. Heart 2013;99:396–400.
3. Osnabrugge RL, Mylotte D, Head SJ, et al. Aortic stenosis in the elderly: disease prevalence and number of candidates for transcatheter aortic valve replacement: a meta-analysis and modeling study. J Am Coll Cardiol 2013;62:1002–12.
4. Lindman BR, Clavel MA, Mathieu P, et al. Calcific aortic stenosis. Nat Rev Dis Primers 2016;2:16006.

Pathophysiology of Aortic Stenosis and Future Perspectives for Medical Therapy

Kang H. Zheng, MD[a], Evangelos Tzolos, MD[b], Marc R. Dweck, MD, PhD[b],*

KEYWORDS

- Aortic valve stenosis • Pathophysiology • Imaging • Treatment targets • Drug development

KEY POINTS

- Calcific aortic valve stenosis is the commonest heart valve disease in high-income countries and set to become a major health care burden.
- Aortic stenosis is a disease of both the valve and the myocardium.
- Currently, there are no medical therapies that have proved to slow down or halt disease progression in aortic stenosis.
- Novel insights in the valvular pathophysiology of aortic stenosis progression have identified numerous molecular targets related to oxidized lipids, calcification, and fibrosis, although only a few have so far been translated to clinical trials.
- Non-invasive imaging modalities such as CT calcium scoring, 18F-NaF PET, and cardiac MRI can assist in risk stratification and the clinical development of drug treatments.

INTRODUCTION

Calcific aortic stenosis (AS) is the most common valve disease in the high-income countries and is set to become a major health care burden with an aging population.[1] It is characterized by fibrocalcific remodeling of the valve leaflets, resulting in progressive narrowing of the aortic valve opening and a hypertrophic response of the left ventricle, which may culminate in heart failure, syncope, angina, and ultimately death.

Although the associated risk factors for AS incidence are similar to atherosclerosis, treatment with statins has failed to slow AS progression in 3 randomized controlled trials.[2–4] Moreover, the optimal timing of valve intervention remains unknown[5]: too early and patients are unnecessarily exposed to the risk of perioperative complications and the long-term risks associated with prosthetic valves; too late and patients are left with irreversible myocardial damage that places them at future risk of heart failure and early mortality. Although optimizing the timing of aortic valve replacement remains an important goal, the development of novel treatments to prevent or slow down AS would be ideal, potentially obviating surgical intervention altogether. An improved understanding of the pathogenesis of AS with respect to both the valve and the myocardium is required to achieve both these aims.

This article discusses the pathophysiology of AS, how noninvasive imaging techniques have improved our understanding of the

[a] Department of Vascular Medicine, Amsterdam UMC, University of Amsterdam, Meibergdreef 9, 1105 AZ Amsterdam, The Netherlands; [b] British Heart Foundation Centre for Cardiovascular Science, University of Edinburgh, The Chancellor's Building, Little France Crescent, Midlothian, Edinburgh EH26 0NL, UK
* Corresponding author.
E-mail address: marc.dweck@ed.ac.uk

Cardiol Clin 38 (2020) 1–12
https://doi.org/10.1016/j.ccl.2019.09.010

underlying biology, and how these emerging insights might translate into potential novel treatments.

PATHOPHYSIOLOGY

AS was long considered a degenerative disease, in which "wear and tear" over the years resulted in gradual accumulation of calcium in the valve leaflets. It is now clear that AS is instead the result of actively regulated and complex cellular processes, coordinated by valve interstitial cells (VICs),[6] a fibroblast-like cell predominantly populating the aortic valve (**Fig. 1**). Over the past decade, compelling evidence from basic science and clinical studies has led us to consider the pathophysiology as occurring in 2 distinct phases: *the initiation phase*, similar to atherosclerosis and characterized by endothelial damage, lipid infiltration, and inflammation; and *the propagation phase*, in which VICs assume an osteoblast-like phenotype and drive a self-

perpetuating cycle of valve calcification with similarities to skeletal bone formation.[7]

Initiation Phase: Lipid Deposition and Inflammation

Early valve lesions are characterized by endothelial damage, lipid deposition, chronic inflammatory infiltrates, and microcalcification.[8] The initiating event is believed to be injury to the valvular endothelium due to mechanical stress or other risk factors, which allows infiltration and retention of lipoproteins and recruitment of inflammatory cells. The importance of mechanical stress is best illustrated by individuals with bicuspid aortic valves (1%–2% in the general population), in whom the altered valve structure results in abnormal hemodynamics and increased mechanical stresses.[9] Patients with bicuspid aortic valves almost invariably develop AS and in general require intervention 1 to 2 decades earlier than patients with tricuspid valves.[10]

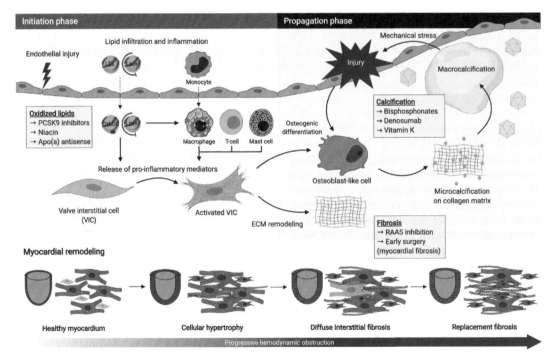

Fig. 1. The pathogenesis of AS. Initiation phase: the initiating event of AS is believed to be injury to the valvular endothelium due to mechanical stress or other risk factors. Low-density lipoprotein (LDL) and lipoprotein(a) [Lp(a)] accumulate and infiltrate the subendothelial fibrosa layer and undergo oxidative modification. This causes a chronic inflammatory response involving recruitment of macrophages, T cells, and mast cells, leading to activation of valve interstitial cells (VICs). Lipid-lowering drugs may reduce AS risk. Propagation phase: activated VICs produce disorganized collagen causing fibrosis and progressive valve thickening and stiffening. RAAS inhibition may have antifibrotic effects. Early surgery may prevent midwall fibrosis. Osteoblast-like cells produce calcifying extracellular vesicles. Calcification of the valve induces compliance mismatch, resulting in increased mechanical stress, injury, apoptosis, and osteoblast activation, which triggers further calcification resulting in a vicious cycle. Bisphosphonates, denosumab, and vitamin K target calcification pathways. RAAS, renin-angiotensin-aldosteron system.

Following endothelial injury, low-density lipoprotein (LDL) and lipoprotein(a) [Lp(a)] particles are able to accumulate in the subendothelial fibrosa layer and undergo oxidative modification,[11,12] promoting a chronic inflammatory response in which macrophages, T cells, and mast cells are recruited through increased expression of endothelial adhesion molecules such as ICAM-1, VCAM-1, and E-selectin.[8,13] These immune cells produce proinflammatory cytokines and proteolytic enzymes that promote and maintain fibrotic and calcific processes in the valve. Concomitantly, oxidized LDLs are cytotoxic[14] and stimulate osteogenic differentiation of VICs via toll-like receptors 2 and 4.[15] Valve explant studies have shown that greater accumulation of oxidized LDLs in the valve and increased levels of circulating oxidized LDLs are associated with worse fibrocalcific remodeling of the valve leaflets.[16,17] In addition, oxidized LDLs and Lp(a) are rich in oxidized phospholipids (OxPL), which have strong proinflammatory and osteogenic properties.[18] Autotaxin, a phospholipase enzyme enriched in the Lp(a) fraction and also produced by VICs, can transform OxPL to the lipid mediator lysophosphatidic acid, which induces calcification of VICs and accelerates development of valvular calcification in a mouse model through an inflammatory nuclear factor-kappa B (NF-κB)/interleukin-6/bone morphogenic protein (BMP) signaling pathway.[19] Lp(a) particles without the presence of OxPL have also been shown to be able to induce osteogenic differentiation of VICs in culture through several putative pathways, including phosphorylation of mitogen-activated protein kinases.[20] Genome-wide association studies have reported associations between genetically elevated levels of LDL cholesterol or Lp(a) with aortic valve calcium measured by computed tomography (CT) and AS incidence, strongly suggesting a causal relationship.[21-24]

Molecular imaging studies have laid the foundation for shaping the paradigm that inflammation leads to calcification.[25] In humans, these concepts were corroborated in vivo using serial PET/CT imaging studies of the aortic valve. In individuals without any aortic valve calcification, increased valvular uptake of glucose analogue fludeoxyglucose F 18 (18F-FDG) (as a marker of inflammation) at baseline was associated with an increased risk of subsequent calcification visible on CT during follow-up.[26] Patients with mild to moderate AS also demonstrated increased valvular uptake of 18F-FDG.[27]

Insights from Genetic Studies

Although early family studies suggested genetic predispositions to the risk of aortic valve surgery[28] and bicuspid aortic valve disease,[29-31] a recent nationwide Swedish registry study established the concept of familial risk for AS incidence in the general population.[32] Having a sibling with AS increases the risk to develop the disease by ~3.5-fold, whereas a spouse history was associated with only a modest increase of risk (hazard ratio ~1.17).

Since the first linkage studies identified mutations in NOTCH1 to be associated with bicuspid aortic valve disease and severe calcification of the valve leaflets,[33] large genome-wide association studies have started to identify genetic variants that infer an increased risk of AS. A multitude of studies have robustly established a highly likely causal relationship between single nucleotide polymorphisms (SNP) in the LPA gene encoding for apolipoprotein(a), elevated plasma levels of Lp(a), and increased risk of aortic valve calcium and AS.[22,24,34-36] Other genomic studies have identified SNPs in RUNX2—confirming its key role in the pathogenesis of aortic valve calcification—and CACNA1C to be associated with AS.[37] Several variants in genes such as MYH6[38] and GATA4/5,[39,40] as well as several mutations causing genetic syndromes,[41] have been reported to associate with bicuspid aortic valves.

Recently, risk variants were identified in the PALMD and TEX41 loci, which were associated with AS.[35,42] Both the PALMD and TEX41 risk variants were also associated with bicuspid aortic valve disease and congenital cardiac septal defects. The risk variant in PALMD was also identified using a transcriptome-wide analysis of explanted tricuspid valves only.[42] The risk alleles in PALMD were associated with lower levels of PALMD gene expression in the explanted valves, but the exact function of PALMD protein is unknown.

Propagation Phase: Fibrosis and Calcification

Histologic and noninvasive imaging studies have established that calcification is a ubiquitous finding during disease progression. However, emerging data on patients with bicuspid aortic valve disease[43] and studies investigating sex differences in AS[44] suggest that fibrosis also plays an important role, particularly in women and younger patients.[45]

In the Multi-Ethnic Study of Atherosclerosis, a longitudinal population study that used repeat CT scans to quantify aortic valve calcium, the presence of valvular calcification at baseline was a strong and independent predictor of progression of aortic valve calcium while traditional cardiovascular risk factors did not predict disease progression when adjusted for baseline calcium.[46]

Prospective cohort studies have shown that disease progressed faster with increasing hemodynamic or calcification severity,[47] whereas severe calcification as measured using CT was strongly associated with increased mortality.[48,49] Nuclear imaging studies that take advantage of 18F-NaF, a radioactive tracer that is incorporated into newly developing hydroxyapatite crystals, have demonstrated that 18F-NaF PET/CT provides a marker of calcification activity in both valve and vasculature, before any macrocalcification is visible on CT.[50–53] Valvular uptake of 18F-NaF was shown to predict progression of calcification during follow-up in patients with AS.[54] In these studies, the strongest predictor of calcification activity (and thus disease progression) was the severity of established calcification and stenosis.

In the inflammatory milieu of valve lesions, VICs are activated and stimulated to proliferate, produce collagen, and secrete proteases including matrix metalloproteinases[55–59] and cathepsins,[60] thus actively regulating the remodeling of the extracellular matrix. This results in accumulation of disorganized fibrous tissue and provides a scaffold on which nucleation of calcium phosphate crystals can start. Macrophages and VICs release calcifying extracellular vesicles[61] resembling matrix vesicles created in the bone—mediated by the multiligand sorting receptor sortilin[62,63]— which may aggregate in the extracellular matrix and form microcalcifications.[64] In addition, apoptosis is promoted by the inflammatory conditions in the valve and mediates calcification by generating apoptotic bodies that can similarly act as a nidus for microcalcification.[65,66] Altered expression of ectonucleotidases such as ectonucleotidase pyrophosphate/phosphodiesterase-1, which regulate phosphate and nucleotide metabolism, are also implicated in promoting calcification mostly through apoptosis.[67,68]

The formation of new hydroxyapatite crystals provides more nucleation sites for calcium deposition and an inflammatory response,[69] resulting in further calcium accumulation and valve leaflet stiffening that in turn increases mechanical stress and injury, prompting further calcium deposition. Thus a self-perpetuating cycle of calcification is established in which pro-osteogenic mechanisms dominate to aggravate calcification and valvular dysfunction.[70]

The hallmark of progressive calcification in the aortic valve is the differentiation of VICs into an osteoblast-like cell type, for which several calcific regulatory pathways have been described,[6] including Notch signaling,[71] the receptor activator of NF-κB ligand (RANKL)/RANK/osteoprotegerin system,[72,73] and Wnt pathway.[74] These pathways converge downstream to upregulate osteogenic differentiation factors such as BMPs[75] and Runt-related transcription factor 2.[37] Osteogenic differentiation also involves mitochondrial changes, which have been shown to be regulated by dynamin-related protein 1 and could potentially be targeted to inhibit calcification.[76] Subsequently, osteoblast-like cells secrete several calcification-regulating proteins that are also highly expressed in bone tissue, including alkaline phosphatase, osteocalcin, and osteopontin.[77]

Fibrosis of the Aortic Valve

An essential feature of AS contributing to the calcification process is fibrotic remodeling, which also contributes to increased stiffness of the valve leaflets. In fact, discordant results between aortic valve calcification (CT) and hemodynamic parameters (echocardiography) have suggested that fibrosis could be the predominant process in driving disease in younger patients with bicuspid aortic valve disease.[43] It has also been corroborated that women need less valvular calcium to develop the same severity of AS and that they are prone to accumulation of more valvular fibrosis.[44,49] These findings illustrate the clinical spectrum of fibrocalcific remodeling in AS.

Although the pathogenesis of aortic valve fibrosis has been understudied, increased production of extracellular matrix proteins such as tenascin-c and proteoglycans have been implicated in this process.[78,79] Experimental mouse models have started to identify proteins that are regulators of the fibrotic process, such as Klotho[80,81] and plasminogen activator inhibitor 1.[82]

Components of the renin-angiotensin-aldosterone system (RAAS) may also directly contribute to the fibrotic remodeling of valve leaflets,[83] as increased local levels of angiotensin-converting enzyme (transported via LDL),[84] chymases,[85] and cathepsin G[86] (both produced by mast cells) result in generation of angiotensin II, a strong promoter of inflammation and fibrosis. Animal studies and nonrandomized clinical studies have suggested that administration of angiotensin-receptor blockers may have beneficial effects on fibrocalcific remodeling of the valve leaflets.[87–90]

Left Ventricular Hypertrophy

Aortic valve narrowing results in an increased afterload, which induces hypertrophy of myocytes and reactive diffuse interstitial fibrosis, restores wall stress, and maintains cardiac function for years or even decades.[91] However, increasing left ventricle hypertrophy is associated with adverse prognosis and over time may transition to heart failure and the development of symptoms and cardiovascular events.[92] The degree of left ventricular hypertrophy is only weakly correlated to the severity of aortic valve narrowing.[93] Instead, gender seems to be the strongest factor associated to the pattern and magnitude of hypertrophy and patient outcomes.[94]

The progression to heart failure is hallmarked by increased myocyte apoptosis, which triggers a healing response leading to development of "replacement" fibrosis, which predominantly occurs in the subendocardial and midwall layers of the left ventricular wall.[95,96] RAAS inhibition has also been suggested as a beneficial therapy to reduce myocyte hypertrophy.[97] Although many small randomized trials suggest that the use of RAAS inhibitors in AS is well tolerated,[98–102] definitive conclusions regarding their efficacy on improving left ventricular function require larger randomized trials with sufficient follow-up time.

Cardiac MRI can detect expansion of the extracellular volume (reflecting diffuse interstitial fibrosis) using T1 mapping and focal (midwall) myocardial fibrosis using late gadolinium enhancement (LGE).[103,104] Longitudinal cardiac MRI studies have established that hypertrophy and diffuse interstitial fibrosis advance with increasing AS severity but reverse after aortic valve replacement.[105] However, once midwall patterns of replacement fibrosis are detected, further accumulation of fibrosis progresses rapidly and is irreversible after valve intervention. Midwall fibrosis serves as a marker of cardiac decompensation and a powerful predictor of increased all-cause and cardiovascular mortality.[106,107] These cardiac MRI techniques hold promise in identifying the early stages of left ventricular decompensation and therefore optimizing timing of aortic valve replacement.[5] The ongoing EVOLVED trial (NCT03094143) aims to address the question whether early aortic valve replacement, compared with routine care, in asymptomatic patients with severe AS and midwall LGE will reduce long-term morbidity and mortality.[108]

POTENTIAL DISEASE-MODIFYING TREATMENTS IN CLINICAL DEVELOPMENT
Targets for Lipid-Lowering Therapy

Despite the failure of statin trials to reduce AS disease progression, targeting atherogenic apolipoprotein B (apoB)-containing lipoproteins has

remained of great interest, in part due to secondary analyses of prospective studies suggesting faster disease progression with increased levels of apoB-containing lipoproteins.[109–111] It has been well established that PCSK9 inhibitors are able to lower both LDL cholesterol (~60%) and Lp(a) (~25%).[112] The *PCSK9* R46L loss-of-function mutation results in lifelong lower exposure to these atherogenic lipoproteins and is associated with reduced risk of aortic valve stenosis and myocardial infarction.[113] In support, experimental data suggested PCSK9 may also directly facilitate calcification in VICs.[114] Whether PCSK9 inhibition therapy could potentially reduce aortic valve stenosis disease progression and valve-related events is currently being investigated in a South Korean clinical trial (NCT03051360; **Table 1**).

Emerging evidence has corroborated that elevated Lp(a) levels are associated not only with incidence of AS but also with disease progression by aggravating calcification in the aortic valve,[115,116] enforcing the notion that lowering Lp(a) may be an effective treatment option in patients with AS. Although not without controversy due to 2 randomized trials that failed to reduce cardiovascular events, niacin is one of the few drugs available in the United States that is able to reduce Lp(a) plasma levels, beyond its effects to increase HDL-cholesterol and lower LDL-cholesterol and triglycerides.[117] The Early Aortic Valve Lipoprotein (a) Lowering (EAVaLL; NCT02109614; see **Table 1**) trial is now investigating the effect of extended-release niacin on progression of aortic valve CT calcium scores in patients with aortic valve sclerosis or mild stenosis.[118] The advent of an antisense oligonucleotide therapy against apolipoprotein(a) has made it possible to specifically lower Lp(a) levels.[119] In a phase IIb trial, AKCEA-APO(a)-Lrx was shown to potently reduce Lp(a) levels (>95%) in patients with established cardiovascular disease (American Heart Association Congress 2018). This drug has been licensed by Novartis and a phase III cardiovascular outcomes trial is in planning. Furthermore, an RNA interference therapeutic targeting apolipoprotein(a) is being developed by Amgen (AMG 890) and is currently undergoing phase I testing.

Bisphosphonates and Denosumab

Given the close links between cardiovascular calcification and bone metabolism, epidemiologic and experimental studies have suggested that drugs targeting osteoporosis may be effective in treating AS. Bisphosphonates, widely used in the

Table 1
Ongoing randomized clinical trials in aortic stenosis

Study	Target	Treatment	Main Inclusion Criteria	Follow-up	Primary Efficacy Endpoints
PCSK9 inhibitors in the progression of aortic stenosis (NCT03051360)	ApoB-containing lipoproteins; PCSK9	Biweekly injection of PCSK9 inhibitor vs placebo	Mild-moderate aortic stenosis (n = 140)	2 years	Change in aortic valve CT calcium score and 18F-NaF uptake
EAVaLL—Early Aortic Valve Lipoprotein (a) Lowering (NCT02109614)	Lipoprotein(a)	Daily extended-release niacin 1500–2000 mg vs Placebo	Aortic sclerosis or mild aortic stenosis + elevated Lp(a) levels (>50 mg/dL) (n = 150)	2 years	Change in aortic valve CT calcium score
SALTIRE II—Study Investigating the Effect of Drugs Used to Treat Osteoporosis on the Progression of Calcific Aortic Stenosis (NCT02132026)	Mineral metabolism	• Alendronic acid (n = 50) vs placebo tablets (n = 25) • Denosumab (n = 50) vs placebo injections (n = 25)	Aortic stenosis (V_{max} >2.5 m/s)	2 years	Change in aortic valve calcium score, aortic valve 18F-NaF uptake
BASIK2—Bicuspid Aortic Valve Stenosis and the Effect of vitamin K2 on calcium metabolism on 18F-NaF PET/MRI (NCT02917525)	Vitamin K2-Matrix Gla protein	Daily vitamin K2 360 µg (n = 22) vs placebo (n = 22)	Bicuspid aortic valve and calcified mild to moderate aortic stenosis	18 months	Change in aortic valve 18F-NaF uptake at 6 mo; change in aortic valve calcium score (secondary endpoint at 6 + 18 mo)
EvoLVeD—Early Valve Replacement Guided by Biomarkers of LV Decompensation in Asymptomatic Patients With Severe AS (NCT03094143)	Midwall fibrosis and timing of intervention	Early aortic valve replacement vs routine care	Asymptomatic severe aortic stenosis (V_{max} >4.0 m/s; or V_{max} >3.5 with AVA <0.6 cm²/m²)	± 3 y (until 88 events accrue)	Composite of all-cause mortality or unplanned aortic stenosis–related hospitalisation

Abbreviations: ApoB, apolipoprotein B; AVA, aortic valve area; V_{max}, peak aortic jet velocity.

management of osteoporosis, are analogues of endogenous inorganic pyrophosphate, an important regulator of extracellular calcification that inhibits hydroxyapatite formation in cardiovascular tissue.[120] Observational studies have suggested that bisphosphonate use is associated with less cardiovascular calcification and slower progression of AS[121–124]; however conflicting results have been reported.[125,126] Another potential therapy in this context is denosumab, a monocloncal antibody against RANKL. Inhibition of RANKL using denosumab was shown to protect against vascular calcification in a mouse model of osteoporosis.[127] In support, denosumab was found to reduce calcification of porcine VICs.[128] Both bisphosphonates and denosumab are now being investigated in the SALTIRE2 randomized clinical trial (NCT02132026; see **Table 1**).

Matrix gla protein depends on vitamin K for its anticalcific effects, and expression is lower in diseased VICs. Nutritional epidemiology studies have reported an inverse association between dietary intake of vitamin K and atherosclerosis,[129] but data on AS are currently lacking. The BASIK2 trial (NCT02917525; see **Table 1**) is now being conducted to investigate the effect of vitamin K2 supplementation on valvular calcification in patients with bicuspid aortic valve disease.[130]

Preclinical Targets Ready for Translation

Several potential drug targets have been investigated in preclinical models and hold promise for clinical translation. Because OxPL are key mediators of the proinflammatory effects of OxLDL and Lp(a), multiple strands of evidence now point toward a potential therapeutic role for inactivating OxPL by specific antibodies such as E06 to improve inflammatory conditions such as atherosclerosis, AS, and steatohepatitis.[131,132] Although the autotaxin-lysophosphatidic acid pathway has been show to interact with Lp(a) to promote valvular calcification,[19] novel insights suggest autotaxin also mediates platelet-induced mineralization of the valve leaflets.[133] Autotaxin inhibitors are currently under clinical development for idiopathic pulmonary fibrosis[134] and are also being explored for cancer treatment.

Valvular endothelial dysfunction leads to nitric oxide depletion, which promotes DPP-4 expression in VICs.[135] In turn, DPP-4 induces VIC calcification by limiting insulin-like growth factor 1 autocrine signaling. Repurposing of DPP-4 inhibitors, now clinically used as oral diabetes drugs, may therefore be a therapeutic strategy in ameliorating AS.

SUMMARY

Despite the fact that AS is a common condition that is set to become a major health care burden, medical therapies are still lacking to prevent or slow down AS. Evolving insights in the pathophysiology of AS progression have resulted in the identification of numerous biological targets related to calcification and fibrosis pathways, although only a handful have reached clinical trials. Development of drugs targeting these pathways can benefit from implementing noninvasive imaging modalities such as CT calcium scoring, 18F-NaF PET, and cardiac MRI, in order to assess efficacy and determine which patients are most likely to benefit from therapy.

ACKNOWLEDGMENTS

Marc R. Dweck is supported by the BHF (FS/14/78/31020) and is the recipient of the Sir Jules Thorn Award for Biomedical Research 2015 (15/JTA).

REFERENCES

1. Iung B, Vahanian A. Degenerative calcific aortic stenosis: a natural history. Heart 2012;98(Suppl 4):iv7–13.
2. Chan KL, Teo K, Dumesnil JG, et al. Effect of Lipid lowering with rosuvastatin on progression of aortic stenosis: results of the aortic stenosis progression observation: measuring effects of rosuvastatin (ASTRONOMER) trial. Circulation 2010;121(2): 306–14.
3. Cowell SJ, Newby DE, Prescott RJ, et al. A randomized trial of intensive lipid-lowering therapy in calcific aortic stenosis. N Engl J Med 2005;352(23):2389–97.
4. Rossebo AB, Pedersen TR, Boman K, et al. Intensive lipid lowering with simvastatin and ezetimibe in aortic stenosis. N Engl J Med 2008;359(13): 1343–56.
5. Everett RJ, Clavel MA, Pibarot P, et al. Timing of intervention in aortic stenosis: a review of current and future strategies. Heart 2018;104(24):2067–76.
6. Rutkovskiy A, Malashicheva A, Sullivan G, et al. Valve interstitial cells: the key to understanding the pathophysiology of heart valve calcification. J Am Heart Assoc 2017;6(9) [pii:e006339].
7. Pawade TA, Newby DE, Dweck MR. Calcification in aortic stenosis: the skeleton key. J Am Coll Cardiol 2015;66(5):561–77.
8. Otto CM, Kuusisto J, Reichenbach DD, et al. Characterization of the early lesion of 'degenerative' valvular aortic stenosis. Histological and immunohistochemical studies. Circulation 1994;90(2): 844–53.

9. Lewin MB, Otto CM. The bicuspid aortic valve: adverse outcomes from infancy to old age. Circulation 2005;111(7):832–4.

10. Roberts WC, Ko JM. Frequency by decades of unicuspid, bicuspid, and tricuspid aortic valves in adults having isolated aortic valve replacement for aortic stenosis, with or without associated aortic regurgitation. Circulation 2005;111(7):920–5.

11. O'Brien KD, Reichenbach DD, Marcovina SM, et al. Apolipoproteins B, (a), and E accumulate in the morphologically early lesion of 'degenerative' valvular aortic stenosis. Arterioscler Thromb Vasc Biol 1996;16(4):523–32.

12. Olsson M, Thyberg J, Nilsson J. Presence of oxidized low density lipoprotein in nonrheumatic stenotic aortic valves. Arterioscler Thromb Vasc Biol 1999;19(5):1218–22.

13. Ghaisas NK, Foley JB, O'Briain DS, et al. Adhesion molecules in nonrheumatic aortic valve disease: endothelial expression, serum levels and effects of valve replacement. J Am Coll Cardiol 2000; 36(7):2257–62.

14. Chisolm GM. Cytotoxicity of oxidized lipoproteins. Curr Opin Lipidol 1991;2(5):311–6.

15. Zeng Q, Song R, Fullerton DA, et al. Interleukin-37 suppresses the osteogenic responses of human aortic valve interstitial cells in vitro and alleviates valve lesions in mice. Proc Natl Acad Sci U S A 2017;114(7):1631–6.

16. Cote C, Pibarot P, Despres JP, et al. Association between circulating oxidised low-density lipoprotein and fibrocalcific remodelling of the aortic valve in aortic stenosis. Heart 2008;94(9): 1175–80.

17. Mohty D, Pibarot P, Despres JP, et al. Association between plasma LDL particle size, valvular accumulation of oxidized LDL, and inflammation in patients with aortic stenosis. Arterioscler Thromb Vasc Biol 2008;28(1):187–93.

18. Boffa MB, Koschinsky ML. Oxidized phospholipids as a unifying theory for lipoprotein(a) and cardiovascular disease. Nat Rev Cardiol 2019;16(5): 305–18.

19. Bouchareb R, Mahmut A, Nsaibia MJ, et al. Autotaxin derived from lipoprotein(a) and valve interstitial cells promotes inflammation and mineralization of the aortic valve. Circulation 2015;132(8):677–90.

20. Yu B, Hafiane A, Thanassoulis G, et al. Lipoprotein(a) induces human aortic valve interstitial cell calcification. JACC Basic Transl Sci 2017;2(4):358–71.

21. Cairns BJ, Coffey S, Travis RC, et al. A replicated, genome-wide significant association of aortic stenosis with a genetic variant for lipoprotein(a): meta-analysis of published and novel data. Circulation 2017;135(12):1181–3.

22. Chen HY, Dufresne L, Burr H, et al. Association of LPA variants with aortic stenosis: a large-scale study using diagnostic and procedural codes from electronic health records. JAMA Cardiol 2017;3(1):18–23.

23. Smith JG, Luk K, Schulz CA, et al. Association of low-density lipoprotein cholesterol-related genetic variants with aortic valve calcium and incident aortic stenosis. JAMA 2014;312(17): 1764–71.

24. Thanassoulis G, Campbell CY, Owens DS, et al. Genetic associations with valvular calcification and aortic stenosis. N Engl J Med 2013;368(6): 503–12.

25. New SE, Aikawa E. Molecular imaging insights into early inflammatory stages of arterial and aortic valve calcification. Circ Res 2011;108(11): 1381–91.

26. Abdelbaky A, Corsini E, Figueroa AL, et al. Early aortic valve inflammation precedes calcification: a longitudinal FDG-PET/CT study. Atherosclerosis 2015;238(2):165–72.

27. Marincheva-Savcheva G, Subramanian S, Qadir S, et al. Imaging of the aortic valve using fluorodeoxyglucose positron emission tomography increased valvular fluorodeoxyglucose uptake in aortic stenosis. J Am Coll Cardiol 2011; 57(25):2507–15.

28. Probst V, Le Scouarnec S, Legendre A, et al. Familial aggregation of calcific aortic valve stenosis in the western part of France. Circulation 2006; 113(6):856–60.

29. Cripe L, Andelfinger G, Martin LJ, et al. Bicuspid aortic valve is heritable. J Am Coll Cardiol 2004; 44(1):138–43.

30. Emanuel R, Withers R, O'Brien K, et al. Congenitally bicuspid aortic valves. Clinicogenetic study of 41 families. Br Heart J 1978;40(12):1402–7.

31. Huntington K, Hunter AG, Chan KL. A prospective study to assess the frequency of familial clustering of congenital bicuspid aortic valve. J Am Coll Cardiol 1997;30(7):1809–12.

32. Martinsson A, Li X, Zoller B, et al. Familial aggregation of aortic valvular stenosis: a nationwide study of sibling risk. Circ Cardiovasc Genet 2017;10(6) [pii:e001742].

33. Garg V, Muth AN, Ransom JF, et al. Mutations in NOTCH1 cause aortic valve disease. Nature 2005;437(7056):270–4.

34. Arsenault BJ, Boekholdt SM, Dube MP, et al. Lipoprotein(a) levels, genotype, and incident aortic valve stenosis: a prospective Mendelian randomization study and replication in a case-control cohort. Circ Cardiovasc Genet 2014;7(3): 304–10.

35. Helgadottir A, Thorleifsson G, Gretarsdottir S, et al. Genome-wide analysis yields new loci associating with aortic valve stenosis. Nat Commun 2018; 9(1):987.

36. Kamstrup PR, Tybjaerg-Hansen A, Nordest-gaard BG. Elevated lipoprotein(a) and risk of aortic valve stenosis in the general population. J Am Coll Cardiol 2014;63(5):470–7.

37. Guauque-Olarte S, Messika-Zeitoun D, Droit A, et al. Calcium signaling pathway genes RUNX2 and CACNA1C are associated with calcific aortic valve disease. Circ Cardiovasc Genet 2015;8(6): 812–22.

38. Bjornsson T, Thorolfsdottir RB, Sveinbjornsson G, et al. A rare missense mutation in MYH6 associates with non-syndromic coarctation of the aorta. Eur Heart J 2018;39(34):3243–9.

39. Alonso-Montes C, Martin M, Martinez-Arias L, et al. Variants in cardiac GATA genes associated with bicuspid aortic valve. Eur J Clin Invest 2018; 48(12):e13027.

40. Yang B, Zhou W, Jiao J, et al. Protein-altering and regulatory genetic variants near GATA4 implicated in bicuspid aortic valve. Nat Commun 2017;8: 15481.

41. Prakash SK, Bosse Y, Muehlschlegel JD, et al. A roadmap to investigate the genetic basis of bicuspid aortic valve and its complications: insights from the International BAVCon (Bicuspid Aortic Valve Consortium). J Am Coll Cardiol 2014; 64(8):832–9.

42. Theriault S, Gaudreault N, Lamontagne M, et al. A transcriptome-wide association study identifies PALMD as a susceptibility gene for calcific aortic valve stenosis. Nat Commun 2018;9(1):988.

43. Shen M, Tastet L, Capoulade R, et al. Effect of age and aortic valve anatomy on calcification and haemodynamic severity of aortic stenosis. Heart 2017; 103(1):32–9.

44. Simard L, Cote N, Dagenais F, et al. Sex-related discordance between aortic valve calcification and hemodynamic severity of aortic stenosis: is valvular fibrosis the explanation? Circ Res 2017; 120(4):681–91.

45. Cartlidge TR, Pawade TA, Dweck MR. Aortic stenosis and CT calcium scoring: is it for everyone? Heart 2017;103(1):8–9.

46. Owens DS, Katz R, Takasu J, et al. Incidence and progression of aortic valve calcium in the Multiethnic Study of Atherosclerosis (MESA). Am J Cardiol 2010;105(5):701–8.

47. Nguyen V, Cimadevilla C, Estellat C, et al. Haemodynamic and anatomic progression of aortic stenosis. Heart 2015;101(12):943–7.

48. Clavel MA, Pibarot P, Messika-Zeitoun D, et al. Impact of aortic valve calcification, as measured by MDCT, on survival in patients with aortic stenosis: results of an international registry study. J Am Coll Cardiol 2014;64(12):1202–13.

49. Pawade T, Clavel MA, Tribouilloy C, et al. Computed tomography aortic valve calcium scoring in patients with aortic stenosis. Circ Cardiovasc Imaging 2018; 11(3):e007146.

50. Creager MD, Hohl T, Hutcheson JD, et al. (18)F-fluoride signal amplification identifies microcalcifications associated with atherosclerotic plaque instability in positron emission tomography/computed tomography images. Circ Cardiovasc Imaging 2019;12(1):e007835.

51. Dweck MR, Jenkins WS, Vesey AT, et al. 18F-sodium fluoride uptake is a marker of active calcification and disease progression in patients with aortic stenosis. Circ Cardiovasc Imaging 2014;7(2): 371–8.

52. Dweck MR, Jones C, Joshi NV, et al. Assessment of valvular calcification and inflammation by positron emission tomography in patients with aortic stenosis. Circulation 2012;125(1):76–86.

53. Irkle A, Vesey AT, Lewis DY, et al. Identifying active vascular microcalcification by (18)F-sodium fluoride positron emission tomography. Nat Commun 2015;6:7495.

54. Jenkins WS, Vesey AT, Shah AS, et al. Valvular (18) F-fluoride and (18)F-fluorodeoxyglucose uptake predict disease progression and clinical outcome in patients with aortic stenosis. J Am Coll Cardiol 2015;66(10):1200–1.

55. Bosse Y, Miqdad A, Fournier D, et al. Refining molecular pathways leading to calcific aortic valve stenosis by studying gene expression profile of normal and calcified stenotic human aortic valves. Circ Cardiovasc Genet 2009;2(5):489–98.

56. Fondard O, Detaint D, Iung B, et al. Extracellular matrix remodelling in human aortic valve disease: the role of matrix metalloproteinases and their tissue inhibitors. Eur Heart J 2005;26(13): 1333–41.

57. Jian B, Jones PL, Li Q, et al. Matrix metalloproteinase-2 is associated with tenascin-C in calcific aortic stenosis. Am J Pathol 2001;159(1):321–7.

58. Jung JJ, Razavian M, Challa AA, et al. Multimodality and molecular imaging of matrix metalloproteinase activation in calcific aortic valve disease. J Nucl Med 2015;56(6):933–8.

59. Kaden JJ, Vocke DC, Fischer CS, et al. Expression and activity of matrix metalloproteinase-2 in calcific aortic stenosis. Z Kardiol 2004;93(2):124–30.

60. Sena BF, Figueiredo JL, Aikawa E. Cathepsin S as an inhibitor of cardiovascular inflammation and calcification in chronic kidney disease. Front Cardiovasc Med 2017;4:88.

61. Bakhshian Nik A, Hutcheson JD, Aikawa E. Extracellular vesicles as mediators of cardiovascular calcification. Front Cardiovasc Med 2017;4:78.

62. Goettsch C, Hutcheson JD, Aikawa M, et al. Sortilin mediates vascular calcification via its recruitment into extracellular vesicles. J Clin Invest 2016; 126(4):1323–36.

63. Goettsch C, Kjolby M, Aikawa E. Sortilin and its multiple roles in cardiovascular and metabolic diseases. Arterioscler Thromb Vasc Biol 2018;38(1):19–25.

64. Hutcheson JD, Goettsch C, Bertazzo S, et al. Genesis and growth of extracellular-vesicle-derived microcalcification in atherosclerotic plaques. Nat Mater 2016;15(3):335–43.

65. Galeone A, Brunetti G, Oranger A, et al. Aortic valvular interstitial cells apoptosis and calcification are mediated by TNF-related apoptosis-inducing ligand. Int J Cardiol 2013;169(4):296–304.

66. Jian B, Narula N, Li QY, et al. Progression of aortic valve stenosis: TGF-beta1 is present in calcified aortic valve cusps and promotes aortic valve interstitial cell calcification via apoptosis. Ann Thorac Surg 2003;75(2):457–65 [discussion: 465–6].

67. Cote N, El Husseini D, Pepin A, et al. Inhibition of ectonucleotidase with ARL67156 prevents the development of calcific aortic valve disease in warfarin-treated rats. Eur J Pharmacol 2012;689(1–3):139–46.

68. Cote N, El Husseini D, Pepin A, et al. ATP acts as a survival signal and prevents the mineralization of aortic valve. J Mol Cell Cardiol 2012;52(5):1191–202.

69. Nadra I, Mason JC, Philippidis P, et al. Proinflammatory activation of macrophages by basic calcium phosphate crystals via protein kinase C and MAP kinase pathways: a vicious cycle of inflammation and arterial calcification? Circ Res 2005;96(12):1248–56.

70. Dweck MR, Pawade TA, Newby DE. Aortic stenosis begets aortic stenosis: between a rock and a hard place? Heart 2015;101(12):919–20.

71. Hadji F, Boulanger MC, Guay SP, et al. Altered DNA methylation of long noncoding RNA H19 in calcific aortic valve disease promotes mineralization by silencing NOTCH1. Circulation 2016;134(23):1848–62.

72. Kaden JJ, Bickelhaupt S, Grobholz R, et al. Receptor activator of nuclear factor kappaB ligand and osteoprotegerin regulate aortic valve calcification. J Mol Cell Cardiol 2004;36(1):57–66.

73. Weiss RM, Lund DD, Chu Y, et al. Osteoprotegerin inhibits aortic valve calcification and preserves valve function in hypercholesterolemic mice. PLoS One 2013;8(6):e65201.

74. Albanese I, Khan K, Barratt B, et al. Atherosclerotic calcification: wnt is the hint. J Am Heart Assoc 2018;7(4) [pii:e007356].

75. Gomez-Stallons MV, Wirrig-Schwendeman EE, Hassel KR, et al. Bone morphogenetic protein signaling is required for aortic valve calcification. Arterioscler Thromb Vasc Biol 2016;36(7):1398–405.

76. Rogers MA, Maldonado N, Hutcheson JD, et al. Dynamin-related protein 1 inhibition attenuates cardiovascular calcification in the presence of oxidative stress. Circ Res 2017;121(3):220–33.

77. Rajamannan NM, Subramaniam M, Rickard D, et al. Human aortic valve calcification is associated with an osteoblast phenotype. Circulation 2003;107(17):2181–4.

78. Hinton RB Jr, Lincoln J, Deutsch GH, et al. Extracellular matrix remodeling and organization in developing and diseased aortic valves. Circ Res 2006;98(11):1431–8.

79. Satta J, Melkko J, Pollanen R, et al. Progression of human aortic valve stenosis is associated with tenascin-C expression. J Am Coll Cardiol 2002;39(1):96–101.

80. Chen J, Fan J, Wang S, et al. Secreted Klotho attenuates inflammation-associated aortic valve fibrosis in senescence-accelerated mice P1. Hypertension 2018;71(5):877–85.

81. Chen J, Lin Y, Sun Z. Deficiency in the anti-aging gene Klotho promotes aortic valve fibrosis through AMPKalpha-mediated activation of RUNX2. Aging Cell 2016;15(5):853–60.

82. Chu Y, Lund DD, Doshi H, et al. Fibrotic aortic valve stenosis in hypercholesterolemic/hypertensive mice. Arterioscler Thromb Vasc Biol 2016;36(3):466–74.

83. Helske S, Lindstedt KA, Laine M, et al. Induction of local angiotensin II-producing systems in stenotic aortic valves. J Am Coll Cardiol 2004;44(9):1859–66.

84. O'Brien KD, Shavelle DM, Caulfield MT, et al. Association of angiotensin-converting enzyme with low-density lipoprotein in aortic valvular lesions and in human plasma. Circulation 2002;106(17):2224–30.

85. Wypasek E, Natorska J, Grudzien G, et al. Mast cells in human stenotic aortic valves are associated with the severity of stenosis. Inflammation 2013;36(2):449–56.

86. Helske S, Syvaranta S, Kupari M, et al. Possible role for mast cell-derived cathepsin G in the adverse remodelling of stenotic aortic valves. Eur Heart J 2006;27(12):1495–504.

87. Arishiro K, Hoshiga M, Negoro N, et al. Angiotensin receptor-1 blocker inhibits atherosclerotic changes and endothelial disruption of the aortic valve in hypercholesterolemic rabbits. J Am Coll Cardiol 2007;49(13):1482–9.

88. Capoulade R, Clavel MA, Mathieu P, et al. Impact of hypertension and renin-angiotensin system inhibitors in aortic stenosis. Eur J Clin Invest 2013;43(12):1262–72.

89. Cote N, Couture C, Pibarot P, et al. Angiotensin receptor blockers are associated with a lower remodelling score of stenotic aortic valves. Eur J Clin Invest 2011;41(11):1172–9.

90. Fujisaka T, Hoshiga M, Hotchi J, et al. Angiotensin II promotes aortic valve thickening independent of elevated blood pressure in apolipoprotein-E deficient mice. Atherosclerosis 2013;226(1):82–7.
91. Lorell BH, Carabello BA. Left ventricular hypertrophy: pathogenesis, detection, and prognosis. Circulation 2000;102(4):470–9.
92. Vakili BA, Okin PM, Devereux RB. Prognostic implications of left ventricular hypertrophy. Am Heart J 2001;141(3):334–41.
93. Dweck MR, Joshi S, Murigu T, et al. Left ventricular remodeling and hypertrophy in patients with aortic stenosis: insights from cardiovascular magnetic resonance. J Cardiovasc Magn Reson 2012; 14:50.
94. Petrov G, Dworatzek E, Schulze TM, et al. Maladaptive remodeling is associated with impaired survival in women but not in men after aortic valve replacement. JACC Cardiovasc Imaging 2014; 7(11):1073–80.
95. Hein S, Arnon E, Kostin S, et al. Progression from compensated hypertrophy to failure in the pressure-overloaded human heart: structural deterioration and compensatory mechanisms. Circulation 2003;107(7):984–91.
96. Travers JG, Kamal FA, Robbins J, et al. Cardiac fibrosis: the fibroblast awakens. Circ Res 2016; 118(6):1021–40.
97. Nadir MA, Wei L, Elder DH, et al. Impact of renin-angiotensin system blockade therapy on outcome in aortic stenosis. J Am Coll Cardiol 2011;58(6): 570–6.
98. Helske-Suihko S, Laine M, Lommi J, et al. Is blockade of the Renin-Angiotensin system able to reverse the structural and functional remodeling of the left ventricle in severe aortic stenosis? J Cardiovasc Pharmacol 2015;65(3):233–40.
99. Bull S, Loudon M, Francis JM, et al. A prospective, double-blind, randomized controlled trial of the angiotensin-converting enzyme inhibitor Ramipril in Aortic Stenosis (RIAS trial). Eur Heart J Cardiovasc Imaging 2015;16(8):834–41.
100. Dahl JS, Videbaek L, Poulsen MK, et al. Effect of candesartan treatment on left ventricular remodeling after aortic valve replacement for aortic stenosis. Am J Cardiol 2010;106(5):713–9.
101. Stewart RA, Kerr AJ, Cowan BR, et al. A randomized trial of the aldosterone-receptor antagonist eplerenone in asymptomatic moderate-severe aortic stenosis. Am Heart J 2008;156(2):348–55.
102. Chockalingam A, Venkatesan S, Subramaniam T, et al. Safety and efficacy of angiotensin-converting enzyme inhibitors in symptomatic severe aortic stenosis: symptomatic Cardiac Obstruction-Pilot Study of Enalapril in Aortic Stenosis (SCOPE-AS). Am Heart J 2004;147(4):E19.
103. Bing R, Cavalcante JL, Everett RJ, et al. Imaging and impact of myocardial fibrosis in aortic stenosis. JACC Cardiovasc Imaging 2019;12(2):283–96.
104. Chin CWL, Everett RJ, Kwiecinski J, et al. Myocardial fibrosis and cardiac decompensation in aortic stenosis. JACC Cardiovasc Imaging 2017;10(11): 1320–33.
105. Everett RJ, Tastet L, Clavel MA, et al. Progression of hypertrophy and myocardial fibrosis in aortic stenosis: a multicenter cardiac magnetic resonance study. Circ Cardiovasc Imaging 2018; 11(6):e007451.
106. Dweck MR, Joshi S, Murigu T, et al. Midwall fibrosis is an independent predictor of mortality in patients with aortic stenosis. J Am Coll Cardiol 2011;58(12): 1271–9.
107. Vassiliou VS, Perperoglou A, Raphael CE, et al. Midwall fibrosis and 5-year outcome in moderate and severe aortic stenosis. J Am Coll Cardiol 2017;69(13):1755–6.
108. Bing R, Everett RJ, Tuck C, et al. Rationale and design of the randomized, controlled early valve replacement guided by biomarkers of left ventricular decompensation in asymptomatic patients with severe aortic stenosis (EVOLVED) trial. Am Heart J 2019;212:91–100.
109. Capoulade R, Yeang C, Chan KL, et al. Association of mild to moderate aortic valve stenosis progression with higher lipoprotein(a) and oxidized phospholipid levels: secondary analysis of a randomized clinical trial. JAMA Cardiol 2018; 3(12):1212–7.
110. Ljungberg J, Holmgren A, Bergdahl IA, et al. Lipoprotein(a) and the apolipoprotein B/A1 ratio independently associate with surgery for aortic stenosis only in patients with Concomitant Coronary Artery disease. J Am Heart Assoc 2017; 6(12) [pii:e007160].
111. Tastet L, Capoulade R, Shen M, et al. ApoB/ApoA-I ratio is associated with faster hemodynamic progression of aortic stenosis: results from the PROGRESSA (metabolic determinants of the progression of aortic stenosis) study. J Am Heart Assoc 2018;7(4) [pii: e007980].
112. O'Donoghue ML, Fazio S, Giugliano RP, et al. Lipoprotein(a), PCSK9 inhibition, and cardiovascular risk. Circulation 2019;139(12):1483–92.
113. Langsted A, Nordestgaard BG, Benn M, et al. PCSK9 R46L loss-of-function mutation reduces lipoprotein(a), LDL cholesterol, and risk of aortic valve stenosis. J Clin Endocrinol Metab 2016; 101(9):3281–7.
114. Poggio P, Songia P, Cavallotti L, et al. PCSK9 involvement in aortic valve calcification. J Am Coll Cardiol 2018;72(24):3225–7.
115. Capoulade R, Chan KL, Yeang C, et al. Oxidized phospholipids, lipoprotein(a), and progression of

calcific aortic valve stenosis. J Am Coll Cardiol 2015;66(11):1236–46.

116. Zheng KH, Tsimikas S, Pawade T, et al. Lipoprotein(a) and oxidized phospholipids promote valve calcification in patients with aortic stenosis. J Am Coll Cardiol 2019;73(17):2150–62.

117. van Capelleveen JC, van der Valk FM, Stroes ES. Current therapies for lowering lipoprotein (a). J Lipid Res 2016;57(9):1612–8.

118. Thanassoulis G. Lipoprotein (a) in calcific aortic valve disease: from genomics to novel drug target for aortic stenosis. J Lipid Res 2016;57(6):917–24.

119. Viney NJ, van Capelleveen JC, Geary RS, et al. Antisense oligonucleotides targeting apolipoprotein(a) in people with raised lipoprotein(a): two randomised, double-blind, placebo-controlled, dose-ranging trials. Lancet 2016;388(10057):2239–53.

120. Rathan S, Yoganathan AP, O'Neill CW. The role of inorganic pyrophosphate in aortic valve calcification. J Heart Valve Dis 2014;23(4):387–94.

121. Innasimuthu AL, Katz WE. Effect of bisphosphonates on the progression of degenerative aortic stenosis. Echocardiography 2011;28(1):1–7.

122. Skolnick AH, Osranek M, Formica P, et al. Osteoporosis treatment and progression of aortic stenosis. Am J Cardiol 2009;104(1):122–4.

123. Elmariah S, Delaney JA, O'Brien KD, et al. Bisphosphonate use and prevalence of valvular and vascular calcification in women MESA (the multi-ethnic study of atherosclerosis). J Am Coll Cardiol 2010;56(21):1752–9.

124. Sterbakova G, Vyskocil V, Linhartova K. Bisphosphonates in calcific aortic stenosis: association with slower progression in mild disease–a pilot retrospective study. Cardiology 2010;117(3):184–9.

125. Aksoy O, Cam A, Goel SS, et al. Do bisphosphonates slow the progression of aortic stenosis? J Am Coll Cardiol 2012;59(16):1452–9.

126. Dweck MR, Newby DE. Osteoporosis is a major confounder in observational studies investigating bisphosphonate therapy in aortic stenosis. J Am Coll Cardiol 2012;60(11):1027 [author reply: 1027].

127. Helas S, Goettsch C, Schoppet M, et al. Inhibition of receptor activator of NF-kappaB ligand by denosumab attenuates vascular calcium deposition in mice. Am J Pathol 2009;175(2):473–8.

128. Lerman DA, Prasad S, Alotti N. Denosumab could be a potential inhibitor of valvular interstitial cells calcification in vitro. Int J Cardiovasc Res 2016;5(1).

129. van Ballegooijen AJ, Beulens JW. The role of vitamin K status in cardiovascular health: evidence from observational and clinical studies. Curr Nutr Rep 2017;6(3):197–205.

130. Peeters F, van Mourik MJW, Meex SJR, et al. Bicuspid aortic valve stenosis and the effect of vitamin K2 on calcification using (18)F-sodium fluoride positron emission tomography/magnetic resonance: the BASIK2 rationale and trial design. Nutrients 2018;10(4) [pii:E386].

131. Ambrogini E, Que X, Wang S, et al. Oxidation-specific epitopes restrain bone formation. Nat Commun 2018;9(1):2193.

132. Que X, Hung MY, Yeang C, et al. Oxidized phospholipids are proinflammatory and proatherogenic in hypercholesterolaemic mice. Nature 2018;558(7709):301–6.

133. Bouchareb R, Boulanger MC, Tastet L, et al. Activated platelets promote an osteogenic programme and the progression of calcific aortic valve stenosis. Eur Heart J 2019;40(17):1362–73.

134. Maher TM, Kreuter M, Lederer DJ, et al. Rationale, design and objectives of two phase III, randomised, placebo-controlled studies of GLPG1690, a novel autotaxin inhibitor, in idiopathic pulmonary fibrosis (ISABELA 1 and 2). BMJ Open Respir Res 2019;6(1):e000422.

135. Choi B, Lee S, Kim SM, et al. Dipeptidyl peptidase-4 induces aortic valve calcification by inhibiting insulin-like growth factor-1 signaling in valvular interstitial cells. Circulation 2017;135(20):1935–50.

Assessment of Aortic Stenosis Severity
A Multimodality Approach

Julien Ternacle, MD, PhD[a,b,c,*], Marie-Annick Clavel, DVM, PhD[a]

KEYWORDS

- Aortic stenosis • Aortic valve calcification • Calcium scoring • Echocardiography
- Computed tomography • Multimodality imaging

KEY POINTS

- Transthoracic echocardiography is the cornerstone to confirm the severity of aortic stenosis.
- In patients with high-gradient severe aortic stenosis, the stroke volume should be evaluated to assess the prognosis.
- In patients with a low-gradient and tight aortic valve area pattern, a multimodality imaging approach should be used to confirm the true severity of aortic stenosis before decision making.

INTRODUCTION

Assessing aortic stenosis (AS) severity is essential in the management of patients. Indeed, class I indications for aortic valve replacement (AVR) are only recommended in patients with severe AS. Doppler-echocardiography is the cornerstone for AS evaluation because of its high performance, low-cost, and large availability. The first-line evaluation after auscultation of a heart sound or in patients at risk, such as patients with known congenitally bicuspid aortic valve, is the transthoracic echocardiography (TTE). In most cases TTE allows to confirm the diagnosis, determine the severity, and evaluate the myocardial repercussion of AS. Moreover, indications for aortic valve intervention in asymptomatic patients are predominantly based on echocardiography. However, a multimodality imaging approach could be mandatory, especially in patients with discordance in echocardiographic parameters used to grade AS severity.

TRANSTHORACIC DOPPLER-ECHOCARDIOGRAPHY: THE FIRST LINE OF AORTIC STENOSIS EVALUATION

Assessment of AS severity is mostly based on three parameters (**Fig. 1**): (1) transaortic valvular peak jet velocity (Vmax), (2) mean pressure gradient (ΔPm) between the left ventricle (LV) and the aorta, and (3) aortic valve area (AVA) calculation. Severe AS is defined by (**Table 1**) a Vmax greater than or equal to 4 m/s, a ΔPm greater than or equal to 40 mm Hg, and an AVA less than 1.0 cm^2 or less than 0.6 cm^2/m^2 after

Disclosures: Dr M.-A. Clavel has Core Lab contracts with Edwards Lifesciences, for which she receives no direct compensation; and research grant with Medtronic. Dr J. Ternacle has no disclosure. J. Ternacle has received a fellowship grant from AREMCAR. M.-A. Clavel is scholar fellow from Fond de recherche du Québec en santé.
[a] Institut Universitaire de Cardiologie et de Pneumologie de Québec, Québec Heart and Lung Institute, Université Laval, 2725 Chemin Sainte-Foy, Québec City, Québec G1V-4G5, Canada; [b] Cardiology Department, Expert Valve Center, Henri Mondor Hospital, 51 Avenue du Maréchal de Lattre de Tassigny, Créteil 94000, France; [c] INSERM Unit U955, Team 8, Paris-Est Creteil University, Val-de-Marne, 51 Avenue du Maréchal de Lattre de Tassigny, Créteil 94000, France
* Corresponding author. Institut Universitaire de Cardiologie et de Pneumologie de Québec, Québec Heart and Lung Institute, Université Laval, 2725 Chemin Sainte-Foy, Québec city, Québec G1V-4G5, Canada
E-mail address: julien.ternacle.hmn@gmail.com

Cardiol Clin 38 (2020) 13–22
https://doi.org/10.1016/j.ccl.2019.09.004
0733-8651/20/© 2019 Elsevier Inc. All rights reserved.

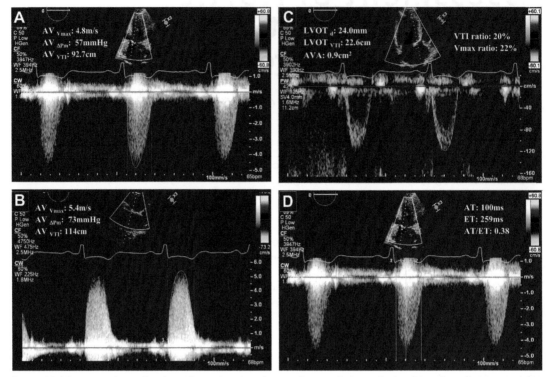

Fig. 1. Multiparametric evaluation of aortic stenosis severity: peak jet velocity (Vmax) and mean pressure gradient (ΔPm) from (*A*) apical and (*B*) right parasternal windows, aortic valve area (AVA), (*C*) velocity and VTI ratio, acceleration time (AT), and its (*D*) ratio over ejection time (AT/ET). AV, aortic valve; LVOT, left ventricular outflow tract; LVOT $_d$, LVOT diameter; VTI, velocity-time integral.

indexation to body surface area.[1] The evolution of these parameters over time is also crucial to identify patients with a rapid AS progression (increase in Vmax ≥0.3 m/s/y).

- Vmax and ΔPm of the antegrade systolic flow across the narrowed aortic valve are measured using continuous-wave Doppler (CWD) ultrasound. The maximum velocity is measured at the outer edge of the dark signal, and the outer edge of the spectral Doppler envelope is traced to provide the velocity-time integral (VTI) for the continuity equation and ΔPm (using the simplified Bernoulli equation) (see **Fig. 1**A). To obtain the highest Vmax, the CWD must be aligned with the ejection flow and Doppler angle correction should be avoided. Hence, a multiple acoustic window exploration including the right parasternal way,[2] if possible with the use of a small dual-crystal CWD transducer (PEDOF), after a careful patient positioning is strongly recommended (see **Fig. 1**B).[1] The window where the highest Vmax is recorded should be mentioned in the TTE report for further evaluations.

- AVA is calculated using the continuity equation, which is based on the concept of flow preservation: the stroke volume (SV) ejected through the left ventricular outflow tract (LVOT) is equal to SV ejected through the aortic valve orifice:

$$SV = LVOT_{area} \times LVOT_{VTI} = AVA \times AV_{VTI}$$

$$AVA = \frac{LVOT_{area} \times LVOT_{VTI}}{AV_{VTI}}$$

$$LVOT_{area} = \pi \left[\frac{LVOT_d}{2} \right]^2$$

Where LVOT $_d$ is the diameter of LVOT.

This equation requires the measurement of two additional echocardiographic parameters: the LVOT VTI (LVOT $_{VTI}$) and the LVOT diameter (LVOT $_d$) to calculate LVOT area. LVOT $_d$ is a key measure to define AS severity. It should be measured at the aortic annulus level (inner edges of leaflet insertion) from a parasternal long axis view zoomed on the aortic valve during the

Table 1
Parameters defining severe aortic stenosis using a multimodality approach

Imaging Modality	Parameters
Echocardiography	
First line (also available for CMR)	
Peak jet velocity	$\geq$4 m/s
Mean pressure gradient	$\geq$40 mm Hg
Aortic valve area	$\leq$1.0 cm^2
Aortic valve area index	$\leq$0.6 cm^2/m^2
Second line	
Velocity or VTI ratio	<0.25
Acceleration time	>110 ms
Acceleration time/ejection time	>0.36
Aortic valve area planimetry	$\leq$1.0 cm^2
Stress echocardiography	
Peak jet velocity at peak	$\geq$4 m/s
Mean pressure gradient at peak	$\geq$40 mm Hg
Aortic valve area at peak	$\leq$1.0 cm^2
Cardiac computed tomography	
Calcium scoring	Men $\geq$2000 AU Women $\geq$1200 AU
Aortic valve area planimetry	$\leq$1.0 cm^2
Hybrid method (LVOT by CT or CMR)	
Aortic valve area	$\leq$1.2 cm^2

Abbreviations: CMR, cardiac magnetic resonance; CT, computed tomography; LVOT, left ventricular outflow tract; VTI, velocity time integral.

systolic phase, when the diameter is maximal (**Fig. 2**A). Although recommended for years, LVOT $_d$ measurement away from the valve should be avoided because of the risk of underestimation (ie, septal bulging and nontubular LVOT). In addition, positioning the LVOT $_d$ within 0.3 to 1.0 cm of the valve may impact the evaluation reproducibility. LVOT $_d$ assessment may be difficult in case of extensive calcifications, and might require the use of transesophageal echocardiography (TEE) or cardiac computed tomography (CT) to accurately define it.[3] LVOT $_{VTI}$ is measured using pulsed-wave Doppler modality from an apical approach. The pulsed-wave Doppler sample is positioned just proximal to the aortic valve, ideally at the same level as the LVOT $_d$ is measured. The recording should show a smooth velocity curve with a well-defined peak, and a narrow band of velocities throughout systole (see **Fig. 1**C). In case of important spectral dispersion, the sample volume should be slowly moved from the valve toward the apex.

Thirty percent to 40% of patients with severe AS may have a discordance between AVA (<1.0 cm^2; ie, in the severe range) and hemodynamic parameters (Vmax <4 m/s and ΔPm <40 mm Hg; ie, in the moderate range). A careful evaluation of LVOT $_d$ measures should be done in these cases, and second-line parameters (see **Fig. 1**, see **Table 1**) should be assessed if the discordance is confirmed: velocity or VTI ratio, acceleration time (AT) and its ratio over ejection time (ET), and AVA planimetry.[1] These parameters reduce the risk of error related to the LVOT $_d$ measurement.

- Velocity or VTI ratio (see **Fig. 1**C) is the ratio Vmax or VTI between LVOT and AV levels. The normal value is 1, whereas in a severe AS the ratio is <0.25 (or 25%). This parameter is particularly interesting when LVOT $_d$-measurement is unclear.

$$\text{Velocity ratio} = \frac{\text{LVOT}_{v_{max}}}{\text{AV}_{v_{max}}}$$

$$\text{VTI ratio} = \frac{\text{LVOT}_{VTI}}{\text{AV}_{VTI}}$$

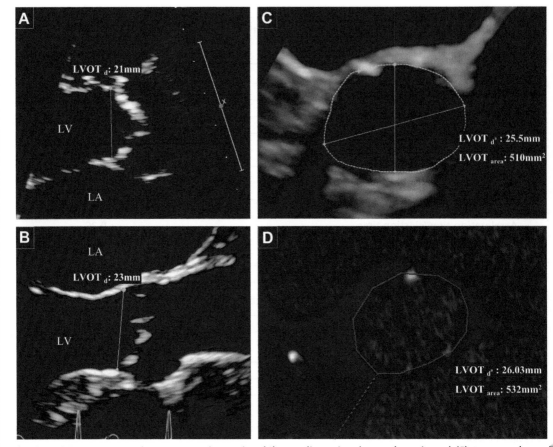

Fig. 2. LVOT $_d$ assessment in a same patient using (*A*) two-dimensional transthoracic and (*B*) transesophageal echocardiography, and (*C*) using three-dimensional multiplanar reconstruction from transesophageal echocardiography and (*D*) contrast cardiac computed tomography. LA, left atrium; LV, left ventricle; LVOT $_d$, LVOT diameter. [a] Indicates that LVOT $_d$ was derived from the LVOT area.

- The analysis of the ejection dynamics transvalvular velocity using CWD may provide additional semiquantitative parameters to better characterize AS severity. AT is the delay between the beginning and the maximal peak of the aortic ejection velocity and ET is the overall ejection duration (see **Fig. 1**D). An AT greater than 110 ms or an AT/ET greater than 0.36 was associated with AS severity and outcomes.[4] However, in low-flow (LF) patients, these parameters could be increased in nonsevere stenosis because of the lack of strength of the flow to open a stenosis that is only moderate.

- AVA planimetry (**Fig. 3**A) is an interesting additional parameter, which offers a direct anatomic visualization of the narrowed AV orifice (cutoff <1.0 cm^2). However, several limits exist: (1) the level of the orifice area assessment must be well positioned at the tips of the leaflets to avoid overestimation and thus positioning should be performed with three-dimensional (3D) imaging modality; (2) planimetry is difficult in case of extensive calcifications (shadows and reverberations); and (3) because of flow contraction, the hemodynamic calculated AVA is could be up to 0.6-fold smaller than the anatomic AVA by planimetry. Thus, severe AS diagnosis should not be challenged on this parameter alone, but it may provide additional information in difficult cases. TEE using two-dimensional (2D) or 3D modalities, and cardiac CT with contrast injection, are more accurate than TTE for AVA planimetry.

All hemodynamic parameters measured by echocardiography are flow dependent: a decrease in flow decreases gradient and velocity but also velocity/VTI ratio and AVA by continuity equation and planimetry.

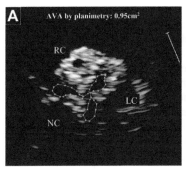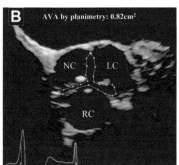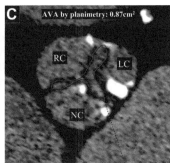

Fig. 3. Aortic valve orifice planimetry in a same patient using transthoracic (*A*) and transesophageal echocardiography (*B*), and contrast cardiac computed tomography (*C*). AVA, aortic valve area; LC, left coronary leaflet; NC, noncoronary leaflet; RC, right coronary leaflet.

Finally, AS severity should also be assessed using a semiquantitative approach based on valvular calcification extension (**Fig. 4**A) because of its strong correlation with the stenosis severity and outcomes.[5] This additional parameter may also help in case of discordant severe AS.

TRANSESOPHAGEAL ECHOCARDIOGRAPHY: AN ANATOMIC EVALUATION

AS severity assessment can require the use of TEE in specific conditions: (1) patient with poor TTE echogenicity, (2) inaccurate LVOT $_d$ measurement, and (3) associated heart valve disease.

In patients with extensive aortic valve calcification, the risk of LVOT $_d$ underestimation by TTE can require the use of TEE.[3] Moreover, the LVOT area calculation is based on the 2D LVOT $_d$ measurement, whereas the aortic annulus has an elliptical shape.[6] This geometric assumption may lead to underestimate AVA in case of misalignment with the larger LVOT diameter (**Fig. 2**B). Thus, a 3D TEE (**Fig. 2**C) may be performed to more accurately assess LVOT dimensions[3] in case of discordance between a small AVA (<1.0 cm²) and a low transvalvular flow (Vmax <4 m/s and ΔPm <40 mm Hg). 3D TEE automated software can provide a rapid and reliable assessment of aortic annulus

and root.[7] However, threshold of AVA used to assess AS severity should probably be modified (discussed elsewhere in this issue).

As previously explained in the TTE section, TEE is used to directly measure the AVA at the tip of leaflets using 2D and 3D planimetry (**Fig. 3**B). In addition, TEE allows a more accurate assessment of the aortic root dimensions and the aortic valve anatomy (ie, bicuspid valve) than TTE.

CARDIAC COMPUTED TOMOGRAPHY: CALCIUM SCORING AND FUSION IMAGING
Noncontrast Computed Tomography: Calcium Scoring

These last years, the quantification of aortic valve calcific burden (ie, calcium scoring) by cardiac CT revolutionized AS evaluation. Calcium scoring (**Fig. 4**B) requires a low-dose (<1 mSv) cardiac CT with electrocardiogram gating but without contrast injection. The quantification of calcific deposition is performed according to the Agatston method using a semiautomated software. Several studies demonstrated the excellent reproducibility and performance of calcium score for the AS severity and prognosis evaluations. Moreover, calcium score may provide a more reliable prognostic evaluation than

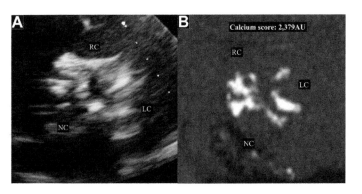

Fig. 4. Calcium scoring evaluation in a patient with severe aortic stenosis using (*A*) a semiquantitative approach by transthoracic echocardiography and (*B*) a quantitative approach by cardiac computed tomography. LC, left coronary leaflet; NC, noncoronary leaflet; RC, right coronary leaflet.

usual hemodynamic parameters.[8–10] According to current guidelines, calcium scoring should be used in patients with discordant parameters of severe AS and both preserved or reduced LV ejection fraction (LVEF <50%), to confirm the severity[11] and avoid unnecessary or delayed intervention. The calcium score cutoff to define severe AS (see **Table 1**) differs according to sex with a lower value in women ($\geq$1200 AU) than in men ($\geq$2000 AU).[9,10] This difference may be explained by the presence of a smaller aortic annulus, in part, and especially a more fibrotic pattern of valve disease in women.[12] In addition, ethnicity may also influence the calcium deposition,[13] but further investigations are required to define additional cutoffs.

Contrast Computed Tomography: Aortic Valve Area and Left Ventricular Outflow Tract Planimetry-Fusion Imaging

The high 3D spatial resolution of contrast cardiac CT allows an accurate evaluation of the anatomy and the dimensions of cardiac structures. Hence, contrast CT may be used in patients with AS to better define LVOT, AV morphology and AVA planimetry, and aortic root dimensions.

As previously explained for TEE, AVA planimetry may be accurately measured by contrast CT (**Fig. 3**C) in case of discordance between AVA and transvalvular flow to better characterize AS severity (AVA <1.0 cm^2, see **Table 1**).

The elliptical shape of the LVOT may lead to AVA underestimation when evaluated by echocardiography, whereas a 3D evaluation by CT using both mean LVOT $_d$ and LVOT area may be more accurate.[3] Hence, some authors evaluated if a hybrid approach to calculate AVA using TTE-derived Doppler parameters and contrast cardiac CT-derived LVOT dimensions (**Fig. 2**D) could reconcile AVA and flow in discordant cases.[14–16] This approach led to find larger LVOT dimensions but the result was not unequivocal because of a similar or even a higher overall percentage of misclassified patients compared with TTE findings.[16] Indeed, some patients with a classical severe AS (AVA <1.0 cm^2 and ΔPm $\geq$40 mm Hg) became discordant (ΔPm $\geq$40 mm Hg but AVA $\geq$1.0 cm^2), whereas patients with a severe discordant AS (AVA <1.0 cm^2 and ΔPm <40 mm Hg) became moderate (AVA $\geq$1.0 cm^2 and ΔPm <40 mm Hg). This could be explained by the fact that the optimal AVA cutoff to predict outcomes was larger than using LVOT measured by TTE (AVA $\leq$1.2 cm^2 vs 1.0 cm^2).[15] Thus, a hybrid approach may be proposed but only in case of discordant severe

AS and using a larger cutoff of AVA (see **Table 1**).[17]

Finally, contrast cardiac CT is essential before transcatheter AVR (TAVR) to define the prosthesis size according to the aortic annulus dimensions, the AV anatomy (bicuspid or tricuspid), and the aortic root characteristics (aortic dimensions and coronary artery position), in addition to the vascular access assessment (Vivian G. Ng and colleagues' article, "Planning For Success: Pre-procedural Evaluation for Transcatheter Aortic Valve Replacement," in this issue).

CARDIAC MRI

Cardiac magnetic resonance (CMR) is the gold standard method for the assessment of ventricular volumes and function, and for the characterization of myocardial abnormality, whereas its use in heart valve disease is recent. Intracardiac flows are evaluated by 2D phase-contrast or more recently by four-dimensional flow imaging acquisitions. The latter has the advantage of analyzing all the components of the flow and not only those perpendicular to the acquisition plane, which is the main limitation of phase-contrast data. The most validated indication is aortic regurgitation in native and prosthetic valves, especially after TAVR.[18] Several publications also reported a good accuracy compared with TTE for assessing AS severity[19] in bicuspid and tricuspid valves. CMR parameters to quantify AS severity are similar to those of TTE: AVA and antegrade systolic flow across the aortic valve. Transvalvular aortic flow parameters (Vmax, ΔPm, and aortic antegrade volume) are obtained from phase-contrast imaging between the leaflet tips and the proximal ascending aorta portion, and AVA is calculated using the continuity equation. LVOT area measurement is obtained from cine-images using the same method as cardiac CT and antegrade LVOT volume is derived from a phase-contrast acquisition at the LVOT level. This method is time consuming and requires a previous TTE analysis (Vmax) to accurately encode CMR velocity. Thus, CMR is not a first-line examination for the evaluation of AS severity but may be used in dedicated conditions as in patients without any correct acoustic window by TTE. In addition, LVOT area by CMR could be used to calculate AVA using a hybrid approach as previously described for cardiac CT. Finally, a phase-contrast acquisition at the tip of aortic leaflets may be used for direct AVA planimetry.

STRESS ECHOCARDIOGRAPHY FOR AORTIC STENOSIS SEVERITY EVALUATION: AN OBSOLETE EXAMINATION?

Two distinct situations should be considered regarding the use of stress echocardiography in patients with AS: the prognostic evaluation of asymptomatic patients with severe AS using exercise-stress echocardiography, and the confirmation of AS severity when TTE at rest is inconclusive.

The first aspect is controversial. Some studies found that exercise-stress echocardiography parameters (LVEF variation, ΔPm increase) might be useful for the prognostic stratification of asymptomatic patients with severe AS to identify patients who would benefit from early surgery.[20,21] However, recent reports did not find any additional value of echocardiography over the stress test alone.[22] In view of the lack of reliable data, the use of exercise-stress echocardiography in asymptomatic severe AS was removed from the latest guidelines.[11]

Conversely, the use of stress echocardiography with low-dose (up to 20 μg/kg/min) dobutamine infusion is recommended by current guidelines to distinguish severe (true-severe) from moderate (pseudosevere) AS (see **Table 1**) in patients with discordant parameters of severe AS (AVA <1.0 cm^2 and ΔPm <40 mm Hg) and reduced LVEF (<50%; ie, classical low-gradient [LG] severe AS). The first step is to determine if the patient has a flow reserve (increase in SV ≥20%). Indeed, AS severity evaluation is complex when the LF state related to LV systolic dysfunction is not corrected by dobutamine infusion. In patients with a flow reserve, the second step is to quantify AVA and transvalvular aortic flow variations at peak stress. Severe AS is confirmed by an increase in Vmax greater than or equal to 4 m/s or ΔPm greater than or equal to 40 mm Hg but with an AVA that remains less than 1.0 cm^2 (**Fig. 5**), whereas moderate AS is defined by an increase in AVA greater than or equal to 1.0 cm^2. However, many patients, even with contractile reserve, do not reach a normal flow rate and remain discordant at peak stress evaluation. To overcome this limitation, the projected AVA calculation may help to identify true-severe AS.[23,24] Finally, in patients without contractile reserve, the projected AVA could be calculated if the increase in flow is higher than 15%. If not, the severity of AS remained undetermined by stress echocardiography. In all of these patients, AS severity could be confirmed/assessed by CT calcium scoring.

These guidelines are mainly based on publications that predate the era of TAVR.[25–27] Patients with a pseudosevere AS had the same prognosis than matched patients with heart failure, whereas patients with a true-severe AS had worse outcomes.[28] In addition, the absence of flow reserve was a major risk marker for postoperative mortality. However, surgical AVR was beneficial in patients with true-severe AS (confirmed by the surgeon) regardless of the presence or absence of flow reserve compared with medical therapy

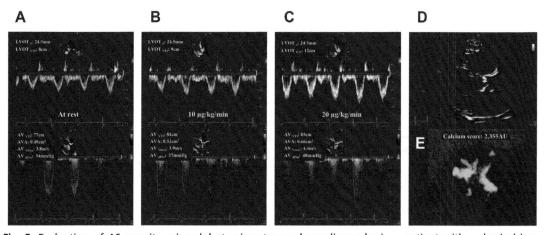

Fig. 5. Evaluation of AS severity using dobutamine stress echocardiography in a patient with a classical low-gradient low-flow severe AS. AVA remained <1 cm^2, whereas transvalvular aortic flow progressively increased with dobutamine infusion (*A*) at rest, (*B*) 10 μg/kg/min, and (*C*) 20 μg/kg/min to reach a peak velocity ≥4 m/s and mean pressure gradient ≥40 mm Hg. AV was severely calcified on (*D*) transthoracic echocardiography and (*E*) computed tomography. AV, aortic valve; LVOT $_d$, LVOT diameter; Vmax, peak jet velocity; ΔPm, mean pressure gradient.

alone.[29] The prognosis impact of flow reserve was not confirmed in surgical AVR[30] patients and after TAVR.[31] To summarize, all patients with a classical LG true-severe AS benefit from AVR, especially using a percutaneous approach, whether or not having a flow reserve. Hence, the current use of dobutamine stress echocardiography is probably less relevant, because the AS severity is directly confirmed by calcium scoring (proposal 1, **Fig. 6**).

CONFIRMATION AND CLASSIFICATION OF SEVERE AORTIC STENOSIS: A MULTIMODALITY APPROACH

AS is classified in different categories according to transvalvular mean pressure gradient (ΔPm cutoff: 40 mm Hg), LVEF (cutoff 50%), and LVOT flow (SVi cutoff: 35 mL/m^2). High-gradient (HG) severe AS corresponds to classical severe AS and requires no further examination to confirm its severity. However, patients with AS with an HG-LF pattern may have a worse prognosis in absence of early treatment compared with HG normal-flow (NF) patients.[32] Conversely, LG (or discordant) severe AS requires a multimodality approach to confirm its true severity before considering AV intervention (see **Fig. 6**). The first step consists in confirming the measurements (especially LVOT $_d$) and in using additional parameters (ie, VTI ratio, AVA planimetry, AT or AT/ET, hybrid AVA) to exclude moderate AS. Next step requires the assessment of LVEF to distinguish LG AS patients with preserved ($\geq$50%) from reduced LVEF (<50%). In patients

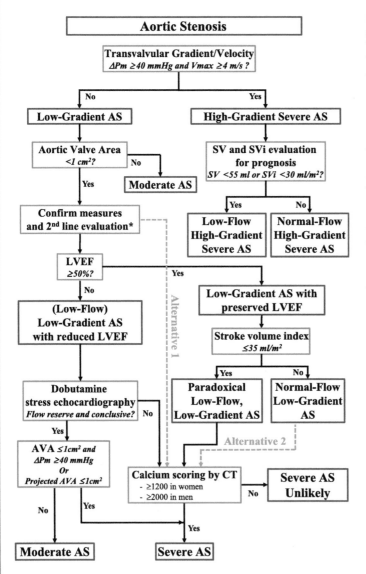

Fig. 6. Algorithm to confirm and classify severe aortic stenosis. Velocity or VTI ratio, AT and AT/ET, AVA planimetry, and AVA using the hybrid method. Alternative 1: AS severity confirmation by calcium scoring in patients with low-gradient pattern, regardless of LVEF and SV levels. Alternative 2: exclude severe AS by calcium scoring in patients with low-gradient normal-flow pattern. ΔPm, mean pressure gradient; SV (SVi), stroke volume (indexed); Vmax, peak jet velocity. *See **Table 1**. (*Adapted from* Baumgartner H, Falk V, Bax JJ, et al. 2017 ESC/EACTS guidelines for the management of valvular heart disease: The Task Force for the management of valvular heart disease of the European Society of Cardiology (ESC) and the European Association for Cardio-Thoracic Surgery (EACTS). *Eur Heart J.* 2017;38(36):2739-2791; with permission.)

with LG AS and reduced LVEF (ie, classical LG-LF AS), the true severity of AS should be confirmed by dobutamine stress echocardiography or by calcium scoring when inconclusive. In patients with LG AS but preserved LVEF, the SV assessment should be used to discriminate NF from paradoxic LF-LG AS. LG-NF AS is classified as severe AS unlikely by the current guidelines, but recent studies suggest that 50% of patients may have a true-severe stenosis and may benefit from AVR.[33] Hence, the use of calcium scoring may help to identify these patients (alternative 2, see **Fig. 6**). Patients with a paradoxic LG-LF AS also require calcium scoring by CT to confirm AS severity. Moreover, their prognosis is darker and interventional risk higher because of the LF state. **Fig. 6** is an adapted version of the different steps reported in the current guidelines to classify and confirm severe AS. In addition, we provide a simplified alternative (alternative 1) to confirm AS severity with calcium scoring in patients with an LG pattern, regardless of the LVEF and SV levels.

SUMMARY

AS is a serious cardiac disease with a significant morbidity and mortality. AS severity confirmation is essential to adequately manage such patients. TTE is the key examination to confirm the diagnosis in most patients. However, parameter discordance is not uncommon and requires a multimodality approach to confirm AS severity.

REFERENCES

1. Baumgartner H, Hung J, Bermejo J, et al. Recommendations on the echocardiographic assessment of aortic valve stenosis: a focused update from the European Association of Cardiovascular Imaging and the American Society of Echocardiography. J Am Soc Echocardiogr 2017;30(4):372–92.
2. de Monchy CC, Lepage L, Boutron I, et al. Usefulness of the right parasternal view and non-imaging continuous-wave Doppler transducer for the evaluation of the severity of aortic stenosis in the modern area. Eur J Echocardiogr 2009;10(3):420–4.
3. Ng AC, Delgado V, van der Kley F, et al. Comparison of aortic root dimensions and geometries before and after transcatheter aortic valve implantation by 2- and 3-dimensional transesophageal echocardiography and multislice computed tomography. Circ Cardiovasc Imaging 2010;3(1):94–102.
4. Ringle Griguer A, Tribouilloy C, Truffier A, et al. Clinical significance of ejection dynamics parameters in patients with aortic stenosis: an outcome study. J Am Soc Echocardiogr 2018;31(5):551–60.e2.
5. Rosenhek R, Binder T, Porenta G, et al. Predictors of outcome in severe, asymptomatic aortic stenosis. N Engl J Med 2000;343(9):611–7.
6. Piazza N, de Jaegere P, Schultz C, et al. Anatomy of the aortic valvar complex and its implications for transcatheter implantation of the aortic valve. Circ Cardiovasc Interv 2008;1:74–81.
7. Prihadi EA, van Rosendael PJ, Vollema EM, et al. Feasibility, accuracy, and reproducibility of aortic annular and root sizing for transcatheter aortic valve replacement using novel automated three dimensional echocardiographic software: comparison with multi-detector row computed tomography. J Am Soc Echocardiogr 2018;31(4):505–14.e3.
8. Cueff C, Serfaty JM, Cimadevilla C, et al. Measurement of aortic valve calcification using multislice computed tomography: correlation with haemodynamic severity of aortic stenosis and clinical implication for patients with low ejection fraction. Heart 2011;97(9):721–6.
9. Clavel MA, Pibarot P, Messika-Zeitoun D, et al. Impact of aortic valve calcification, as measured by MDCT, on survival in patients with aortic stenosis: results of an international registry study. J Am Coll Cardiol 2014;64(12):1202–13.
10. Pawade T, Clavel MA, Tribouilloy C, et al. Computed tomography aortic valve calcium scoring in patients with aortic stenosis. Circ Cardiovasc Imaging 2018; 11(3):e007146.
11. Baumgartner H, Falk V, Bax JJ, et al. 2017 ESC/EACTS guidelines for the management of valvular heart disease: the task force for the management of valvular heart disease of the European Society of Cardiology (ESC) and the European Association for Cardio-Thoracic Surgery (EACTS). Eur Heart J 2017;38(36):2739–91.
12. Simard L, Côté N, Dagenais F, et al. Sex-related discordance between aortic valve calcification and hemodynamic severity of aortic stenosis: is valvular fibrosis the explanation? Circ Res 2017;120(4): 681–91.
13. Patel DK, Green KD, Fudim M, et al. Racial differences in the prevalence of severe aortic stenosis. J Am Heart Assoc 2014;3(3):e000879.
14. Kamperidis V, van Rosendael PJ, Katsanos S, et al. Low gradient severe aortic stenosis with preserved ejection fraction: reclassification of severity by fusion of Doppler and computed tomographic data. Eur Heart J 2015;36(31):2087–96.
15. Clavel MA, Malouf J, Messika-Zeitoun D, et al. Aortic valve area calculation in aortic stenosis by CT and Doppler echocardiography. JACC Cardiovasc Imaging 2015;8(3):248–57.
16. Arangalage D, Laredo M, Ou P, et al. Anatomic characterization of the aortic root in patients with bicuspid and tricuspid aortic valve stenosis does fusion of Doppler-echocardiography and computed

tomography resolve discordant severity grading? JACC Cardiovasc Imaging 2019;12(1):203–19.

17. Delgado V, Clavel MA, Hahn RT, et al. How do we reconcile echocardiography, computed tomography, and hybrid imaging in assessing discordant grading of aortic stenosis severity? JACC Cardiovasc Imaging 2019;12(2):267–82.

18. Ribeiro HB, Orwat S, Hayek SS, et al. Cardiovascular magnetic resonance to evaluate aortic regurgitation after transcatheter aortic valve replacement. J Am Coll Cardiol 2016;68(6):577–85.

19. Mantini C, Di Giammarco G, Pizzicannella J, et al. Grading of aortic stenosis severity: a head-to-head comparison between cardiac magnetic resonance imaging and echocardiography. Radiol Med 2018; 123(9):643–54.

20. Masri A, Goodman AL, Barr T, et al. Predictors of long-term outcomes in asymptomatic patients with severe aortic stenosis and preserved left ventricular systolic function undergoing exercise echocardiography. Circ Cardiovasc Imaging 2016;9(7) [pii: e004689].

21. Maréchaux S, Hachicha Z, Bellouin A, et al. Usefulness of exercise stress echocardiography for risk stratification of true asymptomatic patients with aortic valve stenosis. Eur Heart J 2010;31(11): 1390–7.

22. Goublaire C, Melissopoulou M, Lobo D, et al. Prognostic value of exercise-stress echocardiography in asymptomatic patients with aortic valve stenosis. JACC Cardiovasc Imaging 2018;11(6):787–95.

23. Clavel MA, Burwash IG, Mundigler G, et al. Validation of conventional and simplified methods to calculate projected valve area at normal flow rate in patients with low flow, low gradient aortic stenosis: the multicenter TOPAS (True or Pseudo Severe Aortic Stenosis) study. J Am Soc Echocardiogr 2010;23(4):380–6.

24. Annabi MS, Touboul E, Dahou A, et al. Dobutamine stress echocardiography for management of low-flow, low-gradient aortic stenosis. J Am Coll Cardiol 2018;71(5):475–85.

25. Monin JL, Quere JP, Monchi M, et al. Low-gradient aortic stenosis: operative risk stratification and predictors for long-term outcome: a multicenter study using dobutamine stress hemodynamics. Circulation 2003;108(3):319–24.

26. Monin JL, Monchi M, Gest V, et al. Aortic stenosis with severe left ventricular dysfunction and low transvalvular pressure gradients. J Am Coll Cardiol 2001;37(8):2101–7.

27. Quere JP, Monin JL, Levy F, et al. Influence of preoperative left ventricular contractile reserve on postoperative ejection fraction in low-gradient aortic stenosis. Circulation 2006;113(14):1738–44.

28. Fougères É, Tribouilloy C, Monchi M, et al. Outcomes of pseudo-severe aortic stenosis under conservative treatment. Eur Heart J 2012;33(19): 2426–33.

29. Tribouilloy C, Levy F, Rusinaru D, et al. Outcome after aortic valve replacement for low-flow/low-gradient aortic stenosis without contractile reserve on dobutamine stress echocardiography. J Am Coll Cardiol 2009;53(20):1865–73.

30. Annabi MS, Clavel MA, Pibarot P. Dobutamine stress echocardiography in low-flow, low-gradient aortic stenosis: flow reserve does not matter anymore. J Am Heart Assoc 2019;8(6):e012212.

31. Ribeiro HB, Lerakis S, Gilard M, et al. Transcatheter aortic valve replacement in patients with low-flow, low-gradient aortic stenosis: the TOPAS-TAVI registry. J Am Coll Cardiol 2018;71(12):1297–308.

32. Rusinaru D, Bohbot Y, Ringle A, et al. Impact of low stroke volume on mortality in patients with severe aortic stenosis and preserved left ventricular ejection fraction. Eur Heart J 2018;39(21):1992–9.

33. Zusman O, Pressman GS, Banai S, et al. Intervention versus observation in symptomatic patients with normal flow-low gradient severe aortic stenosis. JACC Cardiovasc Imaging 2018;11(9):1225–32.

Assessment of Cardiac Damage in Aortic Stenosis

Miho Fukui, MD, PhD[a], Philippe Généreux, MD[b], João L. Cavalcante, MD[a,c],*

KEYWORDS

- Aortic stenosis • Aortic valve replacement • Cardiac damage • Classification • Mortality
- Readmission

KEY POINTS

- Severe aortic stenosis (AS) results in progressive cardiac damage, which extends beyond the left ventricle.
- The extent of structural and functional cardiac damage is associated with adverse outcomes after aortic valve replacement in patients with severe AS.
- A new staging system for AS, which classifies according to the extent of cardiac damage, provides incremental risk stratification to conventional systems.
- Additionally, early recognition of subclinical myocardial dysfunction may offer the opportunity to optimize the timing of aortic valve replacement for AS.

INTRODUCTION

Aortic stenosis (AS) is the most common valvular heart disease in developed countries, at 1.7% in the population older than 65 years,[1] and the prevalence is expected to increase with an aging population.[2] Severe AS causes chronic pressure overload of the left ventricle (LV), resulting in the progressive cardiac damage: LV hypertrophy (LVH), LV diastolic dysfunction, left atrium (LA) dilation, development of mitral and tricuspid regurgitation, pulmonary hypertension (PH), and finally right ventricular (RV) dysfunction.[3] Although several previous studies[4–9] have shown an association between the cardiac damage related to (or associated with) AS and the adverse events after aortic valve replacement (AVR) (either surgical or transcatheter), current indications for intervention, risk stratification, and strategies for patient care have not entirely incorporated a systematic assessment of the extent of cardiac damage.

Although AVR is an effective therapy for symptomatic patients with severe AS, when to intervene and how to follow-up these patients after intervention are important metrics to continue improving the outcomes and prognosis for these patients. This review summarizes the current evidences regarding the association of cardiac damage related to AS with clinical outcomes and then introduces a new AS staging classification system characterizing the extent of cardiac damage.

ASSOCIATION OF EACH CARDIAC CHAMBER DAMAGE WITH OUTCOMES IN AORTIC STENOSIS
Left Ventricle

LVH develops as a compensatory mechanism to severe AS to maintain cardiac output and reduce wall stress against progressive chronic pressure overload.[10] Approximately 60% of AS patients undergoing transcatheter AVR (TAVR) have LVH as

Disclosure Statement: The authors have nothing to disclose.
[a] Minneapolis Heart Institute Foundation, Cardiovascular Imaging Research and Valve Science Centers, 920 East 28th Street, Suite 620, Minneapolis, MN 55407, USA; [b] Division of Cardiology, Morristown Medical Center, 100 Madison Avenue, Morristown, NJ 07960, USA; [c] Minneapolis Heart Institute, Abbott Northwestern Hospital, 800 East 28th Street, Suite 300, Minneapolis, MN 55407, USA
* Corresponding author.
E-mail address: Joao.Cavalcante@allina.com
Twitter: @Miho_Fukui_ (M.F.); @philgenereux (P.G.); @JoaoLCavalcante (J.L.C.)

Cardiol Clin 38 (2020) 23–31
https://doi.org/10.1016/j.ccl.2019.09.001
0733-8651/20/© 2019 Elsevier Inc. All rights reserved.

cardiology.theclinics.com

determined by LV mass index (LVMI) and relative wall thickness, in which the majority is in a concentric pattern.[11] The pattern and severity of LVH, however, vary by gender.[12] Although preoperative LVH was associated with an increased risk for adverse in hospital outcomes and mortality in patients with AS who underwent surgical AVR (SAVR),[13,14] in most recent publication,[11] using data from the Society of Thoracic Surgeons (STS)/American College of Cardiology Transcatheter Valve Therapy Registry, showed that preprocedural LVH was not associated with 1-year outcomes post-TAVR in 31,199 patients with severe AS. The difference in the association with outcomes between SAVR and TAVR might be due to the differences in patients' comorbidities, procedural technique, and postprocedural care.

In parallel to LVH development, increased chamber stiffness and delayed active LV relaxation produce LV diastolic dysfunction and increased filling pressures. Diastolic dysfunction has shown to be associated with mortality after SAVR[15,16] and TAVR.[4]

Over time, the long-standing pressure overload of the LV finally causes LV systolic dysfunction. An LVEF of less than 50% currently is a criterion included in the American and European guidelines for triggering AVR,[17,18] regardless of symptoms. This criterion lacks sufficient sensitivity to identify subclinical LV dysfunction. Most recently, Bohbot and colleagues[19] provide further evidence that the current cutoff value of LVEF (<50%) is too low and that a value of less than 55% is more appropriate to identify LV dysfunction and to consider intervention in severe AS. Other recent studies[20,21] even have suggested using an LVEF value of less than 60% for this purpose.

Left Atrium, Mitral Regurgitation, and Atrial Fibrillation

With the progression of LV diastolic dysfunction and increased LV filling pressure, the LA dilates, which facilitates the development of mitral regurgitation (MR) and atrial fibrillation (A-fib). LA dilatation,[5,22] the presence of concomitant significant MR,[6] and A-fib[7] are known to provide prognostic information in patients with severe AS.

Previous studies reported that baseline LA dilation was associated with LVH and increased filling pressure. Furthermore, a greater LA volume index was associated with a higher risk of adverse events in both asymptomatic patients with severe AS[22] and symptomatic patients with severe AS undergoing SAVR.[5]

Various factors can influence the presence and severity of functional MR in patients with severe AS, including the high prevalence of coronary artery disease with subsequent ischemic MR, and/or the LV dilatation seen in end-stage AS. The prevalence rates of concomitant moderate to severe MR in patients with severe AS undergoing TAVR were 19.8% and 22.2% in Placement of Aortic Transcatheter Valve (PARTNER) A[23] and PARTNER B trials,[24] respectively. The exact prevalence of significant MR in the SAVR patient cohort is unclear because these patients might have received double valve surgery. Importantly, the concomitant MR is significantly associated with mortality after SAVR and TAVR.[6]

A-fib is induced not only by LA pressure overload but also directly by the same risk factors of AS (eg, age and hypertension).[7] The prevalence of preexisting A-fib in TAVR cohort ranges from 16% to 51.1%[25] and is higher than those in SAVR cohort, ranging from 8% to 13%.[7,26] This difference may be due to older age and greater number of comorbidities with a worse risk profile of the TAVR patients compared with SAVR patients.[27] New-onset A-fib, defined as the presence of A-fib occurring after intervention, is present in up to 40% of SAVR patients and in up to 32% of TAVR patients[7] and is more frequent in TAVR patients treated transapically (6%–38%) than in those treated transfemorally (<1%–16%).[26,28] Both preexisting and new-onset AF are associated with increased mortality after SAVR[29–31] and TAVR.[32–35]

Pulmonary Hypertension and Tricuspid Regurgitation

PH is common (47%–75%)[36,37] in patients with severe AS due to increased LV filling pressures and has been shown an independent predictor of increased mortality after SAVR and TAVR.[38–41] Approximately 15% to 25% of patients with baseline PH had combined precapillary and postcapillary PH, as defined by invasive hemodynamic parameters,[42] and these patients had higher mortality after SAVR and TAVR than those with no PH or isolated postcapillary PH.[37,43] In addition, persistent PH at 1-month post-TAVR was common (25% of overall TAVR cohort or 37.4% of those with baseline PH) and was associated with a 1.8-fold increased risk of morality, even after adjustment for baseline characteristics.[44]

Concomitant significant TR is also a common finding in patients with AS and associated with worse mortality after SAVR[45] and TAVR.[46] In most patients with severe AS, TR is functional and a consequence of right-side chamber remodeling. PH also may contribute to worsening TR, and differentiating adaptive RV remodeling with poor leaflet coaptation from advanced hemody-namic stress burden secondary to long-standing AS is an important component for future manage-ment of the disease.[8]

Right Ventricular Dysfunction

The long-standing pressure overload in the LV and LA chambers can be transmitted through the pul-monary vascular system and result in RV remodel-ing, dilatation, and finally RV dysfunction.[8] RV dysfunction is identified in up to 1 in 4 patients with severe AS[47,48] and may occur even more frequently among patients with low-flow low-gradient AS.[49] Baseline RV dysfunction has showed to be associated with adverse outcome after SAVR[50] and TAVR[9,49] in patients with severe AS.

A NEW AORTIC STENOSIS STAGING CLASSIFICATION

Although the number of previous studies, dis-cussed previously, clearly documents that the presence of each cardiac chamber damage holds prognostic significance in patients with AS, there have been no data regarding the importance of comprehensive assessment of anatomic or func-tional parameters on outcomes after AVR.

Généreux and colleagues[51] recently proposed a new staging classification system for patients with AS that is based on conventional echocardio-graphic markers of abnormal cardiac structure and function. The new AS staging classification describes 5 stages of cardiac damage (**Fig. 1**):

- Stage 0: no other cardiac damage detected

- Stage 1: LV damage—increased LVMI; early mitral inflow to early diastolic mitral annulus velocity (E/e') >14; or LVEF <50%
- Stage 2: LA or mitral damage—LA volume index >34 mL/m²; moderate to severe MR; or A-fib
- Stage 3: pulmonary artery or tricuspid dam-age—pulmonary artery systolic pressure ≥60 mm Hg or moderate to severe TR
- Stage 4: RV damage—moderate to severe RV dysfunction

This staging classification was initially applied in more than 1600 patients who participated in the randomized clinical trials, PARTNER 2A and PARTNER 2B. This AS staging was found to have important prognostic implications for 1-year mortality after either SAVR or TAVR (**Fig. 2**). For each stage increment, 1-year mortality risk increased by approximately 45%. Even after adjustment for several well-established predictors of worse outcomes after AVR, including patient frailty and the STS Predicted Risk of Mortality (STS-PROM) score, the association of AS staging with 1-year mortality remained significant. More recently, Fukui and colleagues,[52] using a large, single-center cohort of 689 patients with symp-tomatic severe AS undergoing TAVR, confirmed the findings by Généreux and colleagues[51] by demonstrating that the AS staging system had a graded association with all-cause mortality, now up to 2-years post-TAVR follow-up (**Fig. 3**A). In addition, Fukui and colleagues reported the asso-ciation between the staging classification and post-TAVR readmissions for both cardiac and noncardiac causes (Fig. 3B, C), particularly greater

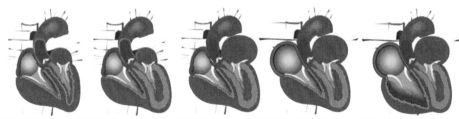

Stages/Criteria	Stage 0	Stage 1	Stage 2	Stage 3	Stage 4
	No Cardiac Damage	LV Damage	LA or Mitral Damage	Pulmonary Vasculature or Tricuspid Damage	RV Damage
Echocardiogram		Increased LV Mass Index >115 g/m² (Male) >95 g/m² (Female)	Indexed left atrial volume >34 mL/m²	Systolic Pulmonary hypertension ≥60 mm Hg	Moderate—Severe right ventricular dysfunction
		'E/e' >14	Moderate—Severe mitral regurgitation	Moderate—Severe tricuspid regurgitation	
		LV Ejection Fraction <50%	Atrial Fibrillation		

Fig. 1. A new AS staging classification, defined by the presence or absence of extra-aortic valve cardiac damage or dysfunction as detected by transthoracic echocardiography.

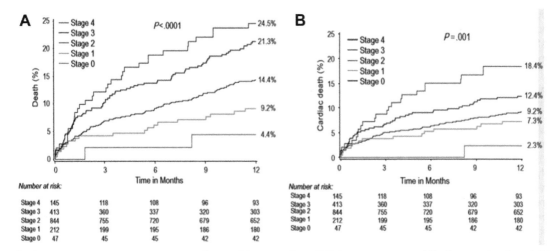

Fig. 2. Post-AVR 1-year outcomes according to AS stages. Post-AVR 1-year outcomes: (*A*) all-cause death and (*B*) cardiac death, which significantly increased with each stage of worsening cardiac damage.

for patients with advanced PH and moderate to severe TR. This association was maintained after adjustment for other traditional risk factors and comorbid conditions through the use of the comprehensive STS-PROM scoring system (**Fig. 4**).

This staging classification provides an opportunity to identify patients who might benefit from a closer follow-up, by continued surveillance of their PH, TR, and RV dysfunctions. Therefore, it raises awareness that such comorbidities could limit the full benefit of TAVR; however, they should not preclude its performance.

SUBCLINICAL MYOCARDIAL DYSFUNCTION IN AORTIC STENOSIS

Use of novel imaging parameters that can detect subclinical myocardial dysfunction beyond conventional echocardiographic parameters[53] might improve the optimal timing of AVR, especially for asymptomatic patients with severe AS and preserved LVEF. Approximately one-third of these patients present with some degree of subclinical dysfunction and have worse outcomes.[1]

Speckle tracking echocardiography (STE)–derived LV global longitudinal strain (GLS) has been shown to detect subclinical myocardial dysfunction beyond LVEF[54,55] in patients with AS.[56,57] Recent studies[58,59] showed that subclinical myocardial dysfunction, detected by impaired STE-GLS, is often present even in asymptomatic patients with severe AS and preserved LVEF. Impaired STE-GLS at baseline seems associated with symptom onset, the need for aortic valve intervention, and higher mortality. Unfortunately, STE-GLS is not feasible in 10% to 20% of patients, most frequently due to inadequate echocardiographic views for analysis. As such, GLS feasibility by not only cardiac magnetic resonance (CMR)[60] but also retrospective gated computed

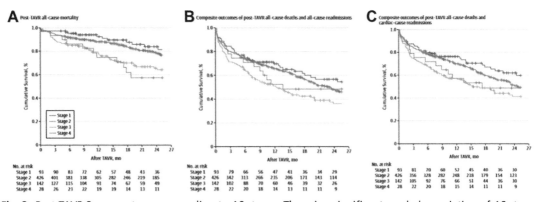

Fig. 3. Post-TAVR 2-year outcomes according to AS stages. There is a significant graded association of AS stages with (*A*) all-cause mortality and (*B*) composite outcomes of all-cause deaths and readmissions for all-cause or (*C*) cardiac-cause after TAVR.

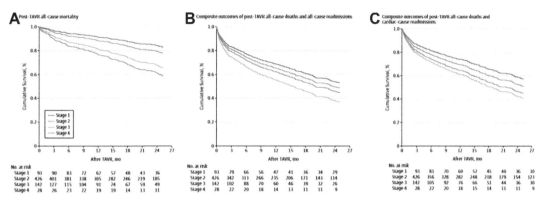

Fig. 4. Adjusted survival curves for post-TAVR 2-year outcomes. (*A*) A strong graded association of AS stages with all-cause mortality after TAVR was unchanged even after adjusting for the STS-PROM score. Regarding post-TAVR readmission rates, patients with stage 3 had the highest risk of composite outcomes of all-cause death and of readmissions for (*B*) all-cause or (*C*) cardiac-cause despite adjustment for STS-PROM score.

tomography angiography,[61] has been recently demonstrated. This might enable evaluation of this important parameter by another imaging modality whenever echocardiography is suboptimal. GLS by STE, CMR, and computed tomography angiography may not be interchangeable,[61] suggesting a potential modality-specific GLS threshold, and outcome studies regarding their utility are needed.

The extent of myocardial fibrosis, as estimated by CMR, has also emerged as a new valuable tool to assess the extent of LV cardiac damage and enhance risk stratification in AS.[62,63] Myocardial fibrosis has 2 categories: replacement fibrosis, which is irreversible and identified using late gadolinium enhancement (LGE) on CMR, and diffuse fibrosis, which tends to occur earlier, is potentially reversible, and can be quantified with CMR T1 mapping techniques (ie, native T1 value, extracellular volume fraction, and indexed extracellular volume).

LGE was observed in approximately 50% in patients with severe AS, and nonischemic patterns of LGE were twice as common as ischemic patterns.[64] The largest multicenter study of CMR in AS to date[64] included 674 patients with severe AS and demonstrated that the presence of LGE doubled all-cause mortality and tripled cardiovascular mortality despite AVR. Whether noninfarct LGE can be used to optimize the timing of valve intervention is currently being tested in the Early Valve Replacement Guided by Biomarkers of LV Decompensation in Asymptomatic Patients With Severe AS trial (NCT03094143).

All 3 parameters of T1 mapping technique have been shown to correlate with collagen volume fraction on histology.[65–71] Recent studies demonstrated that native T1[72] and indexed extracellular volume[65] were significantly higher in patients with AS compared with healthy volunteers and

independently associated with adverse outcomes. Further studies are needed to validate the utility of these parameters in the clinical setting.

BLOOD BIOMARKERS LINKED TO CARDIAC DAMAGES IN AORTIC STENOSIS

Several studies have demonstrated the usefulness of blood biomarkers like brain natriuretic peptides (BNPs), high-sensitivity cardiac troponin, soluble ST2, growth differentiation factor 15, and galectin 3 as markers of the cardiac damage related to AS.[73,74] BNP and its biologically inactive N-terminal (NT) form are by far the most studied in AS. Several studies have reported an additive predictive value of BNP and/or NT-prohormone BNP (NT-proNBP) to predict adverse events; however, thresholds to identify excess risk were highly variable. This is probably because BNP and NT-proBNP are variable according to age and sex of the patient. Clavel and colleagues[75] proposed a new index: the BNP ratio, which is the measured level of BNP divided by the maximal normal reference values. In patients with moderate to severe AS, this new index was associated with excess long-term mortality; it added incremental prognostic value to baseline clinical and echocardiographic characteristics.

High-sensitivity cardiac troponin would be interesting in AS to detect the transition between compensatory LVH to heart failure. In this sense, high-sensitivity cardiac troponin I concentrations were independently associated to indexed LV mass and measures of replacement fibrosis as assessed by late gadolinium enhancement at CMR.[76] High-sensitivity cardiac troponin was also proved an independent prognostic factor in patients with AS.[76,77] In addition, preprocedural and postprocedural troponin levels were associated with poor outcomes in patients undergoing SAVR[78,79] and TAVR.[80]

Numerous other biomarkers of inflammation, apoptosis, fibrosis, and/or tissue remodeling have been linked to adverse outcome in AS, preintervention or postintervention.[81–83] These biomarkers, however, have most of the time been identified in small studies and results were not replicated. Finally, multibiomarker approaches have been proposed with the association of troponin and BNP[84] or multiple biomarkers.[85] Importantly, the role and incremental value of blood biomarkers currently are being investigated further and could bring meaningful information to the clinical management of patients with AS as well as imaging biomarkers.

SUMMARY

The AS staging classification system provides a comprehensive framework for the clinical assessment of cardiac damage associated with AS. This classification can help stratify patients and predict their outcome after TAVR intervention, which can help clinicians better communicate with patients and families to better manage expectations. It not only is easy to do but also gives clinicians an opportunity to learn over time how to adjust or add on management strategies that give patients the best chance at survival and staying out of the hospital.

Given the safety and utility of TAVR in low-risk patients[86,87] and that long-term durability of transcatheter AV prostheses[88] continues to be confirmed, the number of TAVR procedures will continue to grow. Early and accurate recognition of subclinical myocardial dysfunction via assessment of GLS, other CMR markers of myocardial fibrosis, and blood biomarkers can offer the opportunity to optimize the timing for AVR, especially in asymptomatic patients with severe AS and preserved ejection fraction.

REFERENCES

1. Pibarot P, Sengupta P, Chandrashekhar Y. Imaging is the cornerstone of the management of aortic valve stenosis. JACC Cardiovasc Imaging 2019;12(1): 220–3.
2. Bonow RO, Greenland P. Population-wide trends in aortic stenosis incidence and outcomes. Circulation 2015;131(11):969–71.
3. Cavalcante JL. Watchful waiting in aortic stenosis: are we ready for individualizing the risk assessment? Eur Heart J 2016;37(8):724–6.
4. Asami M, Lanz J, Stortecky S, et al. The impact of left ventricular diastolic dysfunction on clinical outcomes after transcatheter aortic valve replacement. JACC Cardiovasc Interv 2018;11(6):593–601.
5. Dahl JS, Videbæk L, Poulsen MK, et al. Noninvasive assessment of filling pressure and left atrial pressure overload in severe aortic valve stenosis: relation to ventricular remodeling and clinical outcome after aortic valve replacement. J Thorac Cardiovasc Surg 2011;142(3):e77–83.
6. Nombela-Franco L, Ribeiro HB, Urena M, et al. Significant mitral regurgitation left untreated at the time of aortic valve replacement: a comprehensive review of a frequent entity in the transcatheter aortic valve replacement era. J Am Coll Cardiol 2014; 63(24):2643–58.
7. Mojoli M, Tarantini G, Vahanian A, et al. Atrial fibrillation in patients undergoing transcatheter aortic valve implantation: epidemiology, timing, predictors, and outcome. Eur Heart J 2016;38(17):1285–93.
8. Cavalcante JL, Simon MA, Chan SY. Comprehensive right-sided assessment for transcatheter aortic valve replacement risk stratification: time for a change. J Am Soc Echocardiogr 2017;30(1): 47–51.
9. Asami M, Stortecky S, Praz F, et al. Prognostic value of right ventricular dysfunction on clinical outcomes after transcatheter aortic valve replacement. JACC Cardiovasc Imaging 2019;12(4):577–87.
10. Rader F, Sachdev E, Arsanjani R, et al. Left ventricular hypertrophy in valvular aortic stenosis: mechanisms and clinical implications. Am J Med 2015; 128(4):344–52.
11. Varshney AS, Manandhar P, Vemulapalli S, et al. Left ventricular hypertrophy does not affect 1-year clinical outcomes in patients undergoing transcatheter aortic valve replacement. JACC Cardiovasc Interv 2019;12(4):373–82.
12. Treibel TA, Kozor R, Fontana M, et al. Sex dimorphism in the myocardial response to aortic stenosis. JACC Cardiovasc Imaging 2018;11(7):962–73.
13. Fuster RG, Argudo JAM, Albarova OG, et al. Left ventricular mass index in aortic valve surgery: a new index for early valve replacement? Eur J Cardiothorac Surg 2003;23(5):696–702.
14. Duncan AI, Lowe BS, Garcia MJ, et al. Influence of concentric left ventricular remodeling on early mortality after aortic valve replacement. Ann Thorac Surg 2008;85(6):2030–9.
15. Dahl JS, Barros-Gomes S, Videbaek L, et al. Early diastolic strain rate in relation to systolic and diastolic function and prognosis in aortic stenosis. JACC Cardiovasc Imaging 2016;9(5):519–28.
16. Chang S-A, Park P-W, Sung K, et al. Noninvasive estimate of left ventricular filling pressure correlated with early and midterm postoperative cardiovascular events after isolated aortic valve replacement in patients with severe aortic stenosis. J Thorac Cardiovasc Surg 2010;140(6):1361–6.

17. Nishimura RA, Otto CM, Bonow RO, et al. 2014 AHA/ACC guideline for the management of patients with valvular heart disease: a report of the American College of Cardiology/American Heart Association Task Force on Practice Guidelines. Circulation 2014; 129(23):e521–643.

18. Baumgartner H, Falk V, Bax JJ, et al. 2017 ESC/EACTS guidelines for the management of valvular heart disease. Eur Heart J 2017;38(36):2739–91.

19. Bohbot Y, de Meester de Ravenstein C, Chadha G, et al. Relationship between left ventricular ejection fraction and mortality in asymptomatic and minimally symptomatic patients with severe aortic stenosis. JACC Cardiovasc Imaging 2019;12(1):38–48.

20. Gu H, Saeed S, Boguslavskyi A, et al. First-phase ejection fraction is a powerful predictor of adverse events in asymptomatic patients with aortic stenosis and preserved total ejection fraction. JACC Cardiovasc Imaging 2019;12(1):52–63.

21. Ito S, Miranda WR, Nkomo VT, et al. Reduced left ventricular ejection fraction in patients with aortic stenosis. J Am Coll Cardiol 2018;71(12):1313–21.

22. Christensen NL, Dahl JS, Carter-Storch R, et al. Relation of left atrial size, cardiac morphology, and clinical outcome in asymptomatic aortic stenosis. Am J Cardiol 2017;120(10):1877–83.

23. Leon MB, Smith CR, Mack M, et al. Transcatheter aortic-valve implantation for aortic stenosis in patients who cannot undergo surgery. N Engl J Med 2010;363(17):1597–607.

24. Smith CR, Leon MB, Mack MJ, et al. Transcatheter versus surgical aortic-valve replacement in high-risk patients. N Engl J Med 2011;364(23):2187–98.

25. Sannino A, Gargiulo G, Schiattarella GG, et al. A meta-analysis of the impact of pre-existing and new-onset atrial fibrillation on clinical outcomes in patients undergoing transcatheter aortic valve implantation. EuroIntervention 2016;12(8):e1047–56.

26. Motloch LJ, Reda S, Rottlaender D, et al. Postprocedural atrial fibrillation after transcatheter aortic valve implantation versus surgical aortic valve replacement. Ann Thorac Surg 2012;93(1):124–31.

27. Tamburino C, Barbanti M, D'Errigo P, et al. 1-Year outcomes after transfemoral transcatheter or surgical aortic valve replacement: results from the Italian OBSERVANT study. J Am Coll Cardiol 2015;66(7):804–12.

28. Urena M, Hayek S, Cheema AN, et al. Arrhythmia burden in elderly patients with severe aortic stenosis as determined by continuous electrocardiographic recording: toward a better understanding of arrhythmic events after transcatheter aortic valve replacement. Circulation 2015;131(5):469–77.

29. Wang TK, Ramanathan T, Choi DH, et al. Preoperative atrial fibrillation predicts mortality and morbidity after aortic valve replacement. Interact Cardiovasc Thorac Surg 2014;19(2):218–22.

30. Levy F, Garayalde E, Quere JP, et al. Prognostic value of preoperative atrial fibrillation in patients with aortic stenosis and low ejection fraction having aortic valve replacement. Am J Cardiol 2006;98(6):809–11.

31. Filardo G, Hamilton C, Hamman B, et al. New-onset postoperative atrial fibrillation and long-term survival after aortic valve replacement surgery. Ann Thorac Surg 2010;90(2):474–9.

32. Siontis GCM, Praz F, Lanz J, et al. New-onset arrhythmias following transcatheter aortic valve implantation: a systematic review and meta-analysis. Heart 2018;104(14):1208–15.

33. Tarantini G, Mojoli M, Windecker S, et al. Prevalence and impact of atrial fibrillation in patients with severe aortic stenosis undergoing transcatheter aortic valve replacement: an analysis from the SOURCE XT prospective multicenter registry. JACC Cardiovasc Interv 2016;9(9):937–46.

34. Chopard R, Teiger E, Meneveau N, et al. Baseline characteristics and prognostic implications of pre-existing and new-onset atrial fibrillation after transcatheter aortic valve implantation: results from the FRANCE-2 registry. JACC Cardiovasc Interv 2015; 8(10):1346–55.

35. Biviano AB, Nazif T, Dizon J, et al. Atrial fibrillation is associated with increased mortality in patients undergoing transcatheter aortic valve replacement: insights from the placement of aortic transcatheter valve (PARTNER) trial. Circ Cardiovasc Interv 2016; 9(1):e002766.

36. D'Ascenzo F, Conrotto F, Salizzoni S, et al. Incidence, predictors, and impact on prognosis of systolic pulmonary artery pressure and its improvement after transcatheter aortic valve implantation: a multicenter registry. J Invasive Cardiol 2015;27(2):114–9.

37. O'Sullivan CJ, Wenaweser P, Ceylan O, et al. Effect of pulmonary hypertension hemodynamic presentation on clinical outcomes in patients with severe symptomatic aortic valve stenosis undergoing transcatheter aortic valve implantation: insights from the new proposed pulmonary hypertension classification. Circ Cardiovasc Interv 2015;8(7):e002358.

38. Lucon A, Oger E, Bedossa M, et al. Prognostic implications of pulmonary hypertension in patients with severe aortic stenosis undergoing transcatheter aortic valve implantation: study from the FRANCE 2 Registry. Circ Cardiovasc Interv 2014;7(2):240–7.

39. Barbash IM, Escarcega RO, Minha S, et al. Prevalence and impact of pulmonary hypertension on patients with aortic stenosis who underwent transcatheter aortic valve replacement. Am J Cardiol 2015;115(10):1435–42.

40. Tang M, Liu X, Lin C, et al. Meta-Analysis of outcomes and evolution of pulmonary hypertension before and after transcatheter aortic valve implantation. Am J Cardiol 2017;119(1):91–9.

41. Lindman BR, Zajarias A, Maniar HS, et al. Risk stratification in patients with pulmonary hypertension undergoing transcatheter aortic valve replacement. Heart 2015;101(20):1656–64.

42. Hoeper MM, Bogaard HJ, Condliffe R, et al. Definitions and diagnosis of pulmonary hypertension. J Am Coll Cardiol 2013;62(25 Suppl):D42–50.

43. Weber L, Rickli H, Haager PK, et al. Haemodynamic mechanisms and long-term prognostic impact of pulmonary hypertension in patients with severe aortic stenosis undergoing valve replacement. Eur J Heart Fail 2019;21(2):172–81.

44. Masri A, Abdelkarim I, Sharbaugh MS, et al. Outcomes of persistent pulmonary hypertension following transcatheter aortic valve replacement. Heart 2018;104(10):821–7.

45. Jeong DS, Sung K, Kim WS, et al. Fate of functional tricuspid regurgitation in aortic stenosis after aortic valve replacement. J Thorac Cardiovasc Surg 2014;148(4):1328–33.e1.

46. Lindman BR, Maniar HS, Jaber WA, et al. Effect of tricuspid regurgitation and the right heart on survival after transcatheter aortic valve replacement: insights from the Placement of Aortic Transcatheter Valves II inoperable cohort. Circ Cardiovasc Interv 2015;8(4) [pii:e002073].

47. Galli E, Mabo P, Donal E, et al. Prevalence and prognostic value of right ventricular dysfunction in severe aortic stenosis. Eur Heart J Cardiovasc Imaging 2014;16(5):531–8.

48. Koifman E, Didier R, Patel N, et al. Impact of right ventricular function on outcome of severe aortic stenosis patients undergoing transcatheter aortic valve replacement. Am Heart J 2017;184:141–7.

49. Cavalcante JL, Rijal S, Althouse AD, et al. Right ventricular function and prognosis in patients with low-flow, low-gradient severe aortic stenosis. J Am Soc Echocardiogr 2016;29(4):325–33.

50. Ternacle J, Berry M, Cognet T, et al. Prognostic value of right ventricular two-dimensional global strain in patients referred for cardiac surgery. J Am Soc Echocardiogr 2013;26(7):721–6.

51. Généreux P, Pibarot P, Redfors B, et al. Staging classification of aortic stenosis based on the extent of cardiac damage. Eur Heart J 2017;38(45):3351–8.

52. Fukui M, Gupta A, Abdelkarim I, et al. Association of structural and functional cardiac changes with transcatheter aortic valve replacement outcomes in patients with aortic stenosis. JAMA Cardiol 2019;4(3):215–22.

53. Fukui M, Cavalcante JL. Strain evaluation in TAVr—current evidence, knowledge gaps, and future directions. Curr Cardiovasc Imaging Rep 2018;11(9):215–22.

54. Potter E, Marwick TH. Assessment of left ventricular function by echocardiography: the case for routinely adding global longitudinal strain to ejection fraction. JACC Cardiovasc Imaging 2018;11(2 Pt 1):260–74.

55. Collier P, Phelan D, Klein A. A test in context: myocardial strain measured by speckle-tracking echocardiography. J Am Coll Cardiol 2017;69(8):1043–56.

56. Ng AC, Delgado V, Bertini M, et al. Alterations in multidirectional myocardial functions in patients with aortic stenosis and preserved ejection fraction: a two-dimensional speckle tracking analysis. Eur Heart J 2011;32(12):1542–50.

57. Ng ACT, Prihadi EA, Antoni ML, et al. Left ventricular global longitudinal strain is predictive of all-cause mortality independent of aortic stenosis severity and ejection fraction. Eur Heart J Cardiovasc Imaging 2018;19(8):859–67.

58. Vollema EM, Sugimoto T, Shen M, et al. Association of left ventricular global longitudinal strain with asymptomatic severe aortic stenosis: natural course and prognostic value. JAMA Cardiol 2018;3(9):839–47.

59. Magne J, Cosyns B, Popescu BA, et al. Distribution and prognostic significance of left ventricular global longitudinal strain in asymptomatic significant aortic stenosis: an individual participant data meta-analysis. JACC Cardiovasc Imaging 2019;12(1):84–92.

60. Hwang JW, Kim SM, Park SJ, et al. Assessment of reverse remodeling predicted by myocardial deformation on tissue tracking in patients with severe aortic stenosis: a cardiovascular magnetic resonance imaging study. J Cardiovasc Magn Reson 2017;19(1):80.

61. Fukui M, Xu J, Abdelkarim I, et al. Global longitudinal strain assessment by computed tomography in severe aortic stenosis patients - feasibility using feature tracking analysis. J Cardiovasc Comput Tomogr 2019;13(2):157–62.

62. Bing R, Cavalcante JL, Everett RJ, et al. Imaging and impact of myocardial fibrosis in aortic stenosis. JACC Cardiovasc Imaging 2019;12(2):283–96.

63. Park SJ, Cho SW, Kim SM, et al. Assessment of myocardial fibrosis using multimodality imaging in severe aortic stenosis: comparison with histologic fibrosis. JACC Cardiovasc Imaging 2018;12(1):109–19.

64. Musa TA, Treibel TA, Vassiliou VS, et al. Myocardial scar and mortality in severe aortic stenosis. Circulation 2018;138(18):1935–47.

65. Chin CWL, Everett RJ, Kwiecinski J, et al. Myocardial fibrosis and cardiac decompensation in aortic stenosis. JACC Cardiovasc Imaging 2017;10(11):1320–33.

66. Bull S, White SK, Piechnik SK, et al. Human non-contrast T1 values and correlation with histology in diffuse fibrosis. Heart 2013;99(13):932–7.

67. Kockova R, Kacer P, Pirk J, et al. Native T1 relaxation time and extracellular volume fraction as accurate markers of diffuse myocardial fibrosis in heart valve

disease- comparison with targeted left ventricular myocardial biopsy. Circ J 2016;80(5):1202–9.

68. Lee SP, Lee W, Lee JM, et al. Assessment of diffuse myocardial fibrosis by using MR imaging in asymptomatic patients with aortic stenosis. Radiology 2015;274(2):359–69.

69. Chin CW, Semple S, Malley T, et al. Optimization and comparison of myocardial T1 techniques at 3T in patients with aortic stenosis. Eur Heart J Cardiovasc Imaging 2014;15(5):556–65.

70. White SK, Sado DM, Fontana M, et al. T1 mapping for myocardial extracellular volume measurement by CMR: bolus only versus primed infusion technique. JACC Cardiovasc Imaging 2013;6(9):955–62.

71. de Meester de Ravenstein C, Bouzin C, Lazam S, et al. Histological Validation of measurement of diffuse interstitial myocardial fibrosis by myocardial extravascular volume fraction from Modified Look-Locker imaging (MOLLI) T1 mapping at 3 T. J Cardiovasc Magn Reson 2015;17:48.

72. Lee H, Park JB, Yoon YE, et al. Noncontrast myocardial T1 Mapping by cardiac magnetic resonance predicts outcome in patients with aortic stenosis. JACC Cardiovasc Imaging 2018;11(7):974–83.

73. Shen M, Tastet L, Bergler-Klein J, et al. Blood, tissue and imaging biomarkers in calcific aortic valve stenosis: past, present and future. Curr Opin Cardiol 2018;33(2):125–33.

74. Généreux P, Stone GW, O'Gara PT, et al. Natural history, diagnostic approaches, and therapeutic strategies for patients with asymptomatic severe aortic stenosis. J Am Coll Cardiol 2016;67(19):2263–88.

75. Clavel MA, Malouf J, Michelena HI, et al. B-type natriuretic peptide clinical activation in aortic stenosis: impact on long-term survival. J Am Coll Cardiol 2014;63(19):2016–25.

76. Chin CW, Shah AS, McAllister DA, et al. High-sensitivity troponin I concentrations are a marker of an advanced hypertrophic response and adverse outcomes in patients with aortic stenosis. Eur Heart J 2014;35(34):2312–21.

77. Røsjø H, Andreassen J, Edvardsen T, et al. Prognostic usefulness of circulating high-sensitivity troponin t in aortic stenosis and relation to echocardiographic indexes of cardiac function and anatomy. Am J Cardiol 2011;108(1):88–91.

78. Saito T, Hojo Y, Hirose M, et al. High-sensitivity troponin T is a prognostic marker for patients with aortic stenosis after valve replacement surgery. J Cardiol 2013;61(5):342–7.

79. Paparella D, Guida P, Caparrotti S, et al. Myocardial damage influences short- and mid-term survival after valve surgery: a prospective multicenter study. J Thorac Cardiovasc Surg 2014;148(5):2373–9.e1.

80. Akodad M, Spaziano M, Chevalier B, et al. Prognostic impact of pre-transcatheter and post-transcatheter aortic valve intervention troponin: a large cohort study. J Am Heart Assoc 2019;8(6):e011111.

81. Lancellotti P, Dulgheru R, Magne J, et al. Elevated plasma soluble ST2 Is associated with heart failure symptoms and outcome in aortic stenosis. PLoS One 2015;10(9):e0138940.

82. Krau NC, Lunstedt NS, Freitag-Wolf S, et al. Elevated growth differentiation factor 15 levels predict outcome in patients undergoing transcatheter aortic valve implantation. Eur J Heart Fail 2015;17(9):945–55.

83. Baldenhofer G, Zhang K, Spethmann S, et al. Galectin-3 predicts short- and long-term outcome in patients undergoing transcatheter aortic valve implantation (TAVI). Int J Cardiol 2014;177(3):912–7.

84. Dahou A, Clavel MA, Capoulade R, et al. B-Type natriuretic peptide and high-sensitivity cardiac troponin for risk stratification in low-flow, low-gradient aortic stenosis. JACC Cardiovasc Imaging 2018;11(7):939–47.

85. Lindman BR, Clavel MA, Abu-Alhayja'a R, et al. Multimarker approach to identify patients with higher mortality and rehospitaliszation rate after surgical aortic valve replacement for aortic stenosis. JACC Cardiovasc Interv 2018;11(21):2172–81.

86. Mack MJ, Leon MB, Thourani VH, et al. Transcatheter aortic-valve replacement with a balloon-expandable valve in low-risk patients. N Engl J Med 2019;380(18):1695–705.

87. Popma JJ, Deeb GM, Yakubov SJ, et al. Transcatheter aortic-valve replacement with a self-expanding valve in low-risk patients. N Engl J Med 2019;380(18):1706–15.

88. Blackman DJ, Saraf S, MacCarthy PA, et al. Long-term durability of transcatheter aortic valve prostheses. J Am Coll Cardiol 2019;73(5):537–45.

Aortic Stenosis with Other Concomitant Valvular Disease

Aortic Regurgitation, Mitral Regurgitation, Mitral Stenosis, or Tricuspid Regurgitation

Philippe Unger, MD, PhD[a],*, Christophe Tribouilloy, MD, PhD[b]

KEYWORDS

- Aortic stenosis • Mitral regurgitation • Tricuspid regurgitation • Mitral stenosis
- Multiple valve disease • Mixed aortic valve disease

KEY POINTS

- Multiple valve disease involving aortic stenosis and mixed aortic valve disease are frequent clinical scenarios.
- Multiple valve disease and mixed aortic valve disease may be associated with diagnostic pitfalls as a result of hemodynamic interactions.
- Mixed aortic valve disease should be managed according to the predominant lesion; however, combined moderate aortic stenosis and regurgitation may have significant clinical impact requiring surgery.
- There is currently no evidence-based management strategy for multiple valve disease, and a case-by-case approach should be adopted by the heart valve team.
- Decision making should include assessment of each individual lesion, global repercussions, operative risk, life expectancy, natural history of the untreated valvular lesion, and suitability for valve repair and/or transcatheter valve procedures.

INTRODUCTION
Prevalence

Aortic stenosis (AS) is often part of multiple valve disease (AS associated with stenosis and/or regurgitation involving 1 or more other heart valves) or mixed valve disease (concurrent AS and aortic regurgitation [AR]). In a Swedish nationwide study, 36,319 patients had a discharge diagnosis of AS based on International Classification of Diseases-10 codes[1]; among these patients, 6.8% had mixed aortic valve disease, and 7.4% had another concomitant valve disease, consisting of mitral regurgitation (MR) in 5.1% of cases, mitral stenosis (MS) in 1.5% of cases, and tricuspid regurgitation (TR) in 0.6% of cases.[1] AS was present in 17.9% of patients with AR, in 9.9% of those with MR, and in 28.3% of those with MS.[1] The prevalence of moderate or severe MR is even higher among patients undergoing transcatheter aortic valve replacement (TAVR) or surgical aortic valve replacement (SAVR), reaching 20% of the patients included in the PARTNER (Placement of Aortic transcatheter Valve Trial) cohort A and B trials.[2,3]

Disclosure: The authors have nothing to disclose.
[a] Department of Cardiology, CHU Saint-Pierre, Université Libre de Bruxelles, 322 rue Haute, B-1000 Brussels, Belgium; [b] Department of Cardiology, Amiens University Hospital, Jules Verne University of Picardie, 1 rue du Professeur Christian Cabrol, 80000 Amiens, France
* Corresponding author.
E-mail address: punger@ulb.ac.be

Moderate or severe TR was diagnosed in up to 16% of patients with severe AS undergoing aortic valve replacement.[4–6] Among patients undergoing TAVR, MS was observed in 11.6% of cases, and was severe in 2.7% of cases.[7] In another series, MS was observed in 18.1% of patients undergoing TAVR and was classified as moderate/severe in 2.9%.[8] Mixed aortic valve disease was observed in 106 (13.4%) of 793 consecutive patients undergoing TAVR.[9] Among the 141,905 patients included in the Society of Thoracic Surgeons (STS) database who had undergone isolated primary SAVR between 2002 and 2010, 19.3% had mixed aortic valve disease.[10]

Cause

AS and the associated valve disease often have the same underlying cause, mostly degenerative calcification or rheumatic heart disease, but they may also be the result of distinct conditions. For example, chordal rupture, endocarditis, or myxomatous mitral valve disease may occur in patients with degenerative or congenital AS (**Fig. 1**). Importantly, the chronic left ventricular (LV) pressure overload of severe AS may considerably alter upstream pressures, decrease ventricular function, and remodel ventricles and atria. These morphologic, hemodynamic, and functional changes are instrumental in the development of secondary MR/TR (**Fig. 2**), with structurally normal valves and with a leaflet coaptation defect mainly resulting from ventricular and/or atrial remodeling.

Diagnosis

Doppler echocardiography is the cornerstone technique for diagnosis and allows quantification

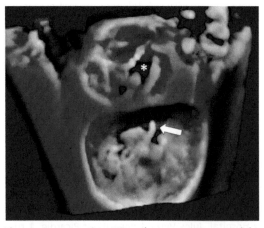

Fig. 1. Degenerative AS and severe MR caused by chordal rupture. Volumetric three-dimensional echocardiography en-face view of the mitral and the aortic valves in a patient with AS (*asterisk*) and ruptured chordae tendineae (*arrow*).

of each valve disease. However, several methods routinely used to assess valvular heart disease have not been validated in the setting of multiple valve disease. Hemodynamic interactions may result in diagnostic pitfalls.[11] AS may affect the diagnosis of other types of valvular disease; conversely, other valve disease may affect the diagnosis of AS (**Table 1**). Diagnostic tools other than echocardiography can also be useful, including exercise testing, MRI, and multidetector computed tomography, but limited data are currently available concerning the specific role of these modalities in patients with multiple valve disease.[12] Occasionally, when noninvasive evaluation remains inconclusive or discordant with clinical findings, cardiac catheterization may be required.[13,14] However, the invasive assessment of cardiac output using thermodilution and Fick methods may prove inaccurate in the presence of severe TR and very low cardiac output, and calculation of aortic valve area by the Gorlin formula may therefore also be inaccurate.[15]

SPECIFIC COMBINATIONS
Aortic Stenosis and Mitral Regurgitation

Concentric LV hypertrophy as a result of the chronic increased afterload induced by severe AS can lead to diastolic dysfunction, left atrial dilatation, and secondary MR.[16] In addition, impaired LV systolic function may also occur as a result of increased afterload and may be associated with eccentric LV remodeling and mitral annular dilatation, also resulting in secondary MR (see **Fig. 2**).[16] MR may be primary, mainly as a result of the high prevalence of mitral annular calcification in the elderly population.[17] Mitral valve chordal rupture occasionally occurs in patients with AS.[18] Coronary artery disease and ischemic MR are also common among patients with AS.[19] In addition, elderly patients with AS can have MR of mixed cause, with both LV dysfunction and mitral leaflet and/or annular calcification.

Multiple quantitative and qualitative echocardiographic parameters should be integrated in order to assess the severity of MR. However, systolic intraventricular pressure is increased in patients with AS, and concomitant MR is therefore characterized by increased transmitral systolic velocity. The resulting regurgitant volume and color-flow jet area are consequently expected to be higher than in patients without AS. Mitral effective regurgitant orifice area and vena contracta are parameters that are not as afterload dependent as regurgitant volume and color-flow jet area and are therefore more representative of the true severity of MR; these parameters are also less

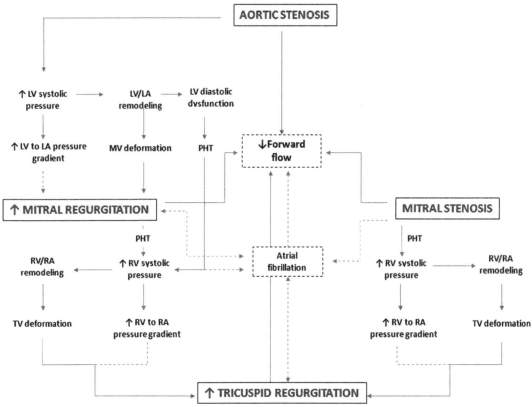

Fig. 2. Pathophysiology of valvular heart disease associated with AS. AS may induce or exacerbate MR by increasing the LV to left atrial (LA) pressure gradient and by mitral valve (MV) deformation. AS may induce or exacerbate TR by inducing pulmonary hypertension either directly or as a result of MR. MR, TR, and MS may all contribute to reducing forward flow and the development of atrial fibrillation (*dotted lines*). Reduced forward flow may prevent the diagnosis of AS (low-flow, low-gradient AS), and atrial fibrillation may also further reduce flow and functional tolerance because of loss of the atrial kick. PHT, pulmonary hypertension; RA, right atrial; RV, right ventricular; TV, tricuspid valve.

affected by aortic valve replacement.[20] MR has a net effect on reducing forward flow and is therefore associated with the development of low-flow low-gradient AS (see **Fig. 2**; **Fig. 3**),[21,22] because the combination of volume overload caused by MR and reduced preload reserve caused by LV hypertrophy resulting from AS further reduces the net forward flow.[22] When the ejection fraction is reduced (classic low-flow low-gradient AS), dobutamine stress echocardiography may be used to increase forward flow and thereby confirm AS severity, although this may be impossible or inconclusive in the presence of MR. Alternatively, assessment of the aortic valve calcium score by multidetector computed tomography may help differentiate between true severe and pseudosevere low-flow low-gradient AS (true severe, >2000 arbitrary units (AU) in men and >1200 in women), in both classic and paradoxic (with preserved ejection fraction) low-flow low-gradient AS.[23]

Whether the presence of preoperative moderate or worse MR independently predicts early and/or late outcomes after SAVR or TAVR remains a matter of debate.[24] However, studies designed to assess prognosis have differed markedly with regard to inclusion criteria, particularly in terms of severity, method of assessment, mechanism and cause of MR, and type of prosthesis used. The acute effect of aortic valve replacement is a decrease in LV systolic pressure, and hence a reduction in MR driving pressure. In addition, reverse LV remodeling may occur, with regression of LV hypertrophy/dilatation and improved LV ejection fraction.[25,26] These changes are instrumental in the improvement in MR observed in most patients after isolated SAVR or TAVR (**Fig. 4**).[27] However, MR does not always improve, and, infrequently, may even worsen. Secondary MR, as opposed to primary MR, is more likely to improve following aortic valve replacement

Table 1
Diagnostic difficulties resulting from the combination of aortic stenosis with another valve disease

	AR	MS	MR	TR
AS Influences the Diagnosis of	AR pressure half-time method is unreliable Peak aortic velocity and mean gradient reflect the severity of both AR and AS; they reflect the severity of the combined disease rather than just the severity of AS	MS pressure half-time method is unreliable Low-flow, low-gradient MS is common	AS increases mitral valve regurgitant volume AS increases MR jet area on color-flow mapping Mitral effective regurgitant orifice is less markedly affected than MR volume and color-flow mapping parameters	—
The Diagnosis of AS is Influenced by the Concomitant Presence of	Simplified Bernoulli equation for gradient determination may not be applicable when left ventricular outflow tract velocity is increased because of high flow Gorlin formula using thermodilution/Fick method is invalid Continuity equation remains applicable to assess AVA, but AVA might be increased at high flow rates	Low-flow, low-gradient AS is common	Mitral regurgitant spectral Doppler signal should not be mistaken for AS spectral Doppler signal Low-flow, low-gradient AS is common	Low-flow, low-gradient AS is common In the presence of severe TR, thermodilution may underestimate cardiac output and consequently overestimate AS severity

Abbreviation: AVA, aortic valve area.

(**Table 2**), because a similar degree of improvement in severe MR caused by flail mitral leaflet is unlikely. Other factors that may predict MR improvement include a potential to reverse LV remodeling, such as dilated LV and reduced ejection fraction, and a large decrease in transaortic pressure gradient, including a high preoperative transvalvular pressure gradient and absence of postoperative prosthesis-patient mismatch (see **Table 2**). Atrial fibrillation, pulmonary hypertension, and atrial and/or mitral annulus dilatation have been associated with more limited improvement in MR. Balloon-expanded aortic prostheses,

as opposed to self-expanded prostheses, may have a more beneficial impact on MR regression.[28]

Accurate prediction of MR improvement in individual patients is difficult. No randomized trials, and therefore no evidence-based recommendations, are available on whether MR should be addressed at the time of SAVR or TAVR. It also remains unclear whether SAVR or TAVR is more effective at reducing MR.

Aortic Stenosis and Tricuspid Regurgitation

The LV hypertrophy and associated diastolic dysfunction present in patients with severe AS

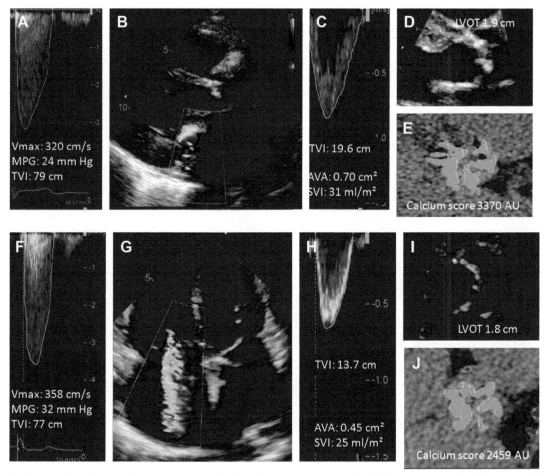

Fig. 3. Low-flow, low-gradient AS associated with other valve disease. (*A–E*) Elderly woman with AS, severe MR, and preserved ejection fraction. (*A*) The mean transaortic pressure gradient (MPG) is 24 mm Hg and the maximal transaortic velocity (Vmax) is 320 cm/s. The large convergence zone of the mitral regurgitant jet is consistent with severe MR. Left ventricular outflow tract (LVOT) pulsed wave Doppler velocity-time integral (TVI) and diameter are 19.6 cm and 1.9 cm, respectively. Calculated stroke volume index (SVI) is 56 mL (31 mL/m²) and aortic valve area (AVA) is 0.70 cm². The aortic valve calcium score is 3370 AU on multidetector computed tomography. (*F–J*) Elderly woman with AS, TR, and preserved ejection fraction. (*A*) The MPG is 32 mm Hg and the Vmax 358 cm/s. Color Doppler flow is consistent with severe TR. LVOT pulsed wave Doppler TVI and diameter are 13.7 cm and 1.8 cm, respectively. Calculated SVI is 35 mL (25 mL/m²) and AVA is 0.45 cm². The aortic valve calcium score is 2459 AU on multidetector computed tomography. These 2 patients have severe AS with a paradoxic low-flow low-gradient pattern, associated with MR (first patient) and TR (second patient). In both cases, quantification of aortic valve calcification confirmed the presence of true severe AS.

may induce pulmonary hypertension, right ventricular remodeling, tricuspid tethering, and annular dilatation, resulting in secondary TR.[29] In addition, increased right ventricular filling pressure may contribute to the development of right atrial dilatation and atrial fibrillation, both of which can cause and exacerbate TR (see **Fig. 2**). Alternatively, patients with AS secondary to rheumatic disease may also have primary tricuspid valve involvement. Severe TR is associated with low flow in patients with AS, but the low flow may also be caused by the associated right ventricular impairment.[21]

Secondary TR is associated with poor prognosis in the presence of severe AS, particularly in patients with concomitant MR.[30,31] TR may be secondary to multiple factors that can have prognostic impact, including LV diastolic dysfunction, pulmonary hypertension, right ventricular dysfunction, and/or atrial fibrillation. It is therefore unclear whether TR per se is an independent prognostic marker or merely a surrogate marker. When left untreated at the time of aortic valve replacement, TR may get worse over time, and can contribute to significant morbidity and mortality.[5,32] The sensitivity of TR to changes in loading

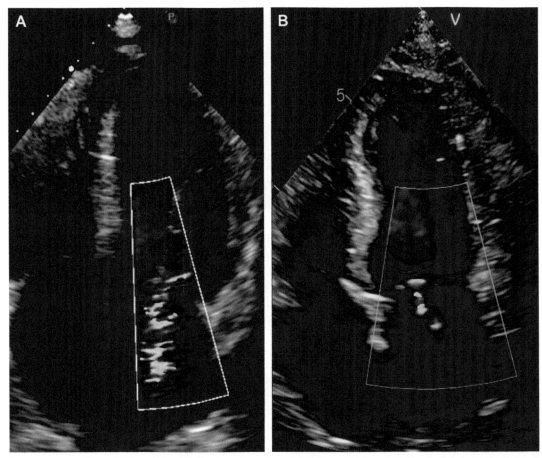

Fig. 4. Downgrading of MR severity following aortic valve replacement. Patient with severe AS undergoing aortic valve replacement. (*A*) Moderate secondary MR is observed preoperatively, but only trivial MR is observed 1 month (*B*) after aortic valve replacement.

conditions has led to the proposal that annular dilatation, rather than the severity of TR, may be predictive of subsequent deterioration. A tricuspid annulus diameter greater than or equal to 40 mm (>21 mm/m^2) has been shown to predict the development of moderate to severe TR during follow-up (**Fig. 5**).[32]

Aortic Stenosis and Mitral Stenosis

MS associated with AS has a degenerative and calcific cause in most cases, and a rheumatic cause in the remaining cases.[7,8]

In patients with concomitant MS and AS, the reduction in cardiac output related to severe MS may be severe and is usually more pronounced than in isolated AS. The aortic and/or mitral pressure gradient may therefore be lower than expected and paradoxic low-flow low-gradient AS is commonly observed. Paradoxic low-flow low-gradient MS (severe MS with a mean pressure

gradient <10 mm Hg) may also be present. It is therefore important not to underestimate the severity of AS and/or MS, which may require aortic valve calcium quantification by multidetector computed tomography and/or mitral planimetry by transesophageal echocardiography. LV filling is altered by the presence of AS, and use of the pressure half-time method to determine mitral valve area should be avoided in this setting. Planimetry of the mitral valve orifice is the method of choice for mitral valve area assessment, but its feasibility is usually limited to rheumatic MS. By providing better alignment of the image plane at the mitral tips, three-dimensional guided planimetry may allow more accurate determination of the mitral valve orifice area.[33] In degenerative MS, mitral valve area assessment using the continuity equation, provided it is not associated with more than mild AR or MR,[34] and direct planimetry with three-dimensional echocardiography and color-flow Doppler are acceptable techniques for

Table 2
Factors associated with postoperative changes in mitral regurgitation severity after surgical or transcatheter aortic valve replacement

Improvement	No Improvement, Deterioration
Secondary MR	Primary MR
Dilated left ventricle, reduced LVEF	Nondilated left ventricle, normal LVEF
Mean transaortic pressure gradient ≥40 mm Hg	Mean transaortic pressure gradient <40 mm Hg
Peak transaortic pressure gradient ≥60 mm Hg	Peak transaortic pressure gradient <60 mm Hg
Absence of prosthesis-patient mismatch	Prosthesis-patient mismatch
Absence of left atrial or mitral annulus dilatation	Left atrial or mitral annulus dilatation
Absence of atrial fibrillation	Atrial fibrillation
Absence of pulmonary hypertension	Pulmonary hypertension
No or mild residual AR	≥ Moderate residual AR
Balloon-expandable prosthesis	Self-expanding prosthesis (particularly when deeply implanted)
Coronary artery disease or previous myocardial infarction	—

Abbreviation: LVEF, left ventricular ejection fraction.

determining mitral valve area.[35] In selected cases, catheterization using the Gorlin-derived method may be used for AS and MS valve area determination, in the absence of concomitant regurgitation.

Severe mitral annular calcification has been associated with conduction abnormalities and increased mortality following TAVR,[36] and MS is an independent risk factor for adverse clinical events following TAVR.[7,8]

Mixed Aortic Valve Disease

Pure AR is characterized by LV enlargement with increased compliance, enabling a large volume overload to be accommodated with no significant increase in LV end-diastolic pressure. In the presence of AR, stroke volume needs to be increased in order to maintain forward cardiac output. In the presence of concomitant AS with consequent

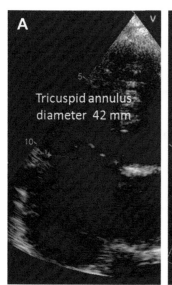
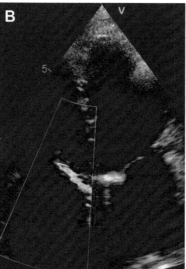
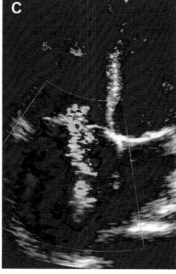

Tricuspid annulus diameter 42 mm

Fig. 5. Development of severe TR following aortic valve replacement. Patient with severe AS undergoing aortic valve replacement without tricuspid annuloplasty. Tricuspid annular dilatation (42 mm, apical 4-chamber view) and mild-to-moderate TR were observed (*A, B*) preoperatively. (*C*) Severe TR was observed 3 years after surgery.

pressure overload, LV hypertrophy, and reduced LV compliance, the AR-induced volume overload leads to LV filling over a steeper portion of the pressure-volume curve, and thereby disproportionally increases LV diastolic pressure and wall stress, which eventually results in poor clinical tolerance (**Figs. 6** and **7**).[37,38] LV concentric hypertrophy secondary to AS may prevent the development of LV dilatation.[38–40] Reduced coronary flow and increased LV filling pressure also contribute to the development of exercise intolerance. The aortic regurgitant volume increases the forward stroke volume and consequently the pressure gradient. In this setting, a significant increase in afterload may occur even in the presence of moderately severe AS.

Several diagnostic pitfalls must be avoided in mixed aortic valve disease. The pressure half-time method is unreliable for the evaluation of AR in the presence of impaired LV relaxation.[41] Increased LV outflow tract velocities may prevent use of the simplified Bernoulli equation for calculation of the aortic valve pressure gradient. Invasive determination of the aortic valve area by the Gorlin formula is inherently inaccurate in patients with mixed aortic valve disease. The hemodynamic burden associated with mixed aortic valve disease is only partially characterized by assessment of the aortic valve area, effective regurgitant orifice area, and regurgitant volume. If cardiac output is preserved, the overall severity and prediction of outcome can be reliably characterized by assessment of peak aortic valve velocity and mean gradient, which increase with the severity of both AS and AR (see **Fig. 7**).[37–39] The assessment of aortic valve area remains accurate using the continuity equation; however, aortic valve area may increase at high transvalvular flow rates, and, in some patients, an aortic valve area greater than 1.0 cm^2 might reflect severe AS.[42] In this setting, the assessment of the aortic valve calcium score by multidetector computed tomography might be considered.

DECISION MAKING

Current guidelines on medical, surgical, and interventional management of patients with multiple valve disease are based on only limited data, as emphasized by the C level of evidence indicated for most recommendations made by the American Heart Association/American College of Cardiology and European Society of Cardiology/European Association for Cardio-Thoracic Surgery guidelines[14,43,44] (**Table 3**).

Clinicians are faced with 2 main scenarios: (1) aortic valve surgery is indicated because of severe AS in the presence of concomitant mitral and/or

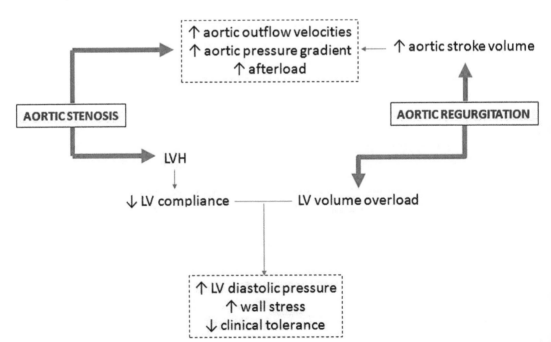

Fig. 6. Pathophysiology of mixed aortic valve disease. In the presence of left ventricular hypertrophy (LVH) and reduced LV compliance secondary to AS, the aortic regurgitant flow disproportionately increases LV diastolic pressure, thereby reducing clinical tolerance. Moreover, AR increases forward stroke volume, which further increases the pressure gradient and LV afterload.

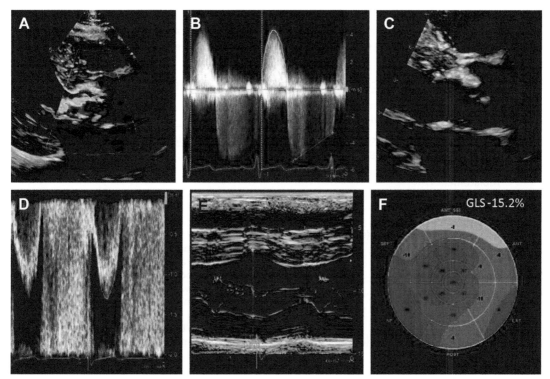

Fig. 7. Example of moderate AS and moderate AR resulting in severe mixed aortic valve disease. (*A*) Parasternal long-axis transthoracic view showing moderate AR (vena contracta, 5 mm). (*B*) Continuous wave Doppler obtained from a right parasternal window showing a maximal forward velocity of 4.15 m/s and a mean gradient of 43 mm Hg. (*C*) The left ventricular outflow tract diameter is 23 mm and the (*D*) velocity-time integral by pulsed wave Doppler is 33.7 cm, giving a calculated stroke volume of 144 mL, and an aortic valve area of 1.35 cm², suggesting a nonsevere AS. Although AS and AR are both moderate, the presence of increased aortic forward velocity, which provides an overall assessment of aortic valve disease, is consistent with severe mixed aortic valve disease. In addition, the typical features of this condition are present, (*E*) including severe left ventricular hypertrophy and absence of LV dilatation. (*F*) Ejection fraction is preserved, but the bull's-eye representation of longitudinal strain is consistent with subclinical LV dysfunction. GLS, global longitudinal strain.

tricuspid valve disease; and (2) mitral and/or tricuspid surgery are indicated in the presence of concomitant AS. In these 2 scenarios, the clinician should follow the current guidelines applicable to the most severe lesion. When both lesions are severe, there is general consensus that they should both be addressed[14,43,44] (see **Table 3**). The management of less-than-severe associated lesions remains more controversial.

Mixed aortic valve disease may present with predominant stenosis or regurgitation, which should be addressed according to current guidelines. However, even moderate AR combined with moderate AS may induce a clinically relevant hemodynamic burden and, although it has not been specifically addressed in current guidelines, intervention should be considered in symptomatic patients with moderate AS and moderate AR with a peak velocity greater than or equal to 4 m/s and a mean gradient greater than or equal to 40 mm Hg (see **Fig. 7**).

Role of the Heart Team and Valve Clinics

The management of each patient must take into account several factors in addition to the patient's symptoms and the severity and effects of the valvular lesions. These factors include the increased operative morbidity and mortality associated with multiple valve surgery. In the EuroHeart Survey and the STS database, the mean operative mortality of double-valve replacement was 2-fold higher than that of single-valve replacement.[13,45–47] In addition, the presence and severity of concomitant coronary artery disease can markedly affect the treatment strategy and operative risk. The expected natural history of a patient with a valve that is left without surgical correction and the risk of redo surgery should be weighed against the patient's life expectancy. The individual surgical risk profile and comorbid conditions are also important determinants of the treatment strategy. The likelihood of spontaneous changes

Table 3
Indications for mitral and/or tricuspid valve surgery in patients undergoing aortic valve replacement, and indications for aortic valve replacement in patients with nonsevere aortic stenosis undergoing other cardiac surgery

	2014–2017 AHA/ACC Guidelines		2017 ESC/EACTS Guidelines	
	Indication	Class (Level of Evidence)	Indication	Class (Level of Evidence)
(1) Surgery for severe AS is indicated. How should concomitant valvular disease be managed?				
MR	Concomitant mitral valve repair or replacement is indicated in patients with chronic severe primary MR	I (B)	Severe primary MR: not mentioned	
	Mitral valve surgery is reasonable for patients with chronic severe secondary MR	IIa (C)	Severe secondary MR: not mentioned However, mitral valve surgery is indicated in patients with severe secondary MR undergoing CABG and with LVEF >30%	I (C)
	Concomitant mitral valve repair is reasonable in patients with chronic moderate primary MR (stage B)	IIa (C)	Moderate primary MR: not mentioned	
	Mitral valve repair may be considered for patients with chronic moderate secondary MR (stage B)	IIb (C)	The potential impact of mitral valve intervention (surgery and catheter intervention) on survival in patients with secondary MR needs to be evaluated	
MS	Concomitant mitral valve surgery is indicated for patients with severe MS	I (C)	Severe concomitant aortic valve disease is a contraindication to percutaneous mitral commissurotomy In patients with severe MS, mitral valve surgery is preferable, when not contraindicated	
	Concomitant mitral valve surgery may be considered for patients with moderate MS (mitral valve area, 1.6–2.0 cm^2)	IIb (C)	Moderate MS: not mentioned	

(continued on next page)

Table 3
(continued)

	2014–2017 AHA/ACC Guidelines		2017 ESC/EACTS Guidelines	
	Indication	Class (Level of Evidence)	Indication	Class (Level of Evidence)
TR	Tricuspid valve surgery is recommended for patients with severe TR (stages C and D)	I (C)	Tricuspid valve surgery is indicated in patients with severe primary or secondary TR	I (C)
	Tricuspid valve repair can be beneficial for patients with mild, moderate, or greater functional TR (stage B) at the time of left-sided valve surgery with either (1) tricuspid annular dilatation or (2) prior evidence of right heart failure	IIa (B)	Tricuspid valve surgery should be considered in patients with moderate primary TR undergoing left-sided valve surgery	IIa (C)
	Tricuspid valve repair may be considered for patients with moderate functional TR (stage B) and pulmonary artery hypertension at the time of left-sided valve surgery	IIb (C)	Tricuspid valve surgery should be considered in patients with mild or moderate secondary TR with dilated annulus ($\geq$40 mm or >21 mm/m^2) undergoing left-sided valve surgery	IIa (C)
			Tricuspid valve surgery may be considered in patients undergoing left-sided valve surgery with mild or moderate secondary TR, even in the absence of annular dilatation when previous recent right heart failure has been documented	IIb (C)
(2) Surgery is indicated on the mitral or tricuspid valve. How should AS be managed?				
—	AVR is reasonable for patients with moderate AS who are undergoing other cardiac surgery	IIa (C)	Surgical AVR should be considered in patients with moderate AS undergoing surgery of the ascending aorta or another valve, after heart team decision	IIa (C)

These indications are according to the AHA/ACC and ESC/EACTS guidelines.
   Abbreviations: ACC, American College of Cardiology; AHA, American Heart Association; AVR, aortic valve replacement; CABG, coronary artery bypass grafting; EACTS, European Association for Cardio-Thoracic Surgery ESC, European Society of Cardiology.
   Data from Refs.[14,42,43]

in MR after aortic valve replacement should be taken into account, remembering that, as mentioned earlier, individual responses are difficult to predict. Tricuspid annular dilatation should also be systematically assessed, because it may predict the development of clinically significant TR during follow-up. Surgical reparability as well as the feasibility of transcatheter approaches should be estimated. Multiple transcatheter procedures have been shown to be feasible in several scenarios,[48] but worldwide clinical experience remains limited. Only 13% of patients with significant persistent MR after TAVR were deemed suitable candidates for percutaneous mitral valve repair with either the MitraClip or balloon-expandable valve.[49] Although TAVR is usually performed for the treatment of degenerative AS, mitral balloon valvuloplasty, indicated in patients with rheumatic valve disease, is only rarely feasible in patients undergoing TAVR. Experience of combined therapy with TR is also currently limited. Technical progress that enables the technique to be used for broader indications is needed before multiple transcatheter valve therapies can be incorporated into routine clinical practice.

The management of patients with multiple or mixed valve disease is challenging and requires an integrated diagnostic approach as well as individually tailored decision making, highlighting the critical role of a collaborative approach between cardiac imagers, interventional cardiologists, and cardiac surgeons. For this purpose, a dedicated heart team–based management strategy in the setting of heart valve centers is required, as recommended by current guidelines,[50,51] in order to identify patients likely to benefit from a double-valve procedure, single aortic valve replacement, or a staged procedure, in which clinical status and lesion severity are reevaluated following aortic valve intervention.

REFERENCES

1. Andell P, Li X, Martinsson A, et al. Epidemiology of valvular heart disease in a Swedish nationwide hospital-based register study. Heart 2017;103: 1696–703.
2. Leon MB, Smith CR, Mack M, et al. Transcatheter aortic-valve implantation for aortic stenosis in patients who cannot undergo surgery. N Engl J Med 2010;363:1597–607.
3. Smith CR, Leon MB, Mack MJ, et al. Transcatheter versus surgical aortic-valve replacement in high-risk patients. N Engl J Med 2011;364:2187–98.
4. Amano M, Izumi C, Taniguchi T, et al, CURRENT AS Registry Investigators. Impact of concomitant tricuspid regurgitation on long-term outcomes in severe aortic stenosis. Eur Heart J Cardiovasc Imaging 2018;20:353–60.
5. Jeong DS, Sung K, Kim WS, et al. Fate of functional tricuspid regurgitation in aortic stenosis after aortic valve replacement. J Thorac Cardiovasc Surg 2014;148:1328–33.
6. Worku B, Valovska MT, Elmously A, et al. Predictors of persistent tricuspid regurgitation after transcatheter aortic valve replacement in patients with baseline tricuspid regurgitation. Innovations (Phila) 2018;13:190–9.
7. Joseph L, Bashir M, Xiang Q, et al. Prevalence and outcomes of mitral stenosis in patients undergoing transcatheter aortic valve replacement: findings from the Society of Thoracic Surgeons/American College of Cardiology Transcatheter Valve Therapies Registry. JACC Cardiovasc Interv 2018;11:693–702.
8. Asami M, Windecker S, Praz F, et al. Transcatheter aortic valve replacement in patients with concomitant mitral stenosis. Eur Heart J 2018. https://doi.org/10.1093/eurheartj/ehy834.
9. Abdelghani M, Cavalcante R, Miyazaki Y, et al. Transcatheter aortic valve implantation for mixed versus pure stenotic aortic valve disease. EuroIntervention 2017;13:1157–65.
10. Thourani VH, Suri RM, Gunter RL, et al. Contemporary real-world outcomes of surgical aortic valve replacement in 141,905 low-risk, intermediate-risk, and high risk patients. Ann Thorac Surg 2015;99: 55–61.
11. Unger P, Rosenhek R, Dedobbeleer C, et al. Management of multiple valve disease. Heart 2011;97: 272–7.
12. Unger P, Pibarot P, Tribouilloy C, et al, On Behalf of the European Society of Cardiology Council on Valvular Heart Disease. Multiple and mixed valvular heart diseases: pathophysiology, imaging, and management. Circ Cardiovasc Imaging 2018;11: e007862.
13. Iung B, Baron G, Butchart EG, et al. A prospective survey of patients with valvular heart disease in Europe: the Euro heart survey on valvular heart disease. Eur Heart J 2003;24:1231–43.
14. Baumgartner H, Falk V, Bax JJ, et al. 2017 ESC/EACTS Guidelines for the management of valvular heart disease: the task force for the management of valvular heart disease of the European Society of Cardiology (ESC) and the European Association for Cardio-Thoracic Surgery (EACTS). Eur Heart J 2017;38:2739–91.
15. Cigarroa RG, Lange RA, Williams RH, et al. Underestimation of cardiac output by thermodilution in patients with tricuspid regurgitation. Am J Med 1989; 86:417–20.
16. Unger P, Dedobbeleer C, Van Camp G, et al. Mitral regurgitation in patients with aortic stenosis undergoing valve replacement. Heart 2010;96:9–14.

17. Abramowitz Y, Jilaihawi H, Chakravarty T, et al. Mitral annulus calcification. J Am Coll Cardiol 2015;66: 1934–41.

18. Effron MK. Aortic stenosis and rupture of mitral chordae tendineae. J Am Coll Cardiol 1983;1:1018–23.

19. Beach JM, Mihaljevic T, Svensson LG, et al. Coronary artery disease and outcomes of aortic valve replacement for severe aortic stenosis. J Am Coll Cardiol 2013;61:837–48.

20. Unger P, Plein D, Van Camp G, et al. Effects of valve replacement for aortic stenosis on mitral regurgitation. Am J Cardiol 2008;102:1378–82.

21. Leong DP, Pizzale S, Haroun MJ, et al. Factors associated with low flow in aortic valve stenosis. J Am Soc Echocardiogr 2016;29:158–65.

22. Benfari G, Clavel MA, Nistri S, et al. Concomitant mitral regurgitation and aortic stenosis: one step further to low-flow preserved ejection fraction aortic stenosis. Eur Heart J Cardiovasc Imaging 2018;19: 569–73.

23. Clavel MA, Pibarot P, Messika-Zeitoun D, et al. Impact of aortic valve calcification, as measured by MDCT, on survival in patients with aortic stenosis: results of an international registry study. J Am Coll Cardiol 2014;64:1202–13.

24. Sannino A, Grayburn PA. Mitral regurgitation in patients with severe aortic stenosis: diagnosis and management. Heart 2018;104:16–22.

25. Clavel MA, Webb JG, Rodés-Cabau J, et al. Comparison between transcatheter and surgical prosthetic valve implantation in patients with severe aortic stenosis and reduced left ventricular ejection fraction. Circulation 2010;122:1928–36.

26. Treibel TA, Kozor R, Schofield R, et al. Reverse myocardial remodeling following valve replacement in patients with aortic stenosis. J Am Coll Cardiol 2018;71:860–71.

27. Nombela-Franco L, Ribeiro HB, Urena M, et al. Significant mitral regurgitation left untreated at the time of aortic valve replacement: a comprehensive review of a frequent entity in the transcatheter aortic valve replacement era. J Am Coll Cardiol 2014;63: 2643–58.

28. Unger P, Dedobbeleer C, Vanden Eynden F, et al. Mitral regurgitation after transcatheter aortic valve replacement: does the prosthesis matter? Int J Cardiol 2013;168:1706–9.

29. Taramasso M, Vanermen H, Maisano F, et al. The growing clinical importance of secondary tricuspid regurgitation. J Am Coll Cardiol 2012;59:703–10.

30. Mascherbauer J, Kammerlander AA, Marzluf BA, et al. Prognostic impact of tricuspid regurgitation in patients undergoing aortic valve surgery for aortic stenosis. PLoS One 2015;10(8):e0136024.

31. Lindman BR, Maniar HS, Jaber WA, et al. Effect of tricuspid regurgitation and the right heart on survival after transcatheter aortic valve replacement: insights from the placement of aortic transcatheter valves II inoperable cohort. Circ Cardiovasc Interv 2015; 8(4) [pii:e002073].

32. Dumont C, Galli E, Oger E, et al. Pre- and postoperative tricuspid regurgitation in patients with severe symptomatic aortic stenosis: importance of preoperative tricuspid annulus diameter. Eur Heart J Cardiovasc Imaging 2018;19:319–28.

33. Wunderlich NC, Beigel R, Siegel RJ. Management of mitral stenosis using 2D and 3D echo-Doppler imaging. JACC Cardiovasc Imaging 2013;6:1191–205.

34. Baumgartner H, Hung J, Bermejo J, et al. Echocardiographic assessment of valve stenosis: EAE/ASE recommendations for clinical practice. J Am Soc Echocardiogr 2009;22:1–23.

35. Oktay AA, Gilliland YE, Lavie CJ, et al. Echocardiographic assessment of degenerative mitral stenosis: a diagnostic challenge of an emerging cardiac disease. Curr Probl Cardiol 2017;42:71–100.

36. Abramowitz Y, Kazuno Y, Chakravarty T, et al. Concomitant mitral annular calcification and severe aortic stenosis: prevalence, characteristics and outcome following transcatheter aortic valve replacement. Eur Heart J 2017;38:1194–203.

37. Egbe AC, Poterucha JT, Warnes CA. Mixed aortic valve disease: midterm outcome and predictors of adverse events. Eur Heart J 2016;37:2671–8.

38. Egbe AC, Luis SA, Padang R, et al. Outcomes in moderate mixed aortic valve disease: is it time for a paradigm shift? J Am Coll Cardiol 2016;67:2321–9.

39. Zilberszac R, Gabriel H, Schemper M, et al. Outcome of combined stenotic and regurgitant aortic valve disease. J Am Coll Cardiol 2013;61:1489–95.

40. Rashedi N, Popovic ZB, Stewart WJ, et al. Outcomes of asymptomatic adults with combined aortic stenosis and regurgitation. J Am Soc Echocardiogr 2014;27:829–37.

41. de Marchi SF, Windecker S, Aeschbacher BC, et al. Influence of left ventricular relaxation on the pressure half time of aortic regurgitation. Heart 1999;82:607–13.

42. Blais C, Burwash IG, Mundigler G, et al. Projected valve area at normal flow rate improves the assessment of stenosis severity in patients with low-flow, low-gradient aortic stenosis: the multicenter TOPAS (Truly or Pseudo-Severe Aortic Stenosis) study. Circulation 2006;113:711–21.

43. Nishimura RA, Otto CM, Bonow RO, et al, ACC/AHA Task Force Members. 2014 AHA/ACC guideline for the management of patients with valvular heart disease: a report of the American College of Cardiology/American Heart Association task force on practice guidelines. Circulation 2014;129:e521–643.

44. Nishimura RA, Otto CM, Bonow RO, et al. 2017 AHA/ACC focused update of the 2014 AHA/ACC guideline for the management of patients with valvular heart disease: a report of the American College of Cardiology/American Heart Association task force

on clinical practice guidelines. Circulation 2017;135: e1159–95.

45. Vassileva CM, Li S, Thourani VH, et al. Outcome characteristics of multiple-valve surgery: comparison with single-valve procedures. Innovations (Phila) 2014;9:27–32.

46. Rankin JS, He X, O'Brien SM, et al. The Society of Thoracic Surgeons risk model for operative mortality after multiple valve surgery. Ann Thorac Surg 2013; 95:1484–90.

47. Lee R, Li S, Rankin JS, et al. Society of Thoracic Surgeons Adult cardiac surgical database. Fifteen-year outcome trends for valve surgery in North America. Ann Thorac Surg 2011;91:677–84.

48. Ando T, Takagi H, Briasoulis A, et al. A systematic review of reported cases of combined transcatheter aortic and mitral valve interventions. Catheter Cardiovasc Interv 2018;91:124–34.

49. Cortes C, Amat-Santos IJ, Nombela-Franco L, et al. Mitral regurgitation after transcatheter aortic valve replacement: prognosis, imaging predictors, and potential management. JACC Cardiovasc Interv 2016;9:1603–14.

50. Lancellotti P, Rosenhek R, Pibarot P, et al. ESC working group on valvular heart disease position paper–heart valve clinics: organization, structure, and experiences. Eur Heart J 2013;34:1597–606.

51. Chambers JB, Prendergast B, Iung B, et al. Standards defining a 'Heart Valve Centre': ESC working group on valvular heart disease and European association for cardiothoracic surgery viewpoint. Eur Heart J 2017;38:2177–83.

Biomarkers Associated with Aortic Stenosis and Structural Bioprosthesis Dysfunction

Cécile Oury, PhD[a],*, Nancy Côté, PhD[b], Marie-Annick Clavel, DVM, PhD[b]

KEYWORDS

• Lipid • Calcium • Hemostasis • Platelets • Aortic stenosis • Biomarkers

KEY POINTS

• Lipoprotein(a) is the most promising lipidic biomarker for identifying patients at risk of developing, or with faster progression of, aortic stenosis (AS).
• Angiotensin II and calcium-phosphorus product may be interesting to identify patients with faster progression of aortic valve remodeling/calcification.
• Platelet-related markers might allow assessment of AS patient hemostatic status both before and after valve replacement and aortic valve calcification.
• Recovery of high molecular weight von Willebrand factor multimers after transcatheter aortic valve replacement may predict patient outcome.
• Cardiovascular risk/comorbid profile (i.e. diabetes, metabolic syndrome, PCSK9) are the main factors contributing to- and serving has circulating biomarkers to identify structural valve degeneration.

The timing of follow-up and intervention in aortic stenosis (AS) is not yet well established and remains controversial. Indeed, the progression of AS is highly variable from one patient to the next. After replacement of the native valve, the prosthesis may also be dysfunctional. The first line of approach for the evaluation of prosthesis is echocardiography, which may be challenging. The use of blood biomarkers to identify patients at risk of AS or faster progression of AS, as well as a dysfunctional bioprosthesis, may have important value in routine clinical practice.

LIPIDIC INFILTRATION

In the early stage of AS, endothelium disruption linked to mechanical stress allows infiltration of lipids. Lipid particles promote inflammation and permeation of inflammatory cells into the valve, which secrete proinflammatory and profibrotic cytokines. Blood levels of low-density lipoprotein (LDL), and especially small and dense LDL and oxidized LDL, have been associated with the presence and faster progression of AS (**Table 1**).[1–3] Atherogenic lipoprotein particles such as LDL contain apolipoprotein B (apoB) (**Fig. 1**) while nonatherogenic lipoprotein particles (high-density lipoprotein) contain apolipoprotein A-I (apoA-I). Recently, the apoB/apoA-I ratio has been found to be independently associated with faster hemodynamic progression of AS in younger patients (<70 years old) (see **Fig. 1**).[4] Accordingly, a strong association was found between increased apoB/apoA-I ratio and the risk

[a] Laboratory of Cardiology, Department of Cardiology, GIGA-Cardiovascular Sciences, University of Liège Hospital, University of Liège, CHU du Sart Tilman, Domaine Universitaire du Sart Tilman, Batiment B35, Liège 4000, Belgium; [b] Institut universitaire de cardiologie et de Pneumologie de Québec, 2725, Chemin Sainte-Foy, A-2047, Québec, Québec G1V 4G5, Canada
* Corresponding author.
E-mail address: cecile.oury@uliege.be

Cardiol Clin 38 (2020) 47–54
https://doi.org/10.1016/j.ccl.2019.09.005
0733-8651/20/© 2019 Elsevier Inc. All rights reserved.

Table 1
Circulating biomarkers and mechanisms implicated in native aortic stenosis and structural valve degeneration of aortic bioprostheses

Mechanisms implicated	Biomarkers	Native Aortic Stenosis	Bioprosthetic aortic valve SVD
Dysregulation of mineral metabolism	↑ Calcium-phosphorus product	✔	✔
	↓ Creatinine clearance	✔	✔
	↑ Total desphosphorylated MGP	✔ (≤57 years)	
	↓ Fetuin-A	✔	
	↑ Osteopontin	✔	
	↑ Osteoprotegerin	✔	
Lipid-mediated inflammation and metabolism processes	↑ HOMA index	✔	✔
	↑ Total cholesterol		✔
	↑ Triglycerides	✔	✔
	↑ ApoB/ApoA-I ratio	✔	✔
	↑ PCSK9	✔	✔
	↑ Lp-PLA2	✔	✔
	↑ Autotaxin	✔	
	↑ small and dense LDLs	✔	
	↑ oxidized LDLs	✔	
	↑ Lp(a)	✔	
Inflammation and macrophage activation	↑ soluble CD14	✔	✔
Tissue remodeling and inflammation	↑ Angiotensin II	✔	
	↑ Angiotensin converting enzyme	✔	
Hemostasis imbalance	↑ Thrombin-antithrombin complexes	✔	
	↑ Prothrombin factor 1+2 (F1+2)	✔	
	↑ Soluble CD40 ligand	✔	
	↑ β-thromboglobulin	✔	
	↑ Plasminogen activator inhibitor-1	✔	
	↑ P-selectin and	✔	
	↑ Activated $\alpha_{IIb}\beta_3$ integrin	✔	
	↑ Serotonin	✔	

Abbreviations: HOMA, homeostatic model assessment; LDLs, low density lipoproteins; Lp(a), lipoprotein (a); Lp-PLA2, lipoprotein-associated phospholipase A2; MGP, Matrix g-carboxyglutamate protein; PCSK9, proprotein convertase subtilisin/kexin 9; SVD, structural valve degeneration.

of developing structural aortic bioprosthetic valve deterioration.[5]

Lipoprotein(a) (Lp(a)) is an LDL-like particle that contains an apo(a) and transports oxidized phospholipids. Lp(a) has been associated with both the presence of AS and faster progression of AS (see **Fig. 1**).[6,7] The blood level of Lp(a) is almost only determined genetically, and one single-nucleotide polymorphism on the Lp(a) locus, associated with elevated level of Lp(a), has been found to be associated with aortic valve calcification (odds ratio per allele, 2.05; $P = 9.0 \times 10^{-10}$).[6] Thus, among lipidic biomarkers associated with AS, Lp(a) is probably the most promising. Around 20% of the population has an increased Lp(a); however, specific thresholds identifying patients at risk of AS or faster progression of AS are as yet not established (75 versus 125 nmol/L).

Going along the Lp(a)/oxidized LDL pathway, the lipoprotein-associated phospholipase A2 (Lp-PLA2) transforms oxidized phospholipids in free fatty acids and lysophosphatidylcholine, which is transformed by autotaxin in lysophosphatidic acid, a phospholipid that promotes inflammation, fibrosis, and calcification. Activity of both Lp-PLA2 and autotaxin has been associated with the presence of AS[8]; however, only Lp-PLA2 activity has been associated with faster progression of AS (see **Table 1**).[9]

Despite inflammation playing an important role in AS initiation and progression, no robust biomarkers linked to inflammation have yet been proposed.

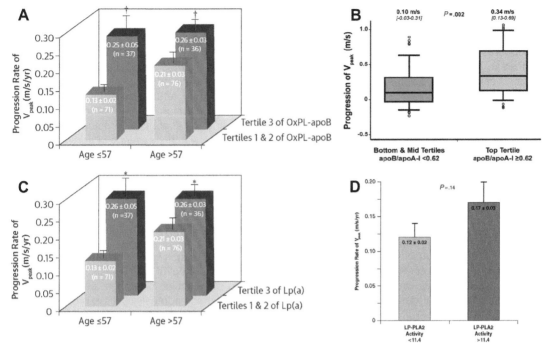

Fig. 1. Annualized progression of aortic valve stenosis according to blood level of lipidic biomarkers. (*A*) Comparison of progression of peak aortic jet velocity according to age and top tertile of oxidized phospholipids on apolipoprotein B-100. † *P* < 0.05 tertile 3 (>5.5 nM) compared with tertiles 1 and 2 (≤5.5 nM) of OxPL-apoB–age ≤57 group. Error bars = SEM. (*B*) Comparison of progression of peak aortic jet velocity in patients younger than 70 years (n = 80) according to top tertile of apoB/apoA-I ratio. (*C*) Comparison of progression of peak aortic jet velocity according to age and top tertile of Lp(a). * *P* < 0.05 tertile 3 (>58.5 mg/dl) compared with tertiles 1 and 2 (≤58.5 mg/dl) of Lp(a)–age ≤57 group. (*D*) Comparison of progression of peak aortic jet velocity according to the level of lipoprotein-associated phospholipase A2. (*From* R. Capoulade, K. L. Chan, C. Yeang, et al., Oxidized Phospholipids, Lioprotein(a), and Progression of Calcific Aortic Valve Stenosis. Journal of the American College of Cardiology 2015; 66:11; with permission.)

EXTRACELLULAR MATRIX REMODELING AND FIBROSIS OF AORTIC VALVE

Remodeling of the extracellular matrix of the aortic valve is mediated through matrix metalloproteinases (MMPs) and tissue inhibitors of metalloproteinases (TIMPs). Indeed, MMPs are endopeptidases that are the most responsible for collagen and other protein degradation of the extracellular matrix. An imbalance between MMP and TIMP activity leads to a pathologic remodeling of the extracellular matrix in the aortic valve.[10,11]

Several MMPs and TIMPs have been identified within the aortic valve, such as MMP2, MMP3, MMP9, and TIMP1. However, correlation between the blood level of these molecules and faster progression of AS is yet to be proved.

In human calcified aortic valves, angiotensin-converting enzyme and chymases are expressed and colocalize with angiotensin II (see **Table 1**).[12,13] The production of angiotensin II within the aortic valve promotes fibrosis and remodeling of valvular tissues owing to the increase in transforming growth factor β, MMP2, and collagen secretion by valvular interstitial cells.[14]

In addition, angiotensin II receptor type 1, which is known to activate vasoconstriction, cell proliferation, inflammation, fibrosis, and thrombosis, is expressed by aortic valve fibroblasts in lesion areas.[12,13] In patients operated on for severe symptomatic AS, the circulating levels of angiotensin II were associated with inflammation and tissue remodeling of the aortic valve.[15] Moreover, higher circulating levels of angiotensin-converting enzyme and angiotensin II have been associated with faster development or progression of AS.[13,16–19]

AORTIC VALVE CALCIFICATION

Aortic valve calcification occurs mostly by accumulation and organization of calcium hydroxyapatite microcrystals in the collagen layer. Serum phosphorus has been proposed as a key regulator of aortic valve calcification. Indeed, the calcium-phosphorus product has been associated with the presence of AS and is correlated with AS severity in patients with and without renal disease (see **Table 1**).[20,21] Moreover, higher calcium-phosphorus product has also been correlated with aortic bioprosthesis calcification.[22] Furthermore, calcium supplements, which are extensively prescribed in older adult patients, are independently associated with higher calcium-phosphorus product.

Matrix γ-carboxyglutamate protein (MGP) is well known to be an inhibitor of cardiovascular calcification. To inhibit ectopic calcification, MGP requires carboxylation and phosphorylation.[23] In the ASTRONOMER (Aortic Stenosis Progression Observation: Measuring Effects of Rosuvastatin) trial, increased circulating levels of total desphosphorylated MGP were associated with a faster progression rate of AS in younger individuals ($\leq$57 years old), whereas older patients experienced a rapid stenosis progression rate of AS, regardless of the total desphosphorylated MGP levels (**Fig. 2**).[24]

Paradoxically, higher levels of total desphosphorylated MGP were observed in the patients with faster AS progression, probably linked to a feedback mechanism increasing the production of uncarboxylated desphosphorylated MGP in response to the ongoing ectopic calcification processes.

Many calcium-binding proteins have been found in stenosed aortic valves; however, the circulating level of these proteins has not always been linked to the presence and/or faster progression rate of AS. Fetuin-A is known to protect against cardiovascular calcification. In AS, a recent meta-analysis confirmed that plasma fetuin-A levels are lower in patients with AS than in those without AS.[25] However, fetuin-A was not associated with slower progression of AS.[26] Accordingly, levels of plasma osteopontin or osteoprotegerin are associated with the presence of aortic valve calcification and/or stenosis,[27,28] although association with AS progression was never demonstrated (see **Table 1**).

A ROLE FOR PLATELETS IN AORTIC STENOSIS PATHOPHYSIOLOGY?

Platelet interaction with vascular endothelial cells is the initial step of hemostasis, which leads to repair of vascular breaches and limits blood loss.[29] Injured endothelial cells express procoagulant and platelet-activating molecules, and components of the subendothelial matrix, mainly collagen, are exposed to flowing blood, which initiates thrombus formation. Under high shear stress, the platelet collagen receptors (glycoprotein VI [GPVI], $\alpha_2\beta_1$) are unable to support platelet adhesion; the initial platelet adhesion to endothelia requires the interaction between immobilized von Willebrand factor (vWF) on the surface of the endothelium or in the subendothelial matrix with its platelet receptor, the GPIb-IX-V complex. When shear force increases, vWF multimers unfold, resulting in the binding of the vWF A1 domain to platelet GPIbα. Two mechanosensitive domains in GPIbα unfold by vWF-mediated pulling force, and the anchoring of GPIbα to actin filaments via filamin-A allows resisting shear force during platelet adhesion.[30] This interaction mediates platelet tethering and translocation on the endothelium. Subsequent $\alpha_{IIb}\beta_3$ integrin inside-out activation and release of platelet granule content leads to platelet arrest and irreversible aggregation.[31] On granule release, the ATP P2X1 receptor and the 2 ADP receptors, P2Y1 and P2Y12, play central roles in the amplification of shear-dependent platelet aggregation.[32] Concomitant activation of the coagulation cascade leads to thrombin generation, which further activates and recruits platelets to the formation of thrombi and produces fibrin that consolidates the clot.

Under normal conditions, endothelial cells produce antithrombotic substances such as nitric oxide (NO) and prostaglandin I$_2$ (PGI$_2$) that inhibit platelet adhesion, activation, and aggregation, and thrombomodulin, which inactivates thrombin. In addition, the ectonucleotidase

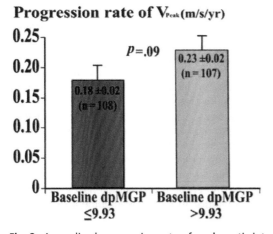

Progression rate of V$_{Peak}$ (m/s/yr)

$p = .09$

0.23 ±0.02 (n = 107)

0.18 ±0.02 (n = 108)

Baseline dpMGP $\leq$9.93   Baseline dpMGP >9.93

Fig. 2. Annualized progression rate of peak aortic jet velocity according to baseline desphosphorylated matrix γ-carboxyglutamate protein level. (*From* R. Capoulade, N. Cote, P. Mathieu, et al., Circulating Levels of Matrix Gla Protein and Progression of Aortic Stenosis: A Substudy of the Aortic Stenosis Progression Observation: Measuring Effects of Rosuvastatin (ASTRONOMER) Trial. Canadian Journal of Cardiology 2014; 1088-1095; with permission.)

CD39 degrades ATP and ADP, 2 main platelet agonists, thereby preventing platelet activation. It is conceivable that such mechanisms also contribute to inhibiting platelet adhesion and activation on aortic valve endothelia. However, the specificities of platelet interactions with aortic valve endothelial cells remain totally unknown. In AS, few available data concur with the new concept that platelets would contribute to the disease through mechanisms that differ from those involved in hemostasis.[33] According to a recent study, platelets may be involved in AS progression by promoting valvular calcification. Activated platelets would participate in valve interstitial cell mineralization through lysophosphatidic acid production and autotaxin activity.[34] In addition, the contribution of platelets to inflammation, including their ability to interact with immune cells, could represent another mechanism underlying the AS-associated osteogenic process.[35] On activation, platelets release soluble mediators from their granules, which further promotes platelet recruitment and activation but also mediates immune and inflammatory responses. Platelet α-granules contain hemostatic factors (ie, coagulation factor V, vWF, fibrinogen), growth factors (ie, platelet-derived growth factor, transforming growth factor β), cytokines and chemokines (ie, interleukin-1β, platelet-activating factor, platelet factor 4, CCL5), and metalloproteinases (ie, MMP9, TIMP1).[36] Dense granules comprise small molecules such as serotonin, calcium, ADP, and ATP. It is therefore possible that on platelet activation, released platelet granule content contributes to valvular extracellular matrix remodeling and fibrosis. Furthermore, inflammation itself might also dictate platelet contribution to AS pathophysiology. Indeed, in addition to platelet contribution to disease pathophysiology, diseases can modify platelets.[37] On the one hand, the disease environment can induce changes in megakaryocytes that produce platelets with modified RNA or protein content. On the other hand, platelet content can also become modified in circulation. Platelets are able to take up proteins and small molecules from blood and release them locally at sites of activation. For instance, platelets accumulate circulating acute-phase proteins, such as C-reactive protein and serum amyloid A, which are produced by the liver during inflammation.[38] Dyslipidemia or hyperglycemia also modifies platelet phospholipid content, which may result in platelet hyperreactivity and subsequent enhanced thrombosis.[39] However, to date, how and when platelets intervene in AS pathophysiology has remained unclear.

HEMOSTASIS IMBALANCE IN AORTIC STENOSIS

In terms of hemostasis, AS patients display both a mild bleeding and a high thrombotic risk.[40] This dual clinical picture is inherent to the disease condition. Indeed, high shear stress through stenosed aortic valve induces vWF unfolding and subsequent GPIbα-mediated platelet activation and release of platelet granule content.[41] Cleavage of unfolded vWF by ADAMTS-13 leads to secondary loss of high molecular weight vWF multimers (HMWM), which results in acquired vWF disease (VWD) and Heyde syndrome (ie, lower gastrointestinal bleeding from angiodysplasia). Indeed, cleaved vWF shows less affinity for platelets and collagen than HMWM, which makes their hemostatic activity much less efficient. Because platelets are very sensitive to and are activated by shear stress, it is likely that, depending on stenosis severity and disease stage, AS differentially alters platelet phenotype, which, in addition to VWD, may contribute to the risk of bleeding or thrombosis. Shear causes shedding of GPIbα and GPVI, resulting in secondary platelet hyporeactivity and potential bleeding.[42] Interestingly it has been shown that in vitro, under high shear stress conditions, GPVI shedding occurs independently of vWF/GPIbα engagement, and does not require $α_{IIb}β_3$ integrin activation or platelet aggregation.[43] GPVI shedding, triggered by brief and transient shear exposure, results in progressive accumulation of circulating soluble GPVI. Thus, these platelet responses to shear might all represent novel markers of AS severity and/or prognosis. Concomitant with the VWD-associated bleeding risk, AS is characterized by increased activation of coagulation with concurrent hypofibrinolysis, which may be responsible for fibrin deposition on the aortic valve. Markers of coagulation, thrombin-antithrombin complexes (TAT) and prothrombin factor 1+2 (F1+2), as well as soluble markers of platelet activation, soluble CD40 ligand and β-thromboglobulin, were found to be elevated in patients with lower percentages of HMWM and more severe stenosis (see **Table 1**).[44] Platelets may thus be activated by thrombin generated as a result of coagulation activation. Markers of impaired systemic fibrinolysis, such as level of plasminogen activator inhibitor-1, the most important regulator of plasminogen activation and plasmin generation, are also elevated.[45] It has also been shown that platelet activation, assessed by measuring surface expression of P-selectin and activated $α_{IIb}β_3$ integrin, increased in parallel with plasma serotonin elevation in patients with severe AS.[41] Overall, these data indicate hemostasis imbalance in AS, leading to both mild bleeding tendency and a high thrombotic risk.[40] However, a clear understanding of platelet contribution to AS and associated bleeding or thrombosis will necessitate detailed investigation of platelet phenotype during disease initiation and progression. Importantly, such studies might reveal new therapeutic avenues of AS and help in defining more tailored antithrombotic management of these patients. The advanced age and comorbidities of most AS patients makes their antithrombotic management highly challenging. Hence, thorough characterization of circulating platelets would seem essential for accurate assessment of patients' hemostatic status.

CIRCULATING BIOMARKERS OF PROSTHESIS VALVE DYSFUNCTION

Bioprosthesis are prone to structural valve deterioration (SVD). Despite major improvements in valve design and surgical procedures, SVD is still a major limiting factor to the durability of bioprostheses. Biomarkers may help to the identification of causal factors for SVD and clinical decision making. Higher calcium-phosphorus product is a strong predictor of bioprosthesis calcification and patients with less than 30 mL/min of preoperative creatinine clearance are at higher risk of SVD compared to patients with a clearance greater than 60 ml/min.[22,46]

Lipid-related biomarkers are other plasma biomarkers implicated in SVD. Patients with total cholesterol of at least 200mg/dL or triglycerides levels higher than 150mg/dL are at greater risk for re-operation for structural valve failure.[47] A study reported that in patients younger than 57 years, total cholesterol level higher than 240mg/dL or triglycerides level higher than 123 mg/dL are predictors of re-intervention for valve failure.[48] Higher levels of Apo-B, ApoB/ApoA-I ratio, Homeostatic model assessment (HOMA) are also associated with increased risk of SVD. High plasma level of the proprotein convertase subtilisin/kenin 9 (PCSK9), a positive regulator of LDL cholesterols, and/or associated with high level of oxidized-LDLs are associated with higher risk of SVD.[49,50] Lipoprotein-associated phospholipase A2 (Lp-PLA2) which enzymatically produce free fatty acids from oxidized-LDLs and promoting inflammation is expressed in explanted bioprostheses for SVD50 in colocation with macrophages (CD68), and oxidized-LDLDs. Plasma Lp-PLA2 activity have also been associated with the occurrence of SVD (see **Table 1**).[49] Lipid insudation found in explanted bioprosthesis for SVD exposed lipid-laden macrophages featuring foam cells that can precipitate SVD in the long-term, even in the absence of mineralization.[51] CD14, a membrane glycoprotein present at the surface of monocytes and macrophages, can be secreted by these cells or the liver, and the circulating soluble form of CD14 has been related to SVD (see **Table 1**).[52]

CIRCULATING BIOMARKER TO IDENTIFY PARAVALVULAR LEAK

Previous studies have shown that loss of HMWM of vWF is observed in patients with AS or regurgitation and is corrected after AVR.40 HMWM defect is predictive of the presence of postprocedural paravalvular regurgitation after TAVI and is associated with increased 1-year mortality.[53] Point-of-care measurement of vWF-dependent platelet function using PFA-200 (Siemens) not only predicted PVAR but also MLTB at 30 days post TAVI.[54] These data are still to be confirmed in larger patient cohorts from independent centers. It is also worth noting that PFA-200 data do not accurately reflect overall platelet reactivity and, because data are influenced by medication, low platelet count, hematocrit, and levels of vWF antigen, the specificity of this technology is a major limitation.

SUMMARY

Lipids, including Lp(a) and the apoB/apoA-I ratio, angiotensin II, and calcium-phosphorus product, may represent valuable markers of AS disease progression and/or bioprosthesis deterioration. However, the implementation of these biomarkers in clinical practice will require further validation in large multicenter patient cohorts. In addition, more basic and translational research is definitely required to clarify AS disease mechanisms to uncover multibiomarker-based diagnostic and prognostic tools that might be useful during the natural progression of AS and after aortic valve replacement. Markers of hemostasis and further demonstration of a role for platelets in aortic valve calcification represent other promising avenues that might not only help the assessment of AS progression but also the management of antithrombotic therapy while preserving hemostasis.

ACKNOWLEDGMENTS

C. Oury is Research Director at the Belgian Funds for Scientific Research (F.R.S.-FNRS). M.-A. Clavel is recipient of a New National Investigator award from the Heart and Stroke Foundation of Canada.

DISCLOSURE

M.-A. Clavel: research grant with Edwards Life-sciences and Medtronic. C. Oury: no disclosures. N. Côté: no disclosures.

REFERENCES

1. Smith JG, Luk K, Schulz CA, et al. Association of low-density lipoprotein cholesterol-related genetic variants with aortic valve calcium and incident aortic stenosis. JAMA 2014;312:1764–71.

2. Mohty D, Pibarot P, Després JP, et al. Association between plasma LDL particle size, valvular accumulation of oxidized LDL, and inflammation in patients with aortic stenosis. Arterioscler Thromb Vasc Biol 2008;28:187–93.

3. Côté C, Pibarot P, Després JP, et al. Association between circulating oxidised low-density lipoprotein and fibrocalcific remodelling of the aortic valve in aortic stenosis. Heart 2008;94:1175–80.

4. Tastet L, Capoulade R, Shen M, et al. ApoB/ApoA-I ratio is associated with faster hemodynamic progression of aortic stenosis: results from the PROGRESSA (Metabolic Determinants of the Progression of Aortic Stenosis) study. J Am Heart Assoc 2018;7. https://doi.org/10.1161/JAHA.117.007980.

5. Mahjoub H, Mathieu P, Sénéchal M, et al. ApoB/ApoA-I ratio is associated with increased risk of bioprosthetic valve degeneration. J Am Coll Cardiol 2013;61:752–61.

6. Thanassoulis G, Campbell CY, Owens DS, et al. Genetic associations with valvular calcification and aortic stenosis. N Engl J Med 2013;368:503–12.

7. Capoulade R, Chan KL, Yeang C, et al. Oxidized phospholipids, lipoprotein(a), and progression of calcific aortic valve stenosis. J Am Coll Cardiol 2015;66:1236–46.

8. Nsaibia MJ, Mahmut A, Boulanger MC, et al. Autotaxin interacts with lipoprotein(a) and oxidized phospholipids in predicting the risk of calcific aortic valve stenosis in patients with coronary artery disease. J Intern Med 2016;280:509–17.

9. Capoulade R, Mahmut A, Tastet L, et al. Impact of plasma Lp-PLA2 activity on the progression of aortic stenosis: the PROGRESSA study. JACC Cardiovasc Imaging 2015;8:26–33.

10. Satta J, Oiva J, Salo T, et al. Evidence for an altered balance between matrix metalloproteinase-9 and its inhibitors in calcific aortic stenosis. Ann Thorac Surg 2003;76:681–8.

11. Kaden JJ, Vocke DC, Fischer CS, et al. Expression and activity of matrix metalloproteinase-2 in calcific aortic stenosis. Z Kardiol 2004;93:124–30.

12. O'Brien KD, Shavelle DM, Caulfield MT, et al. Association of angiotensin-converting enzyme with low-density lipoprotein in aortic valvular lesions and in human plasma. Circulation 2002;106:2224–30.

13. Helske S, Lindstedt KA, Laine M, et al. Induction of local angiotensin II-producing systems in stenotic aortic valves. J Am Coll Cardiol 2004;44:1859–66.

14. O'Brien KD. Pathogenesis of calcific aortic valve disease: a disease process comes of age (and a good deal more). Arterioscler Thromb Vasc Biol 2006;26:1721–8.

15. Côté N, Pibarot P, Pépin A, et al. Oxidized low-density lipoprotein, angiotensin II and increased waist circumference are associated with valve inflammation in prehypertensive patients with aortic stenosis. Int J Cardiol 2010;145:444–9.

16. O'Brien KD, Probstfield JL, Caulfield MT, et al. Angiotensin-converting enzyme inhibitors and change in aortic valve calcium. Arch Intern Med 2005;165:858–62.

17. Fujisaka T, Hoshiga M, Hotchi J, et al. Angiotensin II promotes aortic valve thickening independent of elevated blood pressure in apolipoprotein-E deficient mice. Atherosclerosis 2013;226:82–7.

18. Iwata S, Russo C, Jin Z, et al. Higher ambulatory blood pressure is associated with aortic valve calcification in the elderly: a population-based study. Hypertension 2013;61:55–60.

19. Myles V, Liao J, Warnock JN. Cyclic pressure and angiotensin II influence the biomechanical properties of aortic valves. J Biomech Eng 2014;136:011011.

20. Akat K, Kaden JJ, Schmitz F, et al. Calcium metabolism in adults with severe aortic valve stenosis and preserved renal function. Am J Cardiol 2010;105:862–4.

21. Di Lullo L, Floccari F, Santoboni A, et al. Progression of cardiac valve calcification and decline of renal function in CKD patients. J Nephrol 2013;26:739–44.

22. Mahjoub H, Mathieu P, Larose É, et al. Determinants of aortic bioprosthetic valve calcification assessed by multidetector CT. Heart 2015;101:472–7.

23. Schurgers LJ, Spronk HM, Skepper JN, et al. Posttranslational modifications regulate matrix Gla protein function: importance for inhibition of vascular smooth muscle cell calcification. J Thromb Haemost 2007;5:2503–11.

24. Capoulade R, Côté N, Mathieu P, et al. Circulating levels of matrix gla protein and progression of aortic stenosis: a substudy of the aortic stenosis progression observation: measuring effects of rosuvastatin (ASTRONOMER) trial. Can J Cardiol 2014;30:1088–95.

25. Di Minno A, Zanobini M, Myasoedova VA, et al. Could circulating fetuin A be a biomarker of aortic valve stenosis? Int J Cardiol 2017;249:426–30.

26. Kubota N, Testuz A, Boutten A, et al. Impact of Fetuin-A on progression of calcific aortic valve stenosis—the COFRASA-GENERAC study. Int J Cardiol 2018;265:52–7.

27. Yu PJ, Skolnick A, Ferrari G, et al. Correlation between plasma osteopontin levels and aortic valve calcification: potential insights into the pathogenesis of aortic valve calcification and stenosis. J Thorac Cardiovasc Surg 2009;138:196–9.

28. Borowiec A, Dabrowski R, Kowalik I, et al. Osteoprotegerin in patients with degenerative aortic stenosis and preserved left-ventricular ejection fraction. J Cardiovasc Med (Hagerstown) 2015;16:444–50.

29. Versteeg HH, Heemskerk JW, Levi M, et al. New fundamentals in hemostasis. Physiol Rev 2013;93:327–58.

30. Cranmer SL, Ashworth KJ, Yao Y, et al. High shear-dependent loss of membrane integrity and defective platelet adhesion following disruption of the GPIbalpha-filamin interaction. Blood 2011;117:2718–27.

31. Kulkarni S, Dopheide SM, Yap CL, et al. A revised model of platelet aggregation. J Clin Invest 2000;105:783–91.

32. Oury C, Sticker E, Cornelissen H, et al. ATP augments von Willebrand factor-dependent shear-induced platelet aggregation through Ca^{2+}-calmodulin and myosin light chain kinase activation. J Biol Chem 2004;279:26266–73.

33. Morrell CN, Aggrey AA, Chapman LM, et al. Emerging roles for platelets as immune and inflammatory cells. Blood 2014;123:2759–67.

34. Bouchareb R, Boulanger MC, Tastet L, et al. Activated platelets promote an osteogenic programme and the progression of calcific aortic valve stenosis. Eur Heart J 2019;40(17):1362–73.

35. Foresta C, Strapazzon G, De Toni L, et al. Platelets express and release osteocalcin and co-localize in human calcified atherosclerotic plaques. J Thromb Haemost 2013;11:357–65.

36. Gear AR, Camerini D. Platelet chemokines and chemokine receptors: linking hemostasis, inflammation, and host defense. Microcirculation 2003;10:335–50.

37. Baaten C, Ten Cate H, van der Meijden PEJ, et al. Platelet populations and priming in hematological diseases. Blood Rev 2017;31:389–99.

38. Servais L, Wera O, Dibato Epoh J, et al. Platelets contribute to the initiation of colitis-associated cancer by promoting immunosuppression. J Thromb Haemost 2018;16:762–77.

39. Lepropre S, Kautbally S, Octave M, et al. AMPK-ACC signaling modulates platelet phospholipids and potentiates thrombus formation. Blood 2018;132:1180–92.

40. Vincentelli A, Susen S, Le Tourneau T, et al. Acquired von Willebrand syndrome in aortic stenosis. N Engl J Med 2003;349:343–9.

41. Rouzaud-Laborde C, Delmas C, Pizzinat N, et al. Platelet activation and arterial peripheral serotonin turnover in cardiac remodeling associated to aortic stenosis. Am J Hematol 2015;90:15–9.

42. Al-Tamimi M, Tan CW, Qiao J, et al. Pathologic shear triggers shedding of vascular receptors: a novel mechanism for down-regulation of platelet glycoprotein VI in stenosed coronary vessels. Blood 2012;119:4311–20.

43. Chatterjee M, Gawaz M. Clinical significance of receptor shedding-platelet GPVI as an emerging diagnostic and therapeutic tool. Platelets 2017;28:362–71.

44. Natorska J, Bykowska K, Hlawaty M, et al. Increased thrombin generation and platelet activation are associated with deficiency in high molecular weight multimers of von Willebrand factor in patients with moderate-to-severe aortic stenosis. Heart 2011;97:2023–8.

45. Natorska J, Wypasek E, Grudzien G, et al. Impaired fibrinolysis is associated with the severity of aortic stenosis in humans. J Thromb Haemost 2013;11:733–40.

46. Salaun E, Mahjoub H, Girerd N, et al. Rate, timing, correlates, and outcomes of hemodynamic valve deterioration after bioprosthetic surgical aortic valve replacement. Circulation 2018;138:971–85.

47. Lorusso R, Gelsomino S, Luca F, et al. Type 2 diabetes mellitus is associated with faster degeneration of bioprosthetic valve: results from a propensity score-matched Italian multicenter study. Circulation 2012;125(4):604–14.

48. Nollert G, Miksch J, Kreuzer E, et al. Risk factors for atherosclerosis and the degeneration of pericardial valves after aortic valve replacement. J Thorac Cardiovasc Surg 2003;126(4):965–8.

49. Salaun E, Mahjoub H, Dahou A, et al. Hemodynamic deterioration of surgically implanted bioprosthetic aortic valves. J Am Coll Cardiol 2018;72(3):241–51.

50. Mahmut A, Mahjoub H, Boulanger MC, et al. Lp-PLA2 is associated with structural valve degeneration of bioprostheses. Eur J Clin Invest 2014;44(2):136–45.

51. Bottio T, Thiene G, Pettenazzo E, et al. Hancock II bioprosthesis: a glance at the microscope in mid-long-term explants. J Thorac Cardiovasc Surg 2003;126(1):99–105.

52. Nsaibia MJ, Boulanger MC, Bouchareb R, et al. Soluble CD14 is associated with the structural failure of bioprostheses. Clin Chim Acta 2018;485:173–7.

53. Van Belle E, Rauch A, Vincent F, et al. Von Willebrand factor multimers during transcatheter aortic-valve replacement. N Engl J Med 2016;375(4):335–44.

54. Kibler M, Marchandot B, Messas N, et al. CT-ADP point-of-care assay predicts 30-day paravalvular aortic regurgitation and bleeding events following transcatheter aortic valve replacement. Thromb Haemost 2018;118(5):893–905.

Aortic Stenosis
Guidelines and Evidence Gaps

Andrew W. Harris, MD[a], Philippe Pibarot, DVM, PhD[b], Catherine M. Otto, MD[a],*

KEYWORDS

• Aortic stenosis • Guidelines • Evidence gaps • Controversies

KEY POINTS

- Current guidelines recommend aortic valve replacement for patients with severe aortic stenosis (AS) and symptoms or left ventricular (LV) dysfunction.
- The benefits of aortic valve replacement in patients with asymptomatic, severe AS and moderate AS with LV dysfunction are unknown and currently are being investigated.
- Guidelines recommend transcatheter aortic valve replacement (TAVR) in patients with severe AS with elevated surgical risk; recent trials have demonstrated excellent short-term outcomes in patients with low surgical risk.
- Transcatheter valve durability remains an important uncertainty that currently limits its use in young patients and patients with low surgical risk.

INTRODUCTION

Aortic stenosis (AS) is one of the most common valve diseases and is expected to increase in prevalence due to aging of the world population. The American Heart Association (AHA)/American College of Cardiology (ACC) and European Society of Cardiology (ESC)/European Association for Cardio-Thoracic Surgery (EACTS) Guidelines on the management of valvular heart disease provide comprehensive, evidence-based recommendations for management of patients with valvular AS.[1–3] However, there are significant gaps in the evidence base for optimal management of these patients. The purpose of this article was to review the current Guidelines recommendations and highlight evidence gaps underlying ongoing controversies in patient management.

Diagnosis

Guidelines

The diagnosis of AS frequently is made when routine physical examination reveals a systolic murmur. A transthoracic echocardiogram (TTE) is recommended in patients with an unexplained systolic murmur, a single second heart sound, a history of bicuspid aortic valve, or symptoms that may be due to AS. The diagnosis of AS is based on the presence of a structurally abnormal valve (thickened and calcified or congenitally abnormal) with restricted motion and Doppler evidence of hemodynamic obstruction. When AS is diagnosed in asymptomatic patients, repeat TTEs are recommended for monitoring of progression of disease because of the inevitable progression from mild to moderate and then severe valve obstruction. Patients with mild AS should undergo repeat TTE approximately every 3 to 5 years; those with moderate AS approximately every 1 to 2 years; and those with severe AS approximately every 6 to 12 months, unless earlier imaging is needed for a change in clinical signs or symptoms.

Knowledge gaps

Unfortunately, detection of a systolic murmur is unreliable both for the initial diagnosis of AS and

Disclosure Statement: None.
[a] Department of Medicine, Division of Cardiology, University of Washington, 1959 Northeast Pacific Street, Box 356422, Seattle, WA 98195, USA; [b] Institut Universitaire de Cardiologie et de Pneumologie de Québec (Québec Heart and Lung Institute), Laval University, 2725 Chemin Sainte Foy, Québec, QC G1V-4G5, Canada
* Corresponding author.
E-mail addresses: cmotto@uw.edu; cmotto@u.washington.edu
Twitter: @ottoecho (C.M.O.)

Cardiol Clin 38 (2020) 55–63
https://doi.org/10.1016/j.ccl.2019.09.003

for evaluation of disease severity. One large community-based study demonstrated poor sensitivity and specificity for the diagnosis of significant valvular heart disease based on auscultation by both general practitioners (sensitivity 44%, specificity 69%) and cardiologists (sensitivity 31%, specificity 81%).[4] The accuracy of the physical examination was especially poor for overweight patients (body mass index >25 kg/m^2). Given the increasing prevalence of AS in the aging population as well as the clinical significance of undiagnosed severe AS, screening of elderly populations using office-based TTE, or point-of-care ultrasound, has been proposed. The potential effect on clinical outcomes, the optimal patient groups to screen, and financial implications of an echocardiographic screening program for AS have yet to be established.

Medical Therapy

Guidelines
AS is a slowly progressive condition that does not lead to symptoms or adverse clinical events until late in the disease process. A medical intervention to slow progressive leaflet fibrosis and calcification might slow the disease process or prevent severe stenosis. Prior studies have demonstrated a dose-response relationship between traditional cardiovascular risk factors (hypertension, diabetes, dyslipidemia) and the development of severe AS, and several genetic polymorphisms have been associated with an increased risk of calcific valve disease.[5] However, no medical therapies have proven to be beneficial in preventing or treating AS. Randomized trials of statin therapy in adults with asymptomatic mild to moderate AS demonstrated no benefit for valve-related outcomes, although statin therapy did result in reduced rates of ischemic events.[6–8] However, these trials intervened after the onset of detectable valve obstruction and for relatively short follow-up periods so that the effect of intervening earlier in the disease process or for a longer time interval is unknown. It seems likely, although unproven, that optimal control of cardiovascular risk factors over an individual's lifetime would lead to decreased likelihood or later onset of AS.

Current guidelines focus on management of cardiac comorbid conditions and standard cardiovascular risk reduction in adults with calcific AS, including optimal management of hypertension (**Table 1**). There also may be benefit from angiotensin-converting enzyme inhibitors and angiotensin receptor blockers to decrease left ventricular (LV) fibrosis in the setting of pressure overload from AS. Smoking cessation is strongly advised, as in all patients, given the risk for atherosclerotic disease. Despite the lack of evidence that medical therapies reduce AS progression, optimal control of cardiovascular risk factors remains paramount for improving overall cardiovascular outcomes.

Evidence gaps
Ongoing basic science research into the cellular and molecular basis of calcific valve disease offers the promise that targeted medical therapy might be possible in the future.[9,10] Epidemiologic and genetic studies will help to identify which patients are most at risk of calcific valve disease, allowing intervention to be directed to vulnerable populations. Mendelian randomization studies will help define which conventional risk factors are causal for development of calcific AS,

Guideline Recommendations	AHA/ACC
Optimal treatment of hypertension in patients with AS reduces cardiovascular event rates	I
Lipid lowering therapy has not been shown to be beneficial for valve-related outcomes in patients with mild-moderate AS	III: No benefit
Evidence Gaps	
Does control of cardiovascular risk factors over a patient's lifetime lead to decreased likelihood or later onset of development of AS?	
Are there medical therapies that can target the specific pathophysiology of AS to prevent or slow progression of AS?	

Table 1
Medical therapy: recommendations and evidence gaps

AHA/ACC Recommendations for medical therapy in patients with AS.[1] European Society of Cardiology/European Association for Cardio-Thoracic Surgery Guidelines do not include recommendations for medical therapy in AS.
Abbreviations: ACC, American College of Cardiology; AHA, American Heart Association; AS, aortic stenosis.
Class I (green) indicates a strong recommendation with benefit greatly exceeding risk.
Class III (red) indicates there is no benefit and this treatment is not recommended.

rather than nonspecific associations with valve disease.[11]

Timing of Intervention

Guidelines

The optimal timing of intervention for AS is a complex decision that takes into consideration multiple factors. On one hand, conservative management of asymptomatic severe AS carries a risk of adverse cardiac events, including a risk of sudden cardiac death, as well as progressive LV myocardial remodeling and fibrosis. On the other hand, despite significant advances in the safety and effectiveness of both surgical and transcatheter aortic valve replacement (TAVR), these therapies are not without risk. Furthermore, all bioprosthetic valves have a finite life span due to structural valve deterioration, with the "clock starting" at the time of valve implantation. Mechanical valves require anticoagulation, which increases the risk of bleeding. All prosthetic valves also carry a risk of endocarditis and thromboembolic events. Aortic valve replacement is not a cure for AS but rather trades one medical condition (eg, valve dysfunction) for another (eg, a prosthetic valve). The optimal timing of intervention is best defined as the point in the disease course when the benefits of valve replacement exceed the risks related to native valve disease.

The most recent AHA/ACC and ESC/EACTS guidelines on timing of intervention in AS are summarized in **Table 2** and **Fig. 1**.[1–3] There are several stages of disease in adults with valvular AS defined by clinical symptoms, valve anatomy, severity of outflow obstruction, and LV function. High-gradient severe AS, Stage D1 (mean gradient >40 mm Hg, maximum velocity >4.0 m/s), is the most common phenotype in symptomatic patients and the simplest to diagnose.

However, a low transaortic volume flow rate can mask the presence of severe AS (aortic valve area [AVA] <1.0 cm^2) with a low velocity (or gradient) despite a small valve area. In the AHA/ACC Guidelines, low-gradient severe AS is divided into low-flow, low-gradient (LF-LG) severe AS with a reduced LV ejection fraction (EF <50%) (Stage D2) and LF-LG severe AS with preserved LVEF (Stage D3) (see **Fig. 1**). Both of these conditions are identified by the presence of a low stroke volume indexed to body surface area of less than 35 mL/m^2 resulting in a small calculated AVA less than 1.0 cm^2 despite relatively low aortic valve gradients.

For patients with suspected LF-LG AS with reduced EF, low-dose dobutamine echocardiography is recommended to distinguish severe from pseudo-severe stenosis (in which case the AVA increases to >1.0 cm^2 and mean gradient remains <40 mm Hg with improvement of flow). Patients with LF-LG severe AS with preserved EF typically have LV hypertrophy with a small LV chamber and low stroke volume and are frequently older women. In these patients, computed tomography calcium scoring can be added to the clinical and echocardiographic assessment to identify patients who will benefit from aortic valve intervention. Using a calcium score of greater than 1200 AU in women and greater than 2000 AU in men has been demonstrated to correlate well with severe AS and predict adverse clinical outcomes.

The evidence for timing of aortic valve replacement is strongest for patients with symptoms due to severe high-gradient AS but guideline recommendations for AVR apply to all 3 AS phenotypes, including Stages D1, D2, and D3 (see **Fig. 1**, **Table 2**).

In addition, due to the insidious onset of symptoms, patients may adapt to their physical limitations without recognition of overt symptoms. A careful history is required to elicit symptoms as well as recognize these adaptive lifestyle changes. In patients who have equivocal symptoms or are truly asymptomatic by history, treadmill stress testing can play a helpful role in eliciting symptoms, quantifying aerobic capacity and risk-stratifying patients without overt symptoms. Patients who have symptoms or reduced aerobic capacity on stress testing without another more likely explanation should be considered to have symptomatic valve disease. Event rates are higher in patients with reduced aerobic capacity or an abnormal hemodynamic response to exercise (blood pressure increases by <20 mm Hg or hypotensive response). AVR should be considered in these patients.

Evidence gaps

The benefit of AVR in asymptomatic patients has not been established. Multiple markers have demonstrated the ability to further risk stratify patients with asymptomatic, severe AS. Severely elevated aortic valve peak velocity, rapid increase in peak velocity over time (>0.3 m/s per year), elevated B-type natriuretic peptide levels and pulmonary hypertension have all been shown to be associated with higher event rates.[12] The ESC/EASCTS Guidelines recommend consideration of AVR for asymptomatic patients with any of these high-risk markers, whereas the AHA/ACC only considers peak aortic valve velocity greater than 5.0 m/s to be a potential indication for AVR. These

Table 2
Timing of intervention: recommendations and evidence gaps

Guideline Recommendations	AHA/ACC	ESC/EACTS
AVR is indicated for symptomatic patients with severe AS, plus: • Symptoms or • LVEF <50%	I	I
AVR should be considered at the time of cardiac surgery for other indications in patients with asymptomatic severe AS (Class I) and moderate AS (Class IIa)	I/IIa	I/IIa
AVR should be considered in asymptomatic patients with severe AS who have decreased exercise tolerance or an abnormal BP response to exercise	IIa	IIa
AVR should be considered in asymptomatic patients with severe AS, low procedural risk and one of several high-risk features[a]	IIa	IIa
AVR should be considered in patients with low-flow, low-gradient AS and reduced LVEF showing a mean gradient ≥40 mm Hg at dobutamine stress echocardiography	IIa	I
AVR should be considered in symptomatic patients with low-flow, low-gradient AS and preserved LVEF after confirmation of severe AS	IIa	IIa
Evidence Gaps		
Is there benefit to perform AVR in patients with asymptomatic, severe AS if procedural risk is low?		
Do patients with HFrEF and moderate AS benefit from AVR?		
Should CT aortic valve calcium scoring be included in the guidelines for diagnosis of low-flow, low-gradient, severe AS? What is the role in preserved vs reduced LVEF? What about risk stratification in high gradient AS?		

Abbreviations: ACC, American College of Cardiology; AHA, American Heart Association; AS, aortic stenosis; AVR, aortic valve replacement; BP, blood pressure; CT, computed tomography; EACTS, European Association for Cardio-Thoracic Surgery; ESC, European Society of Cardiology; HFrEF, heart failure with reduced ejection fraction; LVEF, left ventricular ejection fraction.

 Strong Recommendation (Benefit greatly exceeds risk)

Moderate strength Recommendation (Benefit exceeds risk with a moderate strength recommendation)

[a] ACC/AHA guidelines give a Class IIa recommendation for very severe AS with Vmax (peak aortic jet velocity) greater than 5.0 m/s with low surgical risk; severe AS with rapid progression in gradients and low surgical risk is given a Class IIb recommendation. ESC/EACTS recommend Vmax greater than 5.5 m/s, severely calcified valve with rate of progression of greater than 0.3 m/s/y, markedly elevated B-type natriuretic peptide without other explanation or severe pulmonary hypertension as high-risk features; these are given a Class IIa recommendation for AVR. The ESC/EACTS specifically recommends that these patients are limited to those who are candidates for SAVR.

discrepancies are based on clinical studies showing that these factors are markers of more rapid symptom onset but do not necessarily predict adverse outcomes in the absence of symptoms if valve replacement is performed promptly once symptoms develop. Therefore, the benefit of valve replacement versus close outpatient monitoring for the development of symptoms in patients with these adverse markers is uncertain.

Even so, with safer and more effective treatments, it is reasonable to consider whether earlier intervention on AS would improve clinical outcomes by preventing irreversible LV remodeling or sudden cardiac death. Although patients with asymptomatic, severe AS have a better prognosis than those with symptomatic disease, watchful waiting of asymptomatic patients does carry some risk. The risk of sudden death has been reported to be approximately 1% per year, but it is not clear whether these patients were truly asymptomatic preceding sudden death events. In addition, AS causes pressure overload on the LV, which leads to several myocardial changes, including cardiomyocyte hypertrophy; focal, replacement fibrosis; and diffuse, interstitial fibrosis. Although cardiomyocyte hypertrophy and interstitial fibrosis are reversible, replacement fibrosis persists after AVR.[13] It is not known whether these changes have long-term impact on clinical outcomes. Retrospective studies comparing survival in patients with asymptomatic, severe AS have demonstrated better survival in patients undergoing early AVR as compared with waiting for

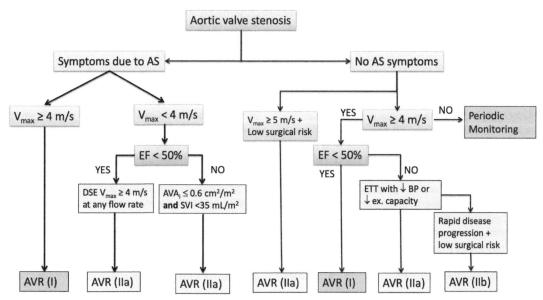

Fig. 1. Guideline recommendations for therapeutic management of AS. AVAi, indexed aortic valve area; AVR, aortic valve replacement; DSE, dobutamine stress echocardiography; ETT, exercise testing; SVI, stroke volume index; V_{max}, peak aortic jet velocity.

the onset of symptoms.[14] As surgery or transcatheter interventions become safer and with improved valve hemodynamics and durability, this may push the risk/benefit equation in favor of earlier intervention. Randomized clinical trials will be necessary to answer this important question. For example, the EARLY TAVR trial (NCT03042104) is currently testing whether patients with asymptomatic, severe AS benefit from TAVR as compared with active surveillance. It will be important to consider long-term outcomes associated with the early intervention approach because earlier timing of intervention leaves patients at risk for structural valve degeneration earlier in the course of their disease process.

Even moderate AS contributes a hemodynamic load on the LV, which can be quantified by valvular-arterial impedance.[15] Patients with heart failure with reduced EF (HFrEF) have significant myocardial dysfunction; LV performance in these patients is more sensitive to changes in afterload conditions than in patients with normal EF. Many pharmacologic therapies in HFrEF benefit LV myocardial performance by decreasing arterial afterload, thereby improving ventriculoarterial coupling. However, in patients with HFrEF and AS, the stenotic valve contributes additional impedance into the system, thereby impairing myocardial performance. Patients with HFrEF and moderate AS may benefit from AVR by reducing afterload imposed on the failing heart.

The TAVR UNLOAD trial (NCT02661451) is an ongoing clinical trial that is randomizing patients with heart failure, LVEF less than 50%, and moderate AS to TAVR with SAPIEN S3 plus optimal therapy for heart failure versus optimal heart failure therapy alone.[16] This trial will provide evidence regarding whether earlier intervention in the course of AS improves clinical outcomes in patients with heart failure with systolic dysfunction.

Choice of Valve Type

Guidelines

After making the decision to intervene on AS, the next question becomes: what is the optimal valve type for our patient? This is also a complex question in which age, comorbidities, valve anatomy, and patient preferences and values are important considerations. The first important dichotomy in decision making is the decision to implant a mechanical versus biologic aortic valve prosthesis. At present, mechanical prostheses can be implanted only surgically, whereas bioprosthetic valves can be placed surgically or via a transcatheter approach. If a bioprosthetic valve is considered to be the most appropriate valve type, the decision for a surgical versus transcatheter approach depends on surgical risk, valve and peripheral vascular anatomy, and need for concomitant interventions, among others.

It is generally recommended that patients younger than 50 years undergo implantation of a mechanical valve due to the high likelihood of bioprosthetic structural valve deterioration over the patient's lifetime. Exceptions would be patients in whom long-term vitamin K antagonist anticoagulation is contraindicated due to bleeding risk or not preferred due to lifestyle choices or a desire for a subsequent pregnancy.

In patients aged 50 to 70 years, either a mechanical or bioprosthetic valve is reasonable; the decision should be based on age, life expectancy, comorbidities, risk of anticoagulation, and patient preferences and values. Patients aged 70 years or older are generally advised to have a bioprosthetic valve. Clearly, age plays an important role in prosthesis selection. In addition to longer life expectancy and need for reintervention on that basis, younger patients with bioprosthetic valves have much higher rates of structural valve deterioration (SVD). At 15 to 20 years from valve implantation, the rate of SVD in a patient

undergoing AVR at 20 years of age is approximately 90% versus 10% in a patient implanted at age 70.[17] Previous randomized trials of mechanical versus bioprosthetic valve implantation have demonstrated improved survival and decreased need for valve reintervention in patients implanted with mechanical valves, with similar rates of thromboembolism; however, this comes at the cost of increased bleeding associated with the attendant anticoagulation for mechanical valves.

If a bioprosthetic valve is most appropriate for the patient, the next decision is whether to pursue surgical versus transcatheter intervention (**Fig. 2**). TAVR has been clearly demonstrated to be superior to medical therapy in patients with severe AS and prohibitive surgical risk and has similar outcomes as surgical AVR (SAVR) in patients with high or intermediate surgical risk.[18] **Table 3** summarizes the most recent guidelines on choice

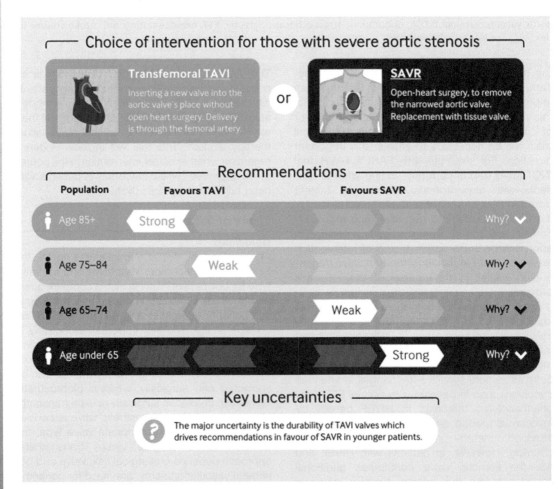

Fig. 2. Choice of intervention for patients with severe AS. TAVI, transcatheter aortic valve implantation. (*From* Vandvik PO, Otto CM, Siemieniuk RA, et al. Transcatheter or surgical aortic valve replacement for patients with severe, symptomatic, aortic stenosis at low to intermediate surgical risk: A clinical practice guideline. BMJ 2016;354:i5085; with permission.)

Table 3
Choice of intervention: guidelines and evidence gaps

Guideline Recommendations[a]	AHA/ACC	ESC/EACTS	BMJ	
Age at which mechanical AVR should be considered in patients without contraindications to anticoagulation	<50 y Maybe: 50–70[b]	<60 y		
Surgical AVR is preferred over TAVR	Low-intermediate surgical risk	Low surgical risk	Age <65	
			Age 65–75	
TAVR is preferred over SAVR	Prohibitive surgical risk	Prohibitive surgical risk	Age >85	
		Elderly patients	Age 75–85	
Either SAVR or TAVR is reasonable	High surgical risk	Increased surgical risk		
	Intermediate surgical risk			
Evidence Gaps				
How does a strategy of mechanical vs bioprosthetic valve compare in modern practice, using modern valves and transcatheter valve-in-valve options? • What are long-term outcomes according to various age strata?				
How do long-term clinical outcomes compare in patients with low and intermediate surgical risk undergoing TAVR vs. SAVR? • How do rates of structural valve deterioration compare? • How do outcomes compare according to age strata?				
Should TAVR recommendations be expanded to low surgical risk patients?				
Should TAVR for intermediate surgical risk be a Class I indication?				
What is the role of TAVR in treatment of bicuspid aortic valves with severe AS • How do long-term outcomes compare between SAVR and TAVR?				

Abbreviations: ACC, American College of Cardiology; AHA, American Heart Association; AS, aortic stenosis; AVR, aortic valve replacement; EACTS, European Association for Cardio-Thoracic Surgery; ESC, European Society of Cardiology; SAVR, surgical AVR; TAVR, transcatheter AVR.

 Strong Recommendation

Moderate Recommendation

[a] ACC/AHA Recommendations reflect 2017 Focused Update[20]; ECS/EACTS reflect 2017 Guidelines, BMJ[6] reflects Rapid Recommendations[17]: recommendations are based on patients with low-intermediate surgical risk.

[b] AHA/ACC guidelines state that it is reasonable to perform mechanical AVR in patients aged 50 y. Individualized approach required for patients aged 50 to 70 y: either mechanical or bioprosthetic valve reasonable.

of valve type. However, recent randomized controlled trials on patients with a low surgical risk have demonstrated similar or better short-term and intermediate-term outcomes in patients undergoing TAVR and these studies became available only after publication of the current guidelines.[19,20] Updated guidelines likely will soon be available.

Patient age, or expected remaining years of life, is an important consideration in deciding on prosthetic valve type (see **Fig. 2**). Several types of surgical bioprosthetic aortic valves have demonstrated good durability for up to 15 to 20 years after implantation.[21] Thus, the absence of long-term durability data for transcatheter valves affects decision making in younger patients. Based on a systematic review of available data for patients with symptoms due to severe AS and a low-intermediate surgical risk, the BMJ Rapid Recommendations strongly recommend TAVR over SAVR for patients older than 85 years with a weak recommendation for those aged 75 to 84 years (see **Fig. 2**). In contrast, SAVR remains strongly recommended over TAVR in patients younger than 65 years and weakly recommended in patients aged 65 to 74 years primarily due to uncertainty about long-term TAVR durability.[22,23]

Other considerations in the choice of TAVR versus SAVR are the presence of suitable peripheral vascular anatomy for TAVR, indications for coronary artery bypass grafting, need for concomitant structural interventions, and relevant medical comorbidities, among others. The complexity of decision making highlights the need for thoughtful evaluation by a Heart Valve Team. Together, the team should weigh the advantages and disadvantages of each approach and counsel the patient to make an informed decision that is right for his or her particular situation. An individualized approach to the care of the patient with AS is essential for optimal patient outcomes.

Evidence gaps

Despite the recommendations for mechanical aortic valve implantation in younger patients, there has been a significant decline in the use of mechanical aortic valves over the past decade. In a large retrospective study of patients aged 45 to 65 undergoing SAVR, the rates of mechanical AVR declined from 89% to 48% from 1996 to 2013.[24] The widespread use of TAVR for treatment of native AS, as well as treatment of structural valve degeneration using valve-in-valve TAVR has likely had a significant influence on these trends. However, these therapeutic approaches have never been directly compared. There is clearly a need for additional modern data comparing an approach for mechanical versus bioprosthetic valves to inform decision making in the era of expanded use of TAVR and valve-in-valve interventions.

Although results from the PARTNER 3 and EVO-LUT low-risk trials on the use of TAVR in patients with low surgical risk have been promising over short-term follow-up, the question of valve durability remains.[25,26] This is an important uncertainty in choosing the optimal procedure for these patients. Patients with low surgical risk and younger patients would be expected to have good short-term outcomes with either approach; however, valve hemodynamics, biocompatibility, and durability are likely to be the major determinants of long-term outcomes in these patients. The mean age in the PARTNER 3 and EVOLUT low-risk trials was 74 years, with only 70 patients (7%) being younger than 65 in the PARTNER 3 trial. In the studied age range, surgical bioprostheses have previously demonstrated excellent durability with SVD generally not developing until 10 years post-implant, and approximately 90% being free from significant SVD at 15 to 20 years. Very little is known about the durability of transcatheter valves over this period. A recent study from the UK TAVR registry provides the largest follow-up out to 5 to 10 years of 241 patients, with a rate of moderate or greater SVD occurring in 9% of patients at a mean of 6.1 years of follow-up.[19] There are no studies with more than 10-year follow-up, which precludes even an indirect comparison of long-

term durability of transcatheter versus surgical valves.[25,26] Certainly, long-term follow-up from the TAVR versus SAVR trials will provide valuable information on comparative rates of SVD between these 2 approaches, but such comparisons are years away. In the absence of randomized trial data to support the use of TAVR over SAVR in young patients, caution must be applied when extrapolating the results of prior trials to younger patients.[27]

Patients with AS due to bicuspid aortic valves are an important special population. Not only are patients with severe AS due to bicuspid aortic valves younger at the time of intervention than their counterparts with degenerative, trileaflet disease, the aortic valve anatomy differs significantly. Patients with bicuspid aortic valves were specifically excluded from the major trials comparing surgical versus transcatheter intervention. Furthermore, the asymmetric valve orifice adds additional anatomic complexity and may lead to a suboptimal hemodynamic result in patients undergoing TAVR and may, in turn, lead to earlier onset of SVD. Randomized controlled trial data are lacking on the use of TAVR for treatment of severe AS due to bicuspid aortic valves. Until further data demonstrate the safety of TAVR compared with SAVR in this population, surgical AVR remains the recommended approach in these patients.

Finally, we have little information on patient-reported outcome or on patient preferences and values in the choice of TAVR versus SAVR.[28]

SUMMARY

AS is the leading cause of valvular heart disease requiring intervention in developed countries. There have been multiple recent advances that have improved the safety and efficacy of our therapies for AS, with TAVR changing the treatment paradigm. Recent advances may lead to recommendations for earlier intervention and an expanded use of TAVR in patients with low and intermediate surgical risk; however, the durability of transcatheter prosthetic valves and long-term outcomes remain important questions that need to be answered. Ultimately, long-term outcomes of well-conducted clinical trials will be necessary to determine optimal management of patients in terms of medical therapies, and timing of and choice of intervention.

REFERENCES

1. Nishimura RA, Otto CM, Bonow RO, et al. 2017 AHA/ACC focused update of the 2014 AHA/ACC guideline for the management of patients with valvular

heart disease: a report of the American College of Cardiology/American Heart Association Task Force on clinical practice guidelines. J Am Coll Cardiol 2017;70(2):252–89.

2. Nishimura RA, Otto CM, Bonow RO, et al. 2014 AHA/ACC guideline for the management of patients with valvular heart disease: a report of the American College of Cardiology/American Heart Association task force on practice guidelines. J Am Coll Cardiol 2014; 63:e57–185.

3. Baumgartner H, Falk V, Bax JJ, et al. 2017 ESC/EACTS guidelines for the management of valvular heart disease. Eur Heart J 2017;38(36):2739–91.

4. Gardezi SKM, Myerson SG, Chambers J, et al. Cardiac auscultation poorly predicts the presence of valvular heart disease in asymptomatic primary care patients. Heart 2018;104(22):1832–5.

5. Koh M, Ko DT, Austin PC, et al. Association between cardiovascular risk factors and aortic stenosis. J Am Coll Cardiol 2017;69:1523–32.

6. Pedersen TR, Egstrup K, Wachtell K, et al. Intensive lipid lowering with simvastatin and ezetimibe in aortic stenosis. N Engl J Med 2008;359:1343–56.

7. Cowell SJ, Reid J, Northridge DB, et al. A randomized trial of intensive lipid-lowering therapy in calcific aortic stenosis. N Engl J Med 2005;352:2389–97.

8. Chan KL, Teo K, Dumesnil JG, et al. Effect of lipid lowering with rosuvastatin on progression of aortic stenosis: results of the aortic stenosis progression observation: measuring effects of rosuvastatin (Astronomer) trial. Circulation 2010;121:306–14.

9. Peeters FECM, Meex SJR, Dweck MR, et al. Calcific aortic valve stenosis: hard disease in the heart: a biomolecular approach towards diagnosis and treatment. Eur Heart J 2018;39(28):2618–24.

10. Weiss RM, Chu Y, Brooks RM, et al. Discovery of an experimental model of unicuspid aortic valve. J Am Heart Assoc 2018;7(13).

11. Rahimi K, Mohseni H, Kiran A, et al. Elevated blood pressure and risk of aortic valve disease: a cohort analysis of 5.4 million UK adults. Eur Heart J 2018; 39(39):3596–603.

12. Nakatsuma K, Taniguchi T, Morimoto T, et al, CURRENT AS Registry Investigators. B-type natriuretic peptide in patients with asymptomatic severe aortic stenosis. Heart 2019;105:384–90.

13. Treibel TA, Kozor R, Schofield R, et al. Reverse myocardial remodeling following valve replacement in patients with aortic stenosis. J Am Coll Cardiol 2018;71:860–71.

14. Taniguchi T, Morimoto T, Shiomi H, et al. Initial surgical versus conservative strategies in patients with asymptomatic severe aortic stenosis. J Am Coll Cardiol 2015;66:2827–38.

15. Pibarot P, Messika-Zeitoun D, Ben-Yehuda O, et al. Moderate aortic stenosis and heart failure with reduced ejection fraction: can imaging guide us to therapy? JACC Cardiovasc Imaging 2019;12(1): 172–84.

16. Spitzer E, Van Mieghem NM, Pibarot P, et al. Rationale and design of the Transcatheter Aortic Valve Replacement to UNload the Left ventricle in patients with ADvanced heart failure (TAVR UNLOAD) trial. Am Heart J 2016;182:80–8.

17. Rahimtoola SH. Choice of prosthetic heart valve in adults. An update. J Am Coll Cardiol 2010;55: 2413–26.

18. Leon MB, Smith CR, Mack MJ, et al. Transcatheter or surgical aortic-valve replacement in intermediate-risk patients. N Engl J Med 2016;374(17):1609–20.

19. Mack MJ, Leon MB, Thourani VH, et al, PARTNER 3 Investigators. Transcatheter aortic-valve replacement with a balloon-expandable valve in low-risk patients. N Engl J Med 2019. https://doi.org/10.1056/NEJMoa1814052.

20. Popma JJ, Deeb GM, Yakubov SJ, et al, Evolut Low Risk Trial Investigators. Transcatheter aortic-valve replacement with a self-expanding valve in low-risk patients. N Engl J Med 2019. https://doi.org/10.1056/NEJMoa1816885.

21. Foroutan F, Guyatt GH, O'Brien K, et al. Prognosis after surgical replacement with a bioprosthetic aortic valve in patients with severe symptomatic aortic stenosis: systematic review of observational studies. BMJ 2016;354:i5065.

22. Vandvik PO, Otto CM, Siemieniuk RA, et al. Transcatheter or surgical aortic valve replacement for patients with severe, symptomatic, aortic stenosis at low to intermediate surgical risk: a clinical practice guideline. BMJ 2016;354.

23. Siemieniuk RA, Agoritsas T, Manja V, et al. Transcatheter versus surgical aortic valve replacement in patients with severe aortic stenosis at low and intermediate risk: systematic review and meta-analysis. BMJ 2016;354:i5130.

24. Patrick WL, Woo YJ, Goldstone AB, et al. Mechanical or biologic prostheses for aortic-valve and mitral-valve replacement. N Engl J Med 2017;377: 1847–57.

25. Foroutan F, Guyatt GH, Otto CM, et al. Structural valve deterioration after transcatheter aortic valve implantation. Heart 2017;103(23):1899–905.

26. Blackman DJ, Saraf S, MacCarthy PA, et al. Long-term durability of transcatheter aortic valve prostheses. J Am Coll Cardiol 2019;73:537–45.

27. Kataruka A, Otto CM. Valve durability after transcatheter aortic valve implantation. J Thorac Dis 2018;10(Suppl 30):S3629–36.

28. Lytvyn L, Guyatt GH, Manja V, et al. Patient values and preferences on transcatheter or surgical aortic valve replacement therapy for aortic stenosis: a systematic review. BMJ Open 2016;6(9): e014327.

Heart Valve Clinics, Centers, and Networks

John B. Chambers, MD, FESC[a],*, Patrizio Lancellotti, MD, FESC[b]

KEYWORDS

- Heart valve center • Valve clinic • Valve disease

KEY POINTS

- Heart valve clinics ensure that patients are cared for by cardiologists and other specialists who undertake to develop and maintain specialist knowledge and experience to improve care.
- Heart valve centers are defined by the standards of the facilities and organization, including individual operator and center volume, to optimize interventional results.
- The key is that every discipline and service, including imaging, has valve-specific expertise.
- Valve disease networks facilitate the transfer of patients across each level of care from community to district hospital to heart valve center.

INTRODUCTION

Specialist valve clinics[1,2] were proposed because of limitations in the care of patients with heart valve disease. They represented a rallying call for developing a specialist interest in valve disease to improve clinical decision making and the organization of care.

A key aim of a valve clinic is to refer to a surgeon or interventional cardiologist appropriately but early in the natural history of the condition before the development of significant adverse left ventricle (LV) geometric and functional changes or major adverse clinical events such as sudden death. If a patient has no or minimal symptoms, it is particularly important that the intervention can be accomplished safely and effectively. This requirement is stated in the guidelines concerning repair of mitral prolapse[3–5] but is equally relevant for patients with class II indications for surgery in aortic stenosis (AS). The need for excellent results led to a consensus statement on standards required for heart valve centers.[3,4,6]

More recently the need to coordinate valve care at cardiac centers, referring hospitals, and the community has led to the concept of a valve care network. This network is intended to rationalize the flow of patients to the center for treatment but then out to the community for follow-up.

This article discusses the makeup of valve clinics, heart valve centers, and valve networks.

WHY ARE SPECIALIST VALVE SERVICES NEEDED?

The prevailing arrangement had been for patients with heart valve disease to be cared for by physicians or cardiologists without specialist competencies in valve disease. Furthermore, there was a general lack of awareness of the frequency and importance of valve disease. These factors led to many limitations to care, which for AS were:

- Reduced detection rate. In the OxVALVE study,[7] 4.9% of people more than 65 years of age had previously known moderate or severe valve disease of all types, but a further 6.4% had disease detected only by population screening. Approximately one-half of cases of severe AS detected at postmortem are known in life.[8]
- Difficulties of assessment. Physicians or cardiologists without specialist competencies may have difficulty in determining whether

[a] Cardiothoracic Center, Guy's and St Thomas' Hospitals, Westminster Bridge Road, London SE1 7EH, UK;
[b] Department of Cardiology, Heart Valve Clinic, CHU Sart Tilman, Rue de l'hôpital 1, 4000 Liège, Belgium
* Corresponding author.
E-mail address: jboydchambers@aol.com

Cardiol Clin 38 (2020) 65–74
https://doi.org/10.1016/j.ccl.2019.09.006

patients are truly asymptomatic. This problem applies particularly in AS, in which the first symptom is often a reduction in exercise capacity rather than overt breathlessness or chest discomfort. Many patients have multiple comorbidities, making it hard to determine whether the AS is the cause of symptoms. These comorbidities may also complicate the decision of when and whether intervention is indicated. The grading of AS is increasingly difficult, especially in patients with discordant echocardiographic results, and there is an increasing need to be aware of the value of nonechocardiographic imaging techniques and biomarkers.[9,10] Decisions about surgery for coexistent mitral regurgitation or the advisability of replacing an aortic valve with mild or moderate stenosis at the time of coronary bypass grafting may also be difficult.

- Timing of surgery. Guidelines are frequently either not known or not followed,[11–13] and about one-third of patients with AS are referred for intervention either too early or too late.[12] Approximately 50% have class III or IV symptoms, which increases the risk and reduces the success of surgery.[14]
- Access to appropriate intervention. In the United Kingdom[15] there is major geographic variation in access to aortic valve replacement (**Fig. 1**). Penetration of transcatheter aortic valve implantation (TAVI) is similarly variable. Access is particularly poor for the elderly, at least one-third of whom with severe AS are not referred for surgery despite clear clinical indications.[16,17] Developing a percutaneous valve program leads to increased rates of conventional surgery, suggesting the prior existence of clinically inappropriate perceptual barriers to referral[18] (see **Fig. 1**).

HEART VALVE CLINIC

A valve clinic is a necessary part of a heart valve center but it is possible and desirable to have a valve clinic at a district general hospital (DGH) without surgery or other intervention. This clinic can refer either to the clinic at the cardiac center or directly to interventional services (**Fig. 2**, **Table 1**).

A cardiac center must have clinics covering all aspects of valve care (see **Table 1**), including surveillance before surgery and care after intervention. It is not appropriate only to have a clinic dedicated, for example, to TAVI assessment, because this does not accommodate the many other types of valve disease.

However, it may not be appropriate to see patients who will never be suitable for intervention and who would be better seen in another clinic; for example, an elderly care clinic. Some patients may be better suited to a heart failure service, although this is more likely for secondary mitral regurgitation than AS.

ROLES OF A VALVE CLINIC

The medical and organizational aims of a heart valve clinic are given in **Table 2**. However, despite its name, its roles extend well beyond the outpatient department. The cardiologist running the valve clinic provides:

- Specialist inpatient opinions and care
- Education and training for doctors and patients, including keeping colleagues up to date
- Valve-specific protocols
- Specialist imaging services
- Links with the community to improve detection or valve disease
- Involvement with multidisciplinary teams

DISCIPLINES AND COMPETENCIES

The core specialist is the cardiologist, but disciplines involved depend on the nature of the clinic

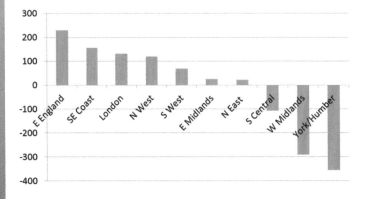

Fig. 1. Predicted versus observed age-adjusted and sex-adjusted aortic valve replacement 2005 to 2008. A comparison of rates of aortic valve replacement in the United Kingdom against estimated need found a variance between observed and expected ranging between −356 and +230. (*Data from* Bridgewater B, Kinsman R, Walton P et al. Demonstrating quality: the sixth National Adult Cardiac Surgery database report. Henley on Thomas UK. Dendrite Clinical Systems Ltd, 2009.)

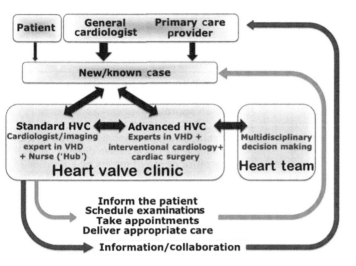

Fig. 2. Organization of a valve clinic. HVC, heart valve center; VHD, valvular heart disease. (*From* Lancellotti P, Rosenhek R, Pibarot P, et al. Heart valve clinics: organisation, structure and experiences. Eur Heart J 2013;34:1597-1606; with permission.)

and might include a surgeon or interventional cardiologist. Large centers are likely to have some clinics for general valve cases and others for patients referred for consideration of surgery or transcatheter procedures. In some countries (eg, the United Kingdom), some roles are devolved to scientist/sonographers or nurses (**Table 3**).[19,20] All should have specialist competencies. As yet, there is no formal qualification to establish competency in valve disease for any medical discipline. However, for all disciplines, competencies should be based on the following areas.[21]

TRAINING

For cardiologists, study at a specialized center during training is useful and an essential criterion is attendance at valve-related training events formally designated by accreditation points from a representative national or international body. Surgeons will have received training in a recognized valve center and must be able to show adequate numbers and quality of results according to standards available in opinion articles and defined by national specialist societies.[12]

Table 1
Clinical and pathologic conditions evaluated in the heart valve clinic

Pathologic Conditions	Priority Criteria[a]
• Moderate or severe native valve regurgitation • Mild, moderate, or severe native valve stenosis • Previous valve repair or replacement • Previous infective endocarditis • Thoracic aortic dilatation • Previous percutaneous valve implantation or repair • Marfan syndrome • Combined valve disease • Bicuspid aortic valve	Patient-related conditions • Unstable condition • Discordance between symptoms and VHD severity • Discordance between VHD severity and LV function • Planned valve repair in asymptomatic patients Valve-related conditions • Severe valvular regurgitation • Severe valvular stenosis • Severe dysfunction of prosthetic valve or valve repair • Previous infective endocarditis • Previous percutaneous valve implantation or repair • Marfan syndrome with any degree of aortic dilatation

Abbreviation: VHD, valvular heart disease.
  [a] The priority criteria may be used to triage the patients eligible for the heart valve center (HVC) in case of limited resources and/or to refer the patients to an advanced HVC.

Table 2
Aims of a specialist heart valve clinic

Medical Aims	Organizational Aims
1. Evaluate patients correctly using multimodality imaging, stress testing, and biomarkers (see **Box 1**, **Table 3**) and communicate a management plan including likely prognosis to all involved in the care of the patient 2. Monitor valve disease at appropriate intervals 3. Determine the correct timing of intervention 4. Determine which type of intervention is needed and refer to the appropriate surgeon or interventional cardiologist 5. Assess results after surgery 6. Importantly, educate and inform patients about valve disease both before and after surgery, including the symptoms of valve disease and of endocarditis	1. Short waiting times appropriate to clinical need 2. A 1-stop approach 3. Clear communication and collaboration with all health care professionals involved in the management of heart valve disease 4. More efficient use of resources; eg, rationalize tests according to international guidelines

Sonographers and nurses must have adequate experience and training; for example, ward-based or laboratory-based experience in cardiology. They should ideally have a higher degree in cardiology and may have attended hospital-based or national clinical skills courses and informal training in consultant-led cardiology clinics.

SPECIALIZED PRACTICE

There is a spectrum in valve-related activity between cardiologists and general practitioners (GPs) who have competencies in valve disease and those, usually at cardiothoracic centers, who subspecialize partly or wholly in valve disease. Specialized practice could be shown by supervision of a valve clinic, being part of the endocarditis

Table 3
Tasks in the standard model of the heart valve clinic

Tasks		Expert in VHD	
	Nurse	Sonographer	Cardiologist
Patient background	+	(+)	+
Blood pressure	+	—	+
Blood sample	+	—	—
12-lead electrocardiogram	+	—	+
Supervise exercise test	—	—	+
Echocardiography	—	+	+
Stress echocardiography	—	(+)	+
Referral to a surgeon/interventional cardiologist	—	—	+
Database entry	+	—	+
Letter to family physician	—	(+)	+
Fix appointments	+	—	+
Organize dental surveillance	+	—	+
Adapt oral anticoagulation therapy	—	—	+
Adapt medical treatment	—	—	+
Follow-up of complex cases	—	—	+

Parentheses indicate tasks that are allowed to be performed by a certified sonographer in some countries; for example, United Kingdom.

team, seeing inpatient referrals with valve disease, and writing departmental protocols. Ideal criteria include research or teaching in valve disease.

CONTINUING PROFESSIONAL DEVELOPMENT

All disciplines attend meetings with valve-specific scientific or educational components, many organized by national or international societies. Membership of a specialist society is encouraged; for example, the European Society of Cardiology Working Group in Valvular Heart Disease, the Society of Heart Valve Disease, or the British Heart Valve Society.

FACILITIES AND LINKS

Echocardiography is the key investigation and should be available as a 1-stop service. Individual operators and departments should be accredited by national or international systems.[22] Other imaging techniques and biomarkers must be available (**Box 1**). Exercise testing is particularly useful in AS[23] for revealing symptoms but remains underused.[12]

DO VALVE CLINICS WORK?

It is obvious that a team with an interest and competencies in valve disease is likely to achieve better results than one without. There is a little published information to support this based on clinical results,[24] cost, and patient satisfaction, as discussed next.

CLINICAL

Specialist valve clinics make watchful waiting safe in severe mitral regurgitation[25] but also deliver better care in severe AS, with symptoms detected earlier and when less severe in a valve clinic compared with those referred from general clinics.[26]

COST

The cost of specialist valve clinics is lower than for conventional clinics, predominantly because of a reduction in unnecessary echocardiograms.[13] In devolved clinics there are also cost savings because salaries for nurses or scientists are less than for physicians.[27] A protocol-driven scientist-led clinic for AS[28] saves money on unnecessary visits, and a multidisciplinary clinic estimated a saving of €45,000 per 100 patients per year.

PATIENT SATISFACTION

Feedback is mainly informal, with patients valuing seeing the same person each time, and 1-stop

---

Box 1
Tests needed for valve clinic

B-type natriuretic peptide (BNP): a BNP level 3 times the upper limit of normal is a class IIa indication for aortic valve replacement,[1] but it is not used routinely. It is most useful when there are multiple causes of breathlessness to help differentiate the effect of valve disease and noncardiac conditions.

Renal function: this is needed to interpret the BNP level because renal dysfunction causes an increase as a result of reduced clearance.

C-reactive protein: as a test for infection if infective endocarditis is suspected.

Hemoglobin: anemia as an alternative cause of breathlessness.

Lung function: for the investigation of breathlessness of uncertain origin.

Stress echocardiogram: this is indicated for a patient with symptoms despite moderate AS.

Computed tomography: this is needed for the assessment of the aorta, particularly if the echocardiographic images are suboptimal.

Magnetic resonance scan: this is useful to assess aortic diameter, branch pulmonary artery stenosis, or right ventricular volumes in severe pulmonary regurgitation. It is occasionally useful if mitral or aortic regurgitation is of uncertain grade.

---

visits with reduced waiting times. Patients also value shared decision making with their surgeons on the type of valve replacement[29] and this leads to better quality of life after surgery.[30] (**Table 4**).

HEART VALVE CENTER

The components of a heart valve center are summarized in **Table 4**. In addition to a heart valve clinic these are discussed next.

MULTIDISCIPLINARY HEART TEAMS

A multidisciplinary approach is recommended for AS as for all types of valve disease, including infective endocarditis.[1,2] Individuals with areas of expertise (eg, TAVI) should be named. Nurses and case managers, depending on local arrangements, are also involved in the multidisciplinary team. Assessment by relevant noncardiac specialists (elderly care physician, pulmonologist and so forth) should be available for patients with significant comorbidities. There should be regular heart team meetings to discuss the indications for and timing of intervention together with necessary procedural details.

Table 4
Requirements of a comprehensive heart valve center

Minimum	Additional at Selected Centers
Specialist valve clinic[3,4]	—
Imaging	
Echocardiography: 2D/3D, stress, transesophageal, intraoperative[5,6] CMR, cardiac CT, CT-PET[7] Departments and individual imagers accredited by recognized national or international systems[8]	—
Procedures Available	
Surgical: replacement of all valves, mitral valve repair, tricuspid valve repair, surgery for aortic root and ascending aorta, atrial fibrillation ablation Percutaneous: TAVI, mitral edge-to-edge procedures (eg, MitraClip) Links with hospitals offering superspecialist techniques	Surgical: Ross procedure, aortic valve repair, robotic mitral valve repair, heart transplant Percutaneous: balloon mitral valvotomy, closure of paraprosthetic regurgitation, developing mitral and tricuspid valve interventions
Collaborative services	
Other specialist cardiac services, including heart failure, and electrophysiology Intensive care (dedicated beds, extracorporeal membrane oxygenation) Extracardiac specialties: vascular surgery, general surgery, neurology, renal, stroke and elderly care medicine, psychology, genetics, and dental surgery	Percutaneous extraction of electronic devices
Processes	
Organization into multidisciplinary teams, including for endocarditis 24-h, 7-d cover allowing for annual leave and sickness Culture of safety (eg, World Health Organization checklist, review of complications) Training Job planning to include valve-related sessions, including continuing education	Research programs
Data Review	
Internal audit processes, including rates of repair and hemodynamic results, complications, durability of repair, and rates of reoperation assessed annually and summarized at 5 and 10 y Involvement in national databases with mandatory external review	—

Abbreviations: 2D, two-dimensional; 3D, three-dimensional; CMR, cardiac magnetic resonance; CT, computed tomography.

Meetings should take place weekly or at a frequency depending on annual hospital volumes. For emergent treatment, ad hoc multidisciplinary consultation should be possible.

The wishes of the patient inform the discussion of treatment options at multidisciplinary meetings. The consensus of the meeting is communicated to the patient and, if desired, informs further discussion about the timing and nature of surgery. It may on occasion be appropriate to invite a patient to a discussion about the procedure.

COLLABORATIVE SERVICES

Centers require cardiologists with all relevant complementary expertise, including adult congenital disease, inherited cardiac diseases, heart failure, and electrophysiology. There must also be noncardiac specialists, including vascular surgery, general surgery, neurology, nephrology, microbiology and infection, stroke and elderly care medicine, and care of psychiatric illness.

The heart valve center must have a dedicated cardiac surgical department, including cardiac anesthesia,[31] intensive care, and step-down unit. The option to use devices such as intra-aortic balloon pump and extracorporeal membrane oxygenation should be available.

PROCEDURES

The following procedures must be available at heart valve centers: replacement of valves in all 4 positions; mitral and tricuspid valve repair; atrial fibrillation ablation; TAVI; and surgery for the aortic root and ascending aorta. It is not possible to perform certain advanced techniques at every cardiac center, including aortic valve repair, the Ross procedure, percutaneous repair of paravalvular regurgitation, and heart transplants. There must be service-level agreements in place to allow transfer to centers that perform these techniques. New designs of valves requiring different implantation techniques should be introduced with the help of a proctor to minimize the learning curve.

PROCESSES

There need to be sufficient physicians and surgeons to allow for leave and sickness. There must also be sufficient beds for swift transfer of patients from peripheral hospitals and sufficient intensive therapy unit capacity to allow urgent surgery when clinically indicated. Operating schedules should allow urgent or emergent operations. There should be a safety checklist at the start of all procedures and a debriefing at the end.

SURGEON AND HOSPITAL VOLUMES

The relationship between case volume and outcomes of surgery and transcatheter interventions is complex. However, the literature suggests that mortalities for aortic valve replacement are lower for surgeons performing more than approximately 25 procedures per year [32,33] and for hospitals performing more than 100 operations per year.[33,34]

For aortic or combined aortic valve and root procedures, 1 study[35] found that mortality increased exponentially in hospitals performing fewer than 40 procedures per annum.

For TAVI, better results (including early mortality and rates of readmission) have been shown for hospitals that undertake more than 20 procedures per year.[36,37] However, all these studies are retrospective and registry data suggest that this threshold may be too low in current practice. Annual center volumes greater than 50 are currently recommended in France and the United Kingdom (and >75 in Holland).

The ability to show good results is more important than mandating volume targets. It is also likely that external audit of results will encourage good outcomes.

DATA REVIEW

Robust internal audit[24] with regular outcome or morbidity and mortality meetings and reporting of near misses are essential. Events should be reported according to available recommendations.[38–40] The center should report at least 30-day, and 1-year and 5-year mortalities (**Box 2**). Echocardiographic follow-up[9] and clinical results must be available for internal and external review and ideally should be presented on the heart valve center Web site and made available to patients and referring clinicians. Universal recording of all valve procedures in an international or national database is essential where these exist. Commonly used risk scores (eg, Society of Thoracic Surgery [STS] score or Euroscore II), including frailty scores for transcatheter valve procedures, should be available to interpret outcome data at the level of individual patient risk despite their limitations. Data collection is a guide to early failure of new designs of replacement valve or repair techniques as well as identifying potential problems at individual centers.

TRAINING

Training is an essential role of heart valve centers and should be established, coordinated, and monitored by national cardiovascular professional societies with provision for surgeons, cardiologists, anesthesiologists, and other disciplines during their initial professional accreditation.

All members of the multidisciplinary heart team, including physicians, surgeons, and nurses, need to be involved in continuing education appropriate to their roles. National societies should organize valve-related training and teaching sessions. There is an expectation of involvement in clinical innovation and research.

Box 2
Example dataset for recording outcomes for audit

Preoperative

  Demographic data, comorbidities

  Grading of valve lesion

  Preoperative risk assessment and stratification using validated multivariate scores

Early clinical results

  Operative mortality and morbidity at 30 days, including stroke, mediastinitis, myocardial infarction, acute kidney injury[26,27]

  Heart valve center repair rates based on preoperative multidisciplinary team classification for repair as likely, unlikely, or not feasible

  Time on intensive therapy unit

In-hospital hemodynamic function[28]

  Transvalve velocity and mean gradient (all positions) and effective orifice area (aortic position) of replacement or transcatheter valves

  Presence and grade of paraprosthetic regurgitation

  Residual regurgitation and new obstruction after surgical or transcatheter repair or systolic anterior motion of the anterior mitral leaflet

Follow-up

  Complications: infection, valve thrombosis

  Mortality: at 1 and 5 years

  Durability of repairs based on routine annual echocardiography (more frequent if significant regurgitation present); proportion per year developing moderate or worse regurgitation

  Incidence and timing of structural valve degeneration and nonstructural valve degeneration

  Rates of redo procedure per year

VALVE NETWORKS

Networks are the organizational mechanism for linking district or local hospitals and cardiac centers with the community. In addition to the roles of the valve clinic, a network is expected to add:

- Improved detection: auscultation is performed variably with higher rates in France compared with Germany and the United Kingdom.[41] However auscultation is insensitive. A survey of open-access studies[42] found that significant valve disease was suspected from a murmur in 127 patients but was unsuspected in 177 cases. Valve disease needs to be suspected in patients with a murmur but also cardiac symptoms, chronic obstructive pulmonary disease with disproportionate breathlessness, atrial fibrillation, and age greater than 75 years. Using these criteria to focus point-of-care scans, AS was found in 2% of patients in a GP practice.[43] A murmur clinic[44] allowing triage of patients to point-of-care echocardiography or standard echocardiography can make the best of scarce resources and also refer directly to a valve clinic.

- Better communication: this must occur at every level and depends on local arrangements. Conventional communication after outpatient meetings, tests, or inpatient visits must occur reliably to all involved with the patient's care in the community, district hospital, and cardiac center as well as to the patient. Some networks have patient passport.

  Case referrals and discussions can occur through regular teleconferences but more immediately using mobile phone–based digital communication systems (eg, MedShr).

- Faster transfers: it is important that patients with severe valve disease, particularly endocarditis or critical AS, are transferred from DGH to cardiac center quickly. It is important that GPs can refer patients directly to the valve service particularly for a new symptom or if endocarditis is suspected.

SUMMARY

Despite a lack of good-quality research there is reasonable consensus on important aspects of valve care. The major challenge is to ensure that these inform direct patient care because physicians and cardiologists in general clinics tend not to follow established guidelines. It is therefore vital that care is delivered by specialists with competencies in valve disease and that interventions are delivered at heart valve centers defined by recognized standards.

DISCLOSURE

The authors have no disclosures.

REFERENCES

1. Lancellotti P, Rosenhek R, Pibarot P, et al. Heart valve clinics: organisation, structure and experiences. Eur Heart J 2013;34:1597–606.
2. Chambers J, Ray S, Prendergast B, et al. Specialist valve clinics: recommendations from the British Heart Valve Society working group on improving

quality in the delivery of care for patients with heart valve disease. Heart 2013;99:1714–6.

3. Baumgartner H, Falk V, Bax JJ, et al. 2017 ESC/EACTS Guidelines for the management of valvular heart disease. Eur Heart J 2017;38(36):2739–91.

4. Nishimura RA, Otto CM, Bonow RO, et al. AHA/ACC Guideline for the management of patients with valvular heart disease. J Am Coll Cardiol 2014;129:2440–92.

5. Nishimura RA, Otto CM, Bonow RO, et al. 2017 AHA/ACC focused update of the 2014 AHA/ACC guideline for the management of patients with valvular heart disease. Circulation 2017;135:e1159–95.

6. Chambers JB, Prendergast B, Iung B, et al. Standards defining a 'Heart Valve Centre'; ESC working group on valvular heart disease and European Association for cardiothoracic surgery viewpoint. Eur Heart J 2017;38:2177–83.

7. d'Arcy JL, Coffey S, Loudon MA, et al. Large-scale community echocardiographic screening reveals a major burden of undiagnosed valvular heart disease in older people: the OxVALVE Population Cohort Study. Eur Heart J 2016. https://doi.org/10.1093/eurheartj/ehw229.

8. Andersen JA, Hansen BF, Lyndborg K. Isolated valvular aortic stenosis. Clinico-pathological findings in an autopsy material of elderly patients. Acta Med Scand 1975;197:61–4.

9. Chambers J, Garbi M, Nieman K, et al. Appropriateness criteria for the use of cardiovascular imaging in heart valve disease in adults: report of literature review and current practice. Eur Heart J Cardiovasc Imaging 2017;18:489–98.

10. Dulgheru R, Pibarot P, Sengupta PP, et al. Multimodality imaging strategies for the assessment of aortic stenosis: viewpoint of the heart valve clinic international database (HAVEC) group. Circ Cardiovasc Imaging 2016;9:e004352.

11. Bach DS, Awaia M, Gurm HS, et al. Valvular heart disease: failure of guideline adherence for intervention in patients with severe mitral regurgitation. J Am Coll Cardiol 2009;54:860–5.

12. Iung B, Baron G, Butchart EG, et al. A prospective survey of patients with valvular heart disease in Europe: the Euro Heart Survey on valvular heart disease. Eur Heart J 2003;24:1231–43.

13. Taggu W, Topham A, Hart L, et al. A cardiac sonographer led follow up clinic for heart valve disease. Int J Cardiol 2009;132:240–3.

14. Pierard S, de Meester C, Seldrum S, et al. Impact of preoperative symptoms on postoperative survival in severe aortic stenosis: implications for the timing of surgery. Ann Thorac Surg 2014;97:803–10.

15. Bridgewater B, Kinsman R, Walton P, et al. Demonstrating quality: the sixth national adult cardiac surgery database report. Henley on Thomas (UK): Dendrite Clinical Systems Ltd; 2009.

16. Bouma BJ, van der Meulen JHP, van den Brink RBA, et al. Variability in treatment advice for elderly patients with aortic stenosis: a nationwide survey in the Netherlands. Heart 2001;85:96–201.

17. Iung B. Management of the elderly patient with aortic stenosis. Heart 2008;94:519–24.

18. Grant SW, Devbhandari MP, Grayson AD, et al. What is the impact of providing a Transcatheter Aortic Valve Implantation (TAVI) service on conventional aortic valve surgical activity, patient risk factors and outcomes in the first two years? Heart 2012;96:1633–7.

19. Chambers JB, Lloyd G, Rimington HM, et al. Multidisciplinary valve clinics with devolved surveillance: a 2 year audit. Br J Cardiol 2011;18:231–2.

20. Parkin D, Chambers J. Routine follow-up for patients with prosthetic valves: the value of a nurse-led valve clinic. Br J Cardiol 2012;19:204–6.

21. Chambers J, Campbell B, Wilson J, et al. How should specialist competencies in heart valve disease be recognised? Q J Med 2015;108:353–4.

22. Nihoyannopoulos P, Fox K, Fraser A, et al. EAE laboratory standards and accreditation. Eur J Echocardiogr 2007;8:80–7.

23. Saeed S, Rajani R, Seifert R, et al. Exercise testing in patients with asymptomatic moderate or severe aortic stenosis. Heart 2018;104:1836–42.

24. Lancellotti P, Magne J, Dulgheru R, et al. Outcomes of patients with asymptomatic aortic stenosis followed up in heart valve clinics. JAMA Cardiol 2018. https://doi.org/10.1001/jamacardio.2018.3152.

25. Rosenhek R, Rader F, Klaar U, et al. Outcome of watchful waiting in asymptomatic severe mitral regurgitation. Circulation 2006;113:2238–44.

26. Zilbersac R, Lancellotti P, Gilon D, et al. Role of a heart valve clinic programme in the management of patients with aortic stenosis. Eur Heart J Cardiovasc Imaging 2017;18:138–44.

27. Ionescu A, McKenzie C, Chambers J. Are valve clinics a sound investment for the health service? A cost-effectiveness model and an automated tool for cost estimation. Open Heart 2015;2:e000275.

28. Turpie D, Maycock M, Crawford C, et al. Establishing an aortic surveillance clinic. Br J Cardiol 2010;17:286–9.

29. Korteland NM, Bras FJ, van Hout FMA, et al. Prosthetic aortic valve selection: current patient experience, preference and knowledge. Open Heart 2015;2:e000237.

30. Rimington HM, Weinman J, Chambers JB. Predicting outcome after valve replacement. Heart 2010;96:118–23.

31. Pagano D, Kappetein AP, Sousa-Uva M, et al, on behalf of the European Association for Cardio-Thoracic Surgery (EACTS) and the EACTS Quality Improvement Programme. EACTS clinical

statement: guidance for the provision of adult cardiac surgery. Eur J Cardiothorac Surg 2016;50:1006–9.

32. Birkmeyer JD, Siewers AE, Finlayson EVA, et al. Hospital volume and surgical mortality in the United States. N Engl J Med 2002;346:1128–37.

33. Patel HJ, Herbert MA, Drake DH, et al. Aortic valve replacement: using a statewide cardiac surgical database identifies a procedural volume hinge point. Ann Thorac Surg 2013;96:1560–5.

34. Goodney PP, Lucas FL, Birkmeyer JD. Should volume standards for cardiovascular surgery focus only on high-risk patients? Circulation 2003;107:384–7.

35. Hughes GC, Zhao Y, Rankin JS, et al. Effects of institutional volumes on operative outcomes for aortic root replacement in North America. J Thorac Cardiovasc Surg 2013;145:166–70.

36. Badheka AO, Patel NJ, Panaich SS, et al. Effect of hospital volume on outcomes of transcatheter aortic valve implantation. Am J Cardiol 2015;116:587–94.

37. Kim LK, Minutello RM, Feldman DN, et al. Association between transcatheter aortic valve implantation volume and outcomes in the United States. Am J Cardiol 2015;116:1910–5.

38. Tommaso CL, Bolman RM, Feldman T, et al. Multisociety (AATS, ACCF, SCAI, and STS) expert consensus statement: operator and institutional requirements for transcatheter valve repair and replacement. Part 1: transcatheter aortic valve replacement. J Am Coll Cardiol 2012;59:2028–42.

39. Tommaso CL, Fullerton DA, Feldman T, et al. SCAI/AATS/ACC/STS operator and institutional requirements for transcatheter valve repair and replacement. Part 2: mitral valve. J Am Coll Cardiol 2014;64:1515–26.

40. Akins CW, Miller DC, Turina MI, et al. Guidelines for reporting mortality and morbidity after cardiac valve interventions. J Thorac Cardiovasc Surg 2008;135:732–8.

41. Webb J, Thoenes M, Chambers J. Identifying heart valve disease in primary care: differences between practice in Germany, France and the United Kingdom. Europ J Cardiovasc Med 2014;III(1):388–92.

42. Chambers JB, Kabir S, Cajeat E. The detection of heart disease by open access echocardiography: a retrospective analysis. Br J Gen Pract 2014;64:86–7.

43. Fabich N, Harrar H, Chambers J. 'Quick scan' cardiac ultrasound in a high-risk general practice population. Br J Cardiol 2016;23:27–9.

44. Draper J, Subbiah S, Bailey R, et al. The murmur clinic. Validation of a new method. Heart 2019;105:56–9.

Prevalence and Prognostic Implications of Frailty in Transcatheter Aortic Valve Replacement

Palina Piankova, MSc[a], Jonathan Afilalo, MD, MSc, FRCPC[a,b],*

KEYWORDS

- Transcatheter aortic valve replacement • Frailty • Older adults

KEY POINTS

- Assessment of frailty is a core element in the preprocedural evaluation of older adults referred for transcatheter aortic valve replacement.
- Prevalent frailty can be elicited in one-third to two-thirds of patients depending on the frailty scale used.
- Addition of frailty to risk scores results in improved discrimination for mortality and identifies patients less likely to be discharged home and more likely to report worsening quality of life.
- Frailty should not be equated with futility, but it should rather inform the shared decision-making process and signal the use of interventions to "defrail" patients to the extent possible.

INTRODUCTION

Aortic valve stenosis is a disease that predominantly afflicts older adults, with the prevalence increasing 50-fold from 0.2% in the sixth decade of life to 10% in the ninth decade of life.[1] In addition to comorbid cardiac and noncardiac diseases, advancing age is associated with subclinical impairments in multiple physiologic systems that can collectively erode a person's homeostatic reserves and bring about the geriatric syndrome known as frailty.[2] Although there is some debate about the operational definition of frailty, there is widespread consensus about its construct validity to identify older adults with reduced resilience who may not tolerate and recover from major stressors arising from illnesses or iatrogenic procedures.

In the setting of surgical or transcatheter aortic valve replacement (TAVR), assessment of frailty has assumed a central role in the preprocedural evaluation and shared decision-making process to gauge risks and benefits in a more individualized fashion.[3] More recently, treatment of frailty has attracted attention in the pre- and postprocedural period to optimize health outcomes and functional recovery. It has become evident that chronologic age and comorbidities are insufficient to accurately predict risk and that successfully correcting the cardiac lesion is insufficient to maximize person-centered benefits.

ASSESSMENT OF FRAILTY
Physical, Cognitive, and Psychosocial Domains

Frailty is the manifestation of cumulative age-related impairments across physical, cognitive, and psychosocial domains. Physical frailty is closely related to sarcopenia, which is defined as

a Centre for Clinical Epidemiology, Jewish General Hospital, McGill University, 3755 Cote Ste Catherine, H-411, Montreal, Quebec H3T1E2, Canada; b Division of Cardiology, Geriatric Cardiology Fellowship Program, Jewish General Hospital, McGill University, 3755 Cote Ste Catherine Road, E-222, Montreal, Quebec H3T 1E2, Canada
* Corresponding author. Division of Cardiology, Geriatric Cardiology Fellowship Program, Jewish General Hospital, McGill University, 3755 Cote Ste Catherine Road, E-222, Montreal, Quebec H3T 1E2, Canada.
E-mail address: jonathan.afilalo@mcgill.ca

Cardiol Clin 38 (2020) 75–87
https://doi.org/10.1016/j.ccl.2019.09.011
0733-8651/20/© 2019 Elsevier Inc. All rights reserved.

age-related loss of muscle mass and strength.[4] Associated symptoms of inactivity and fatigue are assessed by questionnaires, or alternatively, habitual physical activities can be quantified more objectively by actigraphy using step counting devices. Muscle strength is measured by physical performance tests such as handgrip strength using a dynamometer, 5-repetition chair rise time, and 5-m gait speed (5MGS) using a stopwatch. Muscle mass can be suboptimally inferred by body mass index or unintentional weight loss, or preferably measured by imaging tests such as dual x-ray absorptiometry or computed tomography (CT).

The authors' group developed a web-based software (https://www.coreslicer.com/) to simplify the process of analyzing body composition and muscle mass from clinical CT scans.[5] After a representative axial CT image is selected, usually at the top of the fourth lumbar vertebrae, a segmentation tool is used to measure muscle and fat. In particular, psoas muscle area has gained interest as a reproducible and prognostic biomarker of physical frailty and sarcopenia.[6] Women are more likely to have low muscle mass and be physically frail and thus suffer related adverse events or require discharge to rehabilitation facilities.[7,8]

The cognitive domain of frailty is typically assessed by cognitive tests such as the Mini-Mental State Examination,[9] Montreal Cognitive Assessment (MoCA),[10] or the abbreviated Mini-Cog consisting of a 3-word recall and clock-draw test.[11] The psychosocial domain of frailty is assessed by psychological tests such as the Geriatric Depression Scale[12,13] or the Patient Health Questionnaire.[14] In addition, the psychosocial domain includes the patient's living situation, support system, and social engagement. An additional domain of frailty is sensory function, encompassing hearing and vision impairments.

Disentangling Frailty, Disability, and Comorbidity

The Cardiovascular Health Study demonstrated that among frail individuals, 27% had no major comorbidities or disabilities, 46% had comorbidities, 6% had disabilities, and 22% had all three.[15] According to some, comorbidities and disabilities should be broadly integrated into frailty indices to better reflect geriatric risk. According to others, they should be considered as separate interrelated domains with comorbidity as one of the driving causes of frailty and disability is its feared consequence.[16] The International Academy on Nutrition and Aging Task Force sided with the latter, recommending that frailty be viewed as a predisability state.[17] Disabilities are therapeutically less modifiable and prognostically more grim. In the extreme case, disabilities for all or most basic activities of daily living (bathing, toileting, dressing, eating) should raise the concern of futility.[18]

Making Sense of Frailty Scales

Numerous scales have been put forth to operationalize frailty, which is often cited as a source of confusion for clinicians that has hampered clinical applicability. In the absence of a consensus, the spectrum of frailty scales can be distilled as follows. At the narrow end of the spectrum, phenotypic scales focus on physical frailty and sarcopenia. Examples include Fried's frailty scale[15] and Guralnik's short physical performance battery.[19] Gait speed is a component of these scales, and it is also used alone as a screening test for frailty. In the middle of the spectrum, multidomain scales focus on physical and cognitive frailty and at times psychosocial frailty.[20] Examples include our Essential Frailty Toolset (EFT) score[21] and the World Health Organization's Intrinsic Capacity framework.[22] At the broad end of the spectrum, accumulated deficit scales focus on all domains of frailty as well as comorbidities, disabilities, and a variable number of other age-related impairments. Examples include Rockwood's Frailty Index and Clinical Frailty Scale (CFS).[23]

PREVALENCE OF FRAILTY

A systematized review of PubMed was performed to capture original research articles that reported the prevalence or prognostic impact of at least one objective measure of frailty in patients undergoing TAVR (**Table 1**). The search was inclusive of published English-language articles up to May 2019, reflecting studies of mainly high-risk older patients. The pooled prevalence of frailty was computed using random-effects meta-analysis models for each scale that was reported in at least 4 independent studies with the same cut-off. Forest plots are depicted in **Fig. 1**.

For the Fried scale, there were 4 studies representing 3918 patients, and the pooled prevalence of frailty using a cut-off of greater than or equal to 3/5 was 48% (confidence interval [CI] 37% to 58%). For the Rockwood CFS, there were 4 studies representing 4586 patients, and the pooled prevalence of frailty using a cut-off of greater than or equal to 5/9 was 31% (CI 24% to 38%). For 5MGS, there were 8 studies representing 13,845 patients, and the pooled prevalence of frailty using a cut-off of less than or equal to 0.83 m/s (equivalent to $\geq$6 s) was 63% (CI 55%

Table 1
Study characteristics (statistically associated frailty measures and outcomes are bolded)

Study	N	Design	Frailty Measures	Outcomes
Afilalo,[21] 2017	1020 (646 TAVR)	Prospective multicenter (FRAILTY-AVR)	**Bern** **CFS** **Columbia** **EFT** (most predictive) **Fried** **Fried+** **SPPB**	**30-d mortality** **1-y mortality** **1-y disability/mortality**
Alfredsson,[33] 2016	8039	Prospective multicenter (STS/ACC TVT)	**5MGS**	**In-hospital LOS** In-hospital complications **Discharge to facility** 30-d mortality
Arnold,[34] 2017	7014 (1-y subset)	Prospective multicenter (STS/ACC TVT)	**5MGS**	**1-y overall QOL**
Arnold,[35] 2016	2830	Substudy of RCT (CoreValve)	**BADL** **Exhaustion** **Fried scale** **MMSE** **Weight loss**	**6-m poor outcome** **12-m poor outcome**

Assmann,[36] 2016	89	Retrospective single-center	**Frailty scale**
			  4MGS
			  BADL
			  IADL
			  MMSE
			  MNA
			  TUG
			Clinical judgment
				In-hospital delirium
				30-d mortality

Bogdan,[37] 2016	150	Retrospective single-center	**Albumin**	In-hospital complications 30-d mortality **2-y mortality**
Boureau,[38] 2017	150	Prospective multicenter	Frontal assessment Low BMI **Geri Depression Scale** IADL MMSE TUG	6-m physical QOL **6-m mental QOL** 6-m mortality 6-m functioning
Cockburn,[39] 2015	312	Prospective single-center	BADL **Brighton Index** **CFS** Karnofsky Index **Poor mobility**	**30-d mortality** **2.2-y mortality up to 4.8 y**
Codner,[40] 2015	360	Prospective single-center	**Frailty scale (5MGS, Albumin, BADL, Cognition, Home O$_2$, General appearance, Clinical judgment)**	**1.9-y mortality up to 5 y**

Eichler,[41] 2018	344	Prospective multicenter	**Bern scale**
			  BADL
			  IADL
			  MMSE
			  MNA
			  Poor mobility
			  TUG
				1-y mortality

(continued on next page)

Table 1
(continued)

Study	N	Design	Frailty Measures	Outcomes
Eide,[42] 2015	143 (65 TAVR)	Prospective single-center	BADL **MMSE** SOF scale	**In-hospital delirium**
Ewe,[43] 2010	147	Prospective multicenter	**Fried scale**	**9-m composite**
Foldyna,[44] 2018	403	Retrospective single-center	**PMA at L4** **Subcutaneous fat at L4** **Visceral fat at L4**	**1-y mortality**
Forcillo,[45] 2017	361	Retrospective single-center	**5MGS** **Albumin** **BADL** Grip strength	**30-d composite** **30-d readmission** **30-d mortality** **1-y mortality**
Garg,[46] 2017	152	Retrospective single-center	**PMA at L3**	In-hospital LOS In-hospital complications **30-d composite** 30-d mortality 1-y mortality **Resource utilization**
Gassa,[47] 2018	457	Retrospective single-center	**Albumin**	**In-hospital LOS** **In-hospital AKI** **In-hospital infection** **In-hospital transfusion** In-hospital mortality **30-d mortality**
Goudzwaard,[48] 2019	213	Prospective single-center	**Erasmus Frailty Scale** 5MGS **BADL** **IADL** Grip strength **MMSE** **Malnutrition** TUG	**In-hospital delirium** 30-d complications 30-d mortality **1-y mortality**
Green,[49] 2012	159	Prospective single-center	**Columbia scale** 5MGS **Albumin** BADL Grip strength	**In-hospital LOS** **In-hospital bleeding** 30-d composite **1-y mortality**
Green,[50] 2015	244	Substudy of RCT (PARTNER 1A/B)	**Columbia scale** 5MGS Albumin BADL Grip strength	30-d complications 30-d mortality **6-m poor outcome** **1-y mortality**
Grossman,[51] 2017	426	Retrospective single-center	**Albumin**	**1-y mortality**
Hebeler,[52] 2018	470	Prospective single-center	5MGS **Albumin** BADL Grip strength PMA at L3	**1-y mortality**

(continued on next page)

Table 1
(continued)

Study	N	Design	Frailty Measures	Outcomes
Hermiller,[53] 2016	3687	Substudy of RCT (CoreValve)	5MGS **Albumin** **Assisted living** BADL **Falls** Grip strength MMSE Weight loss	**30-d mortality** **1-y mortality**
Honda,[54] 2019	150	Retrospective single-center	**CFS** **CONUT scale**	**In-hospital LOS** In-hospital complications In-hospital mortality **1-y mortality**
Horne,[55] 2018	285	Prospective multicenter (STS/ACC TVT)	**5MGS**	**Discharge to facility**
Hosler,[32] 2019	228	Prospective single-center	5MGS **CFS** CGA-Frailty Index **Chair rises** FRAIL scale Grip strength	**6-m disability/mortality**
Huded,[56] 2016	191	Retrospective single-center	**Frailty scale** **5MGS** **BADL** Grip Weight loss	**Discharge to facility** 30-d complications 30-d mortality 30-d readmission
Kamga,[57] 2013	30	Prospective single-center	ISAR scale **SHERPA scale**	In-hospital composite **1-y mortality**
Kim,[58] 2019	246	Prospective single-center	**CGA-Frailty Index**	**12-m disability**
Kleczynski,[59] 2017	101	Prospective single-center	**5MGS** **BADL** **CFS** **Elderly Mobility Scale** **Grip strength** **ISAR scale**	**1-y mortality**
Koifman,[60] 2015	567	Retrospective single-center	**Albumin**	In-hospital complications **In-hospital mortality** **30-d mortality** **1-y mortality**
Kundi,[61] 2018	52,338	Prospective multicenter	**John Hopkins Claims-based Frailty Indicator**	**4-y mortality**
Mamane,[7] 2016	208	Retrospective multicenter	**PMA at L4**	**In-hospital bleeding males** **1-y mortality females**
Martin,[62] 2018	2624	Retrospective multicenter (UK TAVI registry)	BADL **CFS** Poor mobility	**In-hospital composite** **30-d mortality** **6-m mortality** **>1-y mortality**

(continued on next page)

Table 1
(continued)

Study	N	Design	Frailty Measures	Outcomes
Miura,[63] 2017	112	Prospective single-center (KMH registry)	CFS	30-d mortality 1-y mortality
Mok,[64] 2016	460	Retrospective multicenter	**TMA at L3**	30-d mortality **1-y mortality**
Nemec,[65] 2017	157	Retrospective single-center	Low BMI **TMA at L3** TMA at T7 **TMA at T12** Subcutaneous fat at L3 **Visceral fat at L3**	**In-hospital LOS** In-hospital complications **30-d mortality** **1-y mortality**
Okoh,[66] 2017	75	Retrospective single-center	**Columbia scale**	In-hospital LOS Discharge to facility In-hospital complications **30-d mortality** **1-y mortality** **2-y mortality**
Osnabrugge,[67] 2015	436	Substudy of RCT (CoreValve)	5MGS **Albumin** Grip strength **Wheelchair-bound**	**6-m poor outcome**
Paknikar,[68] 2016	295 (139 TAVR)	Retrospective single-center	**PMA at L4**	**30-d composite** **2-y mortality** **Resource utilization**
Pinheiro,[69] 2017	55	Cross-sectional single-center	**BIA phase angle** CT abdominal fat **CT epicardial fat** CT mediastinal fat	**Frailty (Fried scale)**
Puls,[70] 2014	300	Prospective single-center	**BADL**	**In-hospital LOS** **In-hospital AKI** **In-hospital transfusions** In-hospital bleeding In-hospital vascular In-hospital stroke **Discharge to facility** **30-d mortality** **6-m mortality** **1.5-y mortality**
Rathore,[71] 2017	100	Retrospective single-center	5MGS Edmonton Frail Scale	Next-day discharge 30-d readmission 30-d mortality
Rodes,[72] 2010	345	Retrospective multicenter	Clinical judgment	In-hospital complications 30-d mortality 8-m mortality
Rogers,[73] 2018	544	Prospective single-center	**Frailty scale (5MGS, Albumin, BADL, BMI, Grip strength)**	**30-d mortality** **1-y mortality**
Saji,[74] 2016	232	Retrospective single-center	**PMA at L4**	30-d mortality **6-m mortality**

(continued on next page)

Table 1
(continued)

Study	N	Design	Frailty Measures	Outcomes
Saji,[26] 2018	155	Retrospective single-center	**5MGS** **CFS** **Columbia scale** **Kaigo-Yobo scale** Modified Fried scale **SPPB**	**30-d readmission** **3-y mortality**

Schoenenberger,[75] 2013	119	Prospective single-center	**Bern scale**
			  BADL
			  IADL
			  MMSE
			  MNA
			  Poor mobility
			  TUG
				6-m disability
				6-m disability/death

Seiffert,[76] 2014	347	Prospective multicenter	**Low BMI** **Clinical judgment**	**1-y mortality**
Shi,[77] 2018	228 (137 TAVR)	Prospective single-center	**CGA-Frailty Index** Fried scale	**6-m disability/death**
Shimura,[78] 2017	1215	Prospective multicenter (OCEAN-TAVI)	**Albumin** **CFS**	**30-d mortality** **1-y mortality**

Steinvil,[79] 2018	498	Retrospective single-center	**Frailty scale**
			  5MGS
			  Albumin
			  BADL
			  Low BMI
			  Grip strength
				30-d mortality
				1-y mortality

Stortecky,[80] 2012	100	Prospective single-center	**Bern scale**
			  BADL
			  IADL
			  MMSE
			  MNA
			  Poor mobility
			  TUG
				30-d mortality
				30-d composite
				1-y mortality
				1-y composite

Ungar,[81] 2018	71	Prospective multicenter	**CGA**	**3-m readmit/mortality** **3-m stroke/mortality**
Yamamoto,[82] 2017	1215	Prospective multicenter (OCEAN-TAVI)	**Albumin**	**In-hospital LOS** **In-hospital AKI** **In-hospital bleeding** In-hospital vascular In-hospital stroke **30-d mortality** **1-y mortality**

Abbreviations: 5MGS, 5-m gait speed; AKI, acute kidney injury; BADL, basic activities of daily living; BMI, body mass index; CFS, clinical frailty scale; CGA, comprehensive geriatric assessment; EFT, essential frailty toolset; IADL, instrumental activities of daily living; ISAR, identification of seniors at risk; LOS, length of stay; MMSE, mini-mental state examination; MNA, mini-nutritional assessment; PMA, psoas muscle area on CT; QOL, quality of life; RCT, randomized clinical trial; SHERPA, score hospitalier d'evaluation du risque de perte d'autonomie; SOF, study of osteoporotic fractures; SPPB, short physical performance battery; TMA, total muscle area on CT; TUG, timed up and go.

to 71%). For serum albumin, there were 4 studies representing 2709 patients, and the pooled prevalence of hypoalbuminemia using a cut-off of less than 3.5 mg/dL was 29% (CI 15% to 46%). For disability in activities of daily living (Katz scale[24]), there were 8 studies representing 7024 patients, and the pooled prevalence of greater than or equal to 1 disability was 30% (23% to 39%).

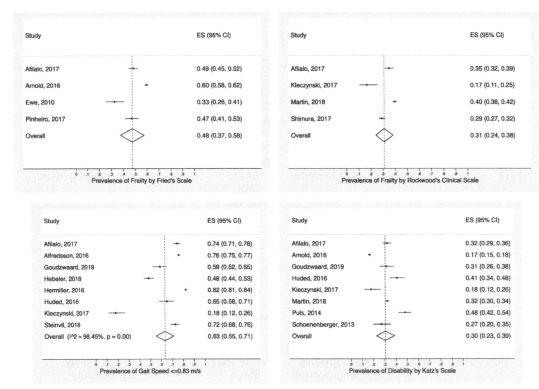

Fig. 1. Pooled prevalence of frailty and disability in older adults undergoing TAVR.

PROGNOSTIC IMPLICATIONS
Short-Term Mortality

Short-term mortality (<6 months) was examined in 30 studies. Frailty was significantly associated with short-term mortality in 20 of 30 studies, with a relative risk ranging from 1.11 to 13.77. The risk of 30-day mortality was 4% to 17% in frail patients as compared with 1% to 6% in nonfrail patients. There was a significant interaction for frail patients undergoing TAVR via a nonfemoral approach (ie, more invasive), with increased procedural mortality in this subgroup.[25]

Mid- and Long-Term Mortality

Midterm mortality (6–36 months) was examined in 37 studies. Frailty was significantly associated with midterm mortality in 29 of 37 studies, with a relative risk ranging from 1.1 to 16.4. The risk of midterm mortality was 14% to 35% in frail patients as compared with 7% to 26% in nonfrail patients. Long-term mortality (>36 months) was examined in 3 studies. In the study published by Kundi and colleagues, the incidence of 4-year mortality was 57% in frail patients as compared with 48% in nonfrail patients.

Procedural Complications

Procedural complications (defined according to the VARC-2 consensus criteria) were examined in 12 studies. Frailty was significantly associated with major bleeding complications in 3 studies, blood transfusions in 3 studies, delirium in 2 studies, acute kidney injury in 2 studies, and infections in 1 study. Frailty was not associated with vascular complications, stroke, or other major complications.

Disposition Outcomes

Discharge to a specialized health care facility was examined in 4 studies, with values ranging from 39% to 53% in frail patients as compared with 9% to 22% in nonfrail patients. Average length of stay was examined in 5 studies, with mean values ranging from 7 to 12 days in frail patients as compared with 5 to 11 days in nonfrail patients. In the study published by Saji and colleagues,[26] the relative risk of 30-day readmissions was between 1.10 and 1.68 using various measures of frailty.

Patient-Centered Outcomes

Disability for basic or instrumental activities of daily living was examined as an outcome in 5 studies, in which 15% to 21% of surviving patients experienced worsening disability at 6 to 12 months. Quality of life was examined in 5 studies, in which 31% to 34% of patients experienced a "poor outcome" (defined as either death,

Kansas City Cardiomyopathy Questionnaire score <45 points, or decline ≤10 points). Frailty was significantly associated with disability and "poor outcome", with a relative risk ranging from 2.13 to 4.21 for the former and 1.33 to 2.40 for the latter.

INCREMENTAL VALUE

Risk assessment typically begins with a risk score that integrates demographic, clinical, and procedural data to compute predicted risks of operative mortality and major morbidity. The most commonly used scores are the Society of Thoracic Surgeons (STS), EuroSCORE II, and STS/ACC TAVR In-Hospital Mortality Risk (http://tools.acc.org/TAVRRisk/). None of these currently contain objective measures of frailty; therefore, frailty scores must be considered in tandem based on their ability to add incremental prognostic value.

The FRAILTY-AVR study was a prospective multicenter cohort study designed to compare the incremental prognostic value of 7 different frailty scales in 1020 older adults undergoing TAVR.[27] The main finding of this study was that the EFT score exhibited the highest C-statistic, Bayesian information criterion, and integrated discrimination improvement above and beyond the STS score for prediction of 1-year mortality and worsening disability.

RECOMMENDATIONS FROM MAJOR SOCIETIES AND GUIDELINES

The 2017 European Society of Cardiology Valvular Heart Disease Guidelines[28] state that frailty should be assessed based "on a combination of different objective estimates … not rely(ing) on a subjective approach such as the eyeball test." Frailty should prompt the heart team's involvement in decision-making, with TAVR being generally favored over SAVR in frail older adults suitable for transfemoral access (Class I, Level B).

The 2017 American College of Cardiology Valvular Heart Disease Guidelines[29] and Expert Consensus Decision Pathway for TAVR[30] highlight (1) 5MGS, (2) disability for activities of daily living, (3) cognitive impairment, (4) depression, and (5) malnutrition as core indicators of frailty that should be routinely assessed pre-TAVR. Irrespective of the STS score, moderate-to-severe frailty should be considered as "high risk" and mild frailty as "intermediate risk."

The 2019 Canadian Cardiovascular Society Position Statement for TAVR endorses that "frailty should be measured using an objective validated tool and integrated into the preprocedural assessment," acknowledging the EFT as a simple and predictive tool. The document cautions not to equate frailty with futility, rather to optimize frailty with interventions such as cardiac rehabilitation, nutritional supplementation, or comprehensive geriatric assessment.

THE AUTHORS' APPROACH

To address the key domains of frailty, the authors use a 2-tiered approach. First, all patients undergo a rapid assessment consisting of the EFT (chair rise test, Mini-Cog test, hemoglobin, albumin) and screening questions for malnutrition,

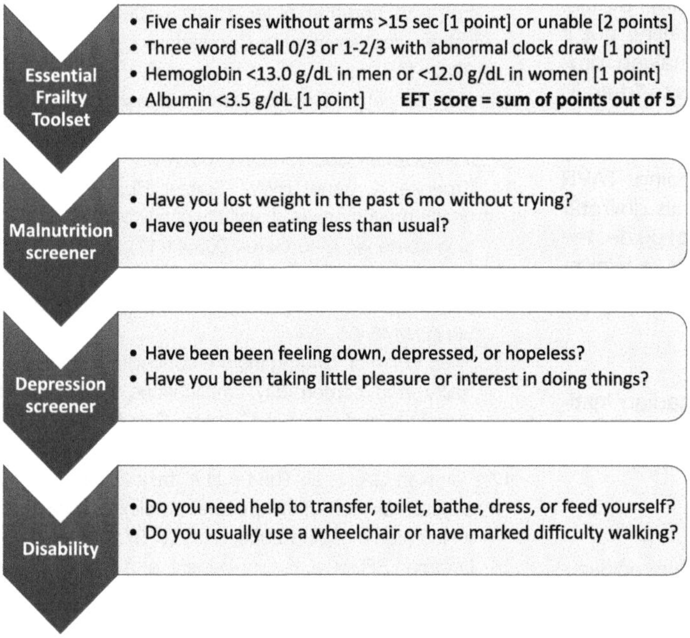

Essential Frailty Toolset
- Five chair rises without arms >15 sec [1 point] or unable [2 points]
- Three word recall 0/3 or 1-2/3 with abnormal clock draw [1 point]
- Hemoglobin <13.0 g/dL in men or <12.0 g/dL in women [1 point]
- Albumin <3.5 g/dL [1 point]   **EFT score = sum of points out of 5**

Malnutrition screener
- Have you lost weight in the past 6 mo without trying?
- Have you been eating less than usual?

Depression screener
- Have been been feeling down, depressed, or hopeless?
- Have you been taking little pleasure or interest in doing things?

Disability
- Do you need help to transfer, toilet, bathe, dress, or feed yourself?
- Do you usually use a wheelchair or have marked difficulty walking?

Fig. 2. Minimum geriatric dataset for pre-TAVR screening.

depression, and disability as shown in **Fig. 2**. The screening questions are borrowed from the validated Canadian Nutrition Screening Tool[31] and the Patient Health Questionnaire.[14] The chair rise test is favored over the 5MGS test because it is easier to administer in a clinical setting and it is more prognostic of adverse events.[32] This screening assessment can be completed in less than 5 minutes with or without the help of a smartphone app (http://frailtytool.com/).

Second, if problematic domains are identified, patients undergo targeted deeper assessments. For example, patients who perform poorly on the chair rise test are further evaluated with the short physical performance battery (and a muscle mass measurement if a CT scan is available) or by a physical therapist. Similarly, patients who do not pass the Mini-Cog test are further evaluated with the MMSE or MoCA or by a geriatrician. Beyond diagnosing frailty, the focus of this assessment is to treat modifiable frailty deficits so as to improve the patient's ability to recover from the TAVR procedure with meaningful gains in quality of life.

SUMMARY

Assessment of frailty has become engrained in the preprocedural evaluation of older adults referred for TAVR. Prevalent frailty can be elicited in one-third to two-thirds of patients depending on the frailty scale used. Addition of frailty to clinical risk scores results in improved discrimination for short- and midterm mortality and identifies patients less likely to be discharged home and more likely to report worsening disability and quality of life. Frailty should not be equated with futility, but it should inform the shared decision-making process and signal the use of interventions to "defrail" patients to the extent possible. Ongoing trials, such as the Protein and Exercise to Reverse Frailty in OldeR women and Men undergoing TAVR (PERFORM-TAVR; https://clinicaltrials.gov/ct2/show/NCT03522454), are awaited to guide the prescription of such interventions and maximize the expected functional benefits of TAVR.

DISCLOSURE

Dr J. Afilalo is supported by the Canadian Institutes of Health Research (CIHR) and the Fonds de recherche en santé du Québec (FRQ-S).

REFERENCES

1. Coffey S, Cairns BJ, Iung B. The modern epidemiology of heart valve disease. Heart 2016;102(1): 75–85.

2. Cesari M, Calvani R, Marzetti E. Frailty in older persons. Clin Geriatr Med 2017;33(3):293–303.

3. Afilalo J, et al. Frailty assessment in the cardiovascular care of older adults. J Am Coll Cardiol 2014; 63(8):747–62.

4. Cruz-Jentoft AJ, Sayer AA. Sarcopenia. Lancet 2019;393(10191):2636–46.

5. Mullie L, Afilalo J. CoreSlicer: a web toolkit for analytic morphomics. BMC Med Imaging 2019;19(1):15.

6. Soud M, et al. Usefulness of skeletal muscle area detected by computed tomography to predict mortality in patients undergoing transcatheter aortic valve replacement: a meta-analysis study. Int J Cardiovasc Imaging 2019;35(6):1141–7.

7. Mamane S, et al. Psoas muscle area and all-cause mortality after transcatheter aortic valve replacement: the montreal-munich study. Can J Cardiol 2016;32(2):177–82.

8. Pighi M, et al. Sex-specific determinants of outcomes after transcatheter aortic valve replacement. Circ Cardiovasc Qual Outcomes 2019;12(3): e005363.

9. Folstein MF, Folstein SE, McHugh PR. "Mini-mental state". A practical method for grading the cognitive state of patients for the clinician. J Psychiatr Res 1975;12(3):189–98.

10. Nasreddine ZS, et al. Brief methodological reports: the montreal cognitive assessment, MoCA: a brief screening tool for mild cognitive impairment. J Am Geriatr Soc 2005;53(4):695–9.

11. Borson S, et al. The Mini-Cog: a cognitive 'vital signs' measure for dementia screening in multilingual elderly. Int J Geriatr Psychiatry 2000;15(11): 1021–7.

12. Goldfarb M, et al. Malnutrition and mortality in frail and non-frail older adults undergoing aortic valve replacement. Circulation 2018;138(20): 2202–11.

13. Hoyl MT, et al. Development and testing of a five-item version of the geriatric depression scale. J Am Geriatr Soc 1999;47(7):873–8.

14. Kroenke K, Janet BWW, Spitzer RL. The patient health questionnaire-2: validity of a two-Item depression screener. Med Care 2003;41(11):1284–92.

15. Fried LP, et al. Frailty in older adults: evidence for a phenotype. J Gerontol A Biol Sci Med Sci 2001; 56(3):M146–56.

16. Fried LP, et al. Untangling the concepts of disability, frailty, and comorbidity: implications for improved targeting and care. J Gerontol Ser A 2004;59(3): M255–63.

17. Van Kan GA, et al. The I.A.N.A. task force on frailty assessment of older people in clinical practice. J Nutr Health Aging 2008;12(1):29–37.

18. Lindman BR, et al. Futility, benefit, and transcatheter aortic valve replacement. JACC Cardiovasc Interv 2014;7(7):707–16.

19. Guralnik JM, et al. A short physical performance battery assessing lower extremity function: association with self-reported disability and prediction of mortality and nursing home admission. J Gerontol 1994;49(2):M85.

20. Bergman H, et al. Frailty: an emerging research and clinical paradigm–issues and controversies. J Gerontol A Biol Sci Med Sci 2007;62(7):731–7.

21. Afilalo J, et al. Frailty in older adults undergoing aortic valve replacement: the FRAILTY-AVR study. J Am Coll Cardiol 2017;70(6):689–700.

22. Cesari M, et al. Evidence for the domains supporting the construct of intrinsic capacity. J Gerontol A Biol Sci Med Sci 2018;73(12):1653–60.

23. Rockwood K, et al. A global clinical measure of fitness and frailty in elderly people. CMAJ 2005; 173(5):489–95.

24. Katz S. Studies of illness in the aged the index of ADL: a standardized measure of biological and psychosocial function. JAMA 1963;185(12):914.

25. Drudi LM, et al. Interaction between frailty and access site in older adults undergoing transcatheter aortic valve replacement. JACC Cardiovasc Interv 2018;11(21):2185–92.

26. Saji M, et al. Impact of frailty markers for unplanned hospital readmission following transcatheter aortic valve implantation. Circ J 2018;82(8):2191–8.

27. Afilalo J. The clinical frailty scale: upgrade your eyeball test. Circulation 2017;135(21):2025–7.

28. Baumgartner H, et al. 2017 ESC/EACTS Guidelines for the management of valvular heart disease. Eur Heart J 2017;38(36):2739–91.

29. Nishimura RA, et al. 2017 AHA/ACC focused Update of the 2014 AHA/ACC Guideline for the management of patients with valvular heart disease: a report of the American College of Cardiology/ American heart association task force on clinical practice Guidelines. Circulation 2017;135(25): e1159–95.

30. Otto CM, et al. 2017 ACC Expert consensus decision Pathway for transcatheter aortic valve replacement in the management of adults with aortic stenosis: a report of the American College of Cardiology task force on clinical Expert consensus documents. J Am Coll Cardiol 2017; 69(10):1313–46.

31. Laporte M, Teterina A. Validity and reliability of the new Canadian Nutrition Screening Tool in the 'real-world' hospital setting. Eur J Clin Nutr 2015;69(7): 865.

32. Hosler QP, Maltagliati AJ, Shi SM, et al. A practical two-stage frailty assessment for older adults undergoing aortic valve replacement. J Am Geriatr Soc 2019;67(10):2031–7.

33. Alfredsson J, et al. Gait speed predicts 30-day mortality after transcatheter aortic valve replacement: results from the society of thoracic surgeons/

34. Arnold SV, et al. Quality-of-Life outcomes after transcatheter aortic valve replacement in an unselected population: a report from the STS/ACC transcatheter valve therapy registry. JAMA Cardiol 2017;2(4): 409–16.

35. Arnold SV, et al. Prediction of poor outcome after transcatheter aortic valve replacement. J Am Coll Cardiol 2016;68(17):1868–77.

36. Assmann P, et al. Frailty is associated with delirium and mortality after transcatheter aortic valve implantation. Open Heart 2016;3(2):e000478.

37. Bogdan A, et al. Albumin correlates with all-cause mortality in elderly patients undergoing transcatheter aortic valve implantation. EuroIntervention 2016;12(8):e1057–64.

38. Boureau AS, et al. Predictors of health-related quality of life decline after transcatheter aortic valve replacement in older patients with severe aortic stenosis. J Nutr Health Aging 2017;21(1):105–11.

39. Cockburn J, et al. Poor mobility predicts adverse outcome better than other frailty indices in patients undergoing transcatheter aortic valve implantation. Catheter Cardiovasc Interv 2015;86(7):1271–7.

40. Codner P, et al. Long-term outcomes for patients with severe symptomatic aortic stenosis treated with transcatheter aortic valve implantation. Am J Cardiol 2015;116(9):1391–8.

41. Eichler S, et al. Nutrition and mobility predict all-cause mortality in patients 12 months after transcatheter aortic valve implantation. Clin Res Cardiol 2018;107(4):304–11.

42. Eide LS, et al. Comparison of frequency, risk factors, and time course of postoperative delirium in octogenarians after transcatheter aortic valve implantation versus surgical aortic valve replacement. Am J Cardiol 2015;115(6):802–9.

43. Ewe SH, et al. Impact of left ventricular systolic function on clinical and echocardiographic outcomes following transcatheter aortic valve implantation for severe aortic stenosis. Am Heart J 2010;160(6): 1113–20.

44. Foldyna B, et al. Computed tomography-based fat and muscle characteristics are associated with mortality after transcatheter aortic valve replacement. J Cardiovasc Comput Tomogr 2018;12(3): 223–8.

45. Forcillo J, et al. Assessment of commonly used frailty markers for high- and extreme-risk patients undergoing transcatheter aortic valve replacement. Ann Thorac Surg 2017;104(6):1939–46.

46. Garg L, et al. Psoas muscle area as a predictor of outcomes in transcatheter aortic valve implantation. Am J Cardiol 2017;119(3):457–60.

47. Gassa A, et al. Effect of preoperative low serum albumin on postoperative complications and early

mortality in patients undergoing transcatheter aortic valve replacement. J Thorac Dis 2018;10(12):6763–70.

48. Goudzwaard JA, et al. The erasmus frailty score is associated with delirium and 1-year mortality after transcatheter aortic valve implantation in older patients. The TAVI care & cure program. Int J Cardiol 2019;276:48–52.

49. Green P, et al. The impact of frailty status on survival after transcatheter aortic valve replacement in older adults with severe aortic stenosis: a single-center experience. JACC Cardiovasc Interv 2012;5(9):974–81.

50. Green P, et al. Relation of frailty to outcomes after transcatheter aortic valve replacement (from the PARTNER trial). Am J Cardiol 2015;116(2):264–9.

51. Grossman Y, et al. Addition of albumin to traditional risk score improved prediction of mortality in individuals undergoing transcatheter aortic valve replacement. J Am Geriatr Soc 2017;65(11):2413–7.

52. Hebeler KR, et al. Albumin is predictive of 1-year mortality after transcatheter aortic valve replacement. Ann Thorac Surg 2018;106(5):1302–7.

53. Hermiller JB Jr, et al. Predicting early and late mortality after transcatheter aortic valve replacement. J Am Coll Cardiol 2016;68(4):343–52.

54. Honda Y, et al. Prognostic value of objective nutritional status after transcatheter aortic valve replacement. J Cardiol 2019;73(5):401–7.

55. Horne CE, et al. Factors associated with discharge to a skilled nursing facility after transcatheter aortic valve replacement surgery. Int J Environ Res Public Health 2018;16(1) [pii:E73].

56. Huded CP, et al. Frailty status and outcomes after transcatheter aortic valve implantation. Am J Cardiol 2016;117(12):1966–71.

57. Kamga M, et al. Impact of frailty scores on outcome of octogenarian patients undergoing transcatheter aortic valve implantation. Acta Cardiol 2013;68(6):599–606.

58. Kim DH, et al. Evaluation of changes in functional status in the year after aortic valve replacement. JAMA Intern Med 2019;179(3):383–91.

59. Kleczynski P, et al. Impact of frailty on mortality after transcatheter aortic valve implantation. Am Heart J 2017;185:52–8.

60. Koifman E, et al. Impact of pre-procedural serum albumin levels on outcome of patients undergoing transcatheter aortic valve replacement. Am J Cardiol 2015;115(9):1260–4.

61. Kundi H, et al. Impact of a claims-based frailty indicator on the prediction of long-term mortality after transcatheter aortic valve replacement in medicare beneficiaries. Circ Cardiovasc Qual Outcomes 2018;11(10):e005048.

62. Martin GP, et al. Do frailty measures improve prediction of mortality and morbidity following transcatheter aortic valve implantation? An analysis of the UK TAVI registry. BMJ Open 2018;8(6):e022543.

63. Miura M, et al. Early safety and efficacy of transcatheter aortic valve implantation for Asian nonagenarians (from KMH registry). Int Heart J 2017;58(6):900–7.

64. Mok M, et al. Prognostic value of fat mass and skeletal muscle mass determined by computed tomography in patients who underwent transcatheter aortic valve implantation. Am J Cardiol 2016;117(5):828–33.

65. Nemec U, et al. Diagnosing sarcopenia on thoracic computed tomography: quantitative assessment of skeletal muscle mass in patients undergoing transcatheter aortic valve replacement. Acad Radiol 2017;24(9):1154–61.

66. Okoh AK, et al. The impact of frailty status on clinical and functional outcomes after transcatheter aortic valve replacement in nonagenarians with severe aortic stenosis. Catheter Cardiovasc Interv 2017;90(6):1000–6.

67. Osnabrugge RL, et al. Health status after transcatheter aortic valve replacement in patients at extreme surgical risk: results from the CoreValve U.S. trial. JACC Cardiovasc Interv 2015;8(2):315–23.

68. Paknikar R, et al. Psoas muscle size as a frailty measure for open and transcatheter aortic valve replacement. J Thorac Cardiovasc Surg 2016;151(3):745–51.

69. Pinheiro M, et al. Frailty syndrome: visceral adipose tissue and frailty in patients with symptomatic severe aortic stenosis. J Nutr Health Aging 2017;21(1):120–8.

70. Puls M, et al. Impact of frailty on short- and long-term morbidity and mortality after transcatheter aortic valve implantation: risk assessment by Katz Index of activities of daily living. EuroIntervention 2014;10(5):609–19.

71. Rathore S, et al. Safety and predictors of next-day discharge after elective transfemoral transcatheter aortic valve replacement. Cardiovasc Revasc Med 2017;18(8):583–7.

72. Rodés-Cabau J, et al. Transcatheter aortic valve implantation for the treatment of severe symptomatic aortic stenosis in patients at very high or prohibitive surgical risk: acute and late outcomes of the multicenter Canadian experience. J Am Coll Cardiol 2010;55(11):1080–90.

73. Rogers T, et al. Clinical frailty as an outcome predictor after transcatheter aortic valve implantation. Am J Cardiol 2018;121(7):850–5.

74. Saji M, et al. Usefulness of psoas muscle area to predict mortality in patients undergoing transcatheter aortic valve replacement. Am J Cardiol 2016;118(2):251–7.

75. Schoenenberger AW, et al. Predictors of functional decline in elderly patients undergoing transcatheter aortic valve implantation (TAVI). Eur Heart J 2013; 34(9):684–92.

76. Seiffert M, et al. Development of a risk score for outcome after transcatheter aortic valve implantation. Clin Res Cardiol 2014;103(8):631–40.

77. Shi S, Afilalo J, Lipsitz LA, et al. Frailty phenotype and deficit accumulation frailty index in predicting recovery after transcatheter and surgical aortic valve replacement. J Gerontol A Biol Sci Med Sci 2018. [Epub ahead of print].

78. Shimura T, et al. Impact of the clinical frailty scale on outcomes after transcatheter aortic valve replacement. Circulation 2017;135(21):2013–24.

79. Steinvil A, et al. Utility of an additive frailty tests index score for mortality risk assessment following transcatheter aortic valve replacement. Am Heart J 2018;200:11–6.

80. Stortecky S, et al. Evaluation of multidimensional geriatric assessment as a predictor of mortality and cardiovascular events after transcatheter aortic valve implantation. JACC Cardiovasc Interv 2012; 5(5):489–96.

81. Ungar A, et al. Comprehensive geriatric assessment in patients undergoing transcatheter aortic valve implantation - results from the CGA-TAVI multicentre registry. BMC Cardiovasc Disord 2018; 18(1):1.

82. Yamamoto M, et al. Prognostic value of hypoalbuminemia after transcatheter aortic valve implantation (from the Japanese multicenter OCEAN-TAVI registry). Am J Cardiol 2017;119(5):770–7.

Procedures and Outcomes of Surgical Aortic Valve Replacement in Adults

Amine Mazine, MD, MSc[a,b], Ismail El-Hamamsy, MD, PhD[c],*

KEYWORDS

- Aortic valve replacement • Bioprosthesis • Mechanical valve • Homograft • Ross procedure
- Pulmonary autograft

KEY POINTS

- Although in elderly patients, bioprosthetic valves are durable and associated with low rates of valve-related complications, in non-elderly adults, they are associated with reduced durability and lower than expected survival, both of which are worsened by the presence of patient-prosthesis mismatch.
- In young adults, mechanical valves are associated with lower rates of prosthesis degeneration and need for reoperation compared with bioprosthetic valves, at the cost of higher rates of anticoagulation-related bleeding and thromboembolic events.
- Nevertheless, both mechanical and bioprosthetic valves are associated with excess mortality compared with the general population when implanted in non-elderly patients.
- The Ross procedure is the only operation that can restore a normal life expectancy in young and middle-aged adults undergoing aortic valve replacement.

INTRODUCTION

Aortic stenosis is the most prevalent form of valvular heart disease in Western countries.[1,2] In the absence of treatment, severe aortic stenosis is a fatal condition, with a mortality rate of about 25% per year after symptom onset.[3] No medical therapy has been shown to alter the natural history of severe symptomatic aortic stenosis,[4] and mechanical relief of left ventricular outflow obstruction is the only effective treatment.[3] This can be achieved percutaneously with transcatheter aortic valve implantation or surgically with aortic valve replacement (AVR). When surgically replacing an aortic valve, several options for valve substitutes are available: mechanical valves, bioprosthetic

valves, aortic valve homografts, and pulmonary autografts (Ross procedure). Although less prevalent, severe aortic regurgitation also requires surgical intervention when symptoms or signs of left ventricular dysfunction or dilatation are observed. Furthermore, recent evidence supports early intervention in asymptomatic patients with chronic severe aortic regurgitation.[5] Although aortic valve repair and valve-sparing techniques represent the option of choice in these patients, in a significant proportion of cases, valve replacement is mandated because of leaflet calcification, extensive fibrosis, or retraction.

When choosing a valve substitute, it is important to remember that the aortic valve does more than passively open and close in response to changes

[a] Division of Cardiac Surgery, University of Toronto, Toronto, Ontario, Canada; [b] Montreal Heart Institute, 5000 Belanger Street East, Montreal, Quebec H1T 1C8, Canada; [c] Division of Cardiac Surgery, Montreal Heart Institute, Université de Montréal, 5000 Belanger Street East, Montreal, Quebec H1T 1C8, Canada
* Corresponding author.
E-mail address: i.elhamamsy@icm-mhi.org
Twitter: @AmineMazineMD (A.M.); @IHamamsy (I.E.-H.)

Cardiol Clin 38 (2020) 89–102
https://doi.org/10.1016/j.ccl.2019.09.012

in pressure across the root. The aortic valve and root is a highly complex and sophisticated structure, which performs complex functions, all of which have a direct impact on left ventricular dynamics, coronary flow reserve, and dynamic movements of the leaflets themselves.[6] Therefore, the optimal replacement option must be carefully tailored to the individual patient, as the choice of aortic valve substitute has been shown to affect long-term outcomes and quality of life. In addition to providing patients with complete information, it is crucial to factor their values and preferences into the choice of surgical option (**Table 1**). In this article, the authors review the various options for surgical AVR and examine their contemporary applications and outcomes and then summarize the literature comparing these options in various patient populations and provide a framework for selecting the optimal valve substitute based on patient characteristics and preferences. They conclude with a perspective on the future of aortic valve disease management.

MECHANICAL VALVES

Because of their proven durability and ease of implantation, mechanical valves have long been the preferred option for AVR in young adults. Since the introduction of the caged ball valve in the early 1960s, significant strides have been made in mechanical valve design and engineering, culminating in the bileaflet mechanical prosthesis, which represents the most recent generation of mechanical valves.[7] Despite these improvements, mechanical valves remain thrombogenic and require lifelong anticoagulation with warfarin. This exposes patients to a continuous hazard of thromboembolic and hemorrhagic complications. Studies with long-term follow-up (>20 years)

report linearized rates of thromboembolic and hemorrhagic complications ranging from 1.1% to 4.5% per patient-year.[8,9] In addition, the use of mechanical valves is particularly problematic in women of childbearing potential who are contemplating pregnancy.[10–13] Furthermore, although mechanical valves are widely considered the most durable valve substitute available, rates of reoperation after mechanical AVR are not trivial, with prospective studies showing reoperation rates of 0.6% to 1.8% per patient-year.[14–16] Thus, although structural valve deterioration of mechanical valves is virtually unheard of, a significant proportion of patients still undergo reoperation due to thrombosis, infection, or nonstructural valve dysfunction (eg, pannus or paravalvular leak).

The continuous hazard of valve-related complications in patients with mechanical AVR translates into excess mortality compared with the age- and sex-matched general population, including in carefully selected low-risk patients undergoing isolated AVR[17] (**Fig. 1**). Furthermore, studies have shown that this excess mortality is inversely proportional to patient age at surgery (ie, younger patients have the highest observed to expected mortality rates).[18] A recently published meta-analysis, which included a microsimulation analysis, estimated that a 45-year-old patient undergoing mechanical AVR has an estimated life expectancy of 19 years, whereas the age-matched general population has a life expectancy of 34 years.[19]

Because the burden of anticoagulation is the main drawback of mechanical valves, several strategies have been proposed to mitigate the thromboembolic and hemorrhagic risks associated with the use of mechanical prostheses. Given warfarin's narrow therapeutic index and

Table 1
Benefits and drawbacks of the various surgical options for aortic valve replacement in non-elderly adults

	Mechanical AVR	Bioprosthetic AVR	Aortic Homograft	Ross Procedure
Long-term survival[17,19,29,31,36,43,51–57,85,86]	+	+	+	+++
Durability[37,43,51–57]	+++	+	+	++
Freedom from valve-related complications[16,36,63,86,88,96]	+	+	+	+++
Quality of life[58–60]	+	++	++	+++
Hemodynamics[49]	+	+	++	+++
Technical complexity[62]	+	+	++	+++
Risk of reoperation[55,63,70,71]	+	+	+++	++

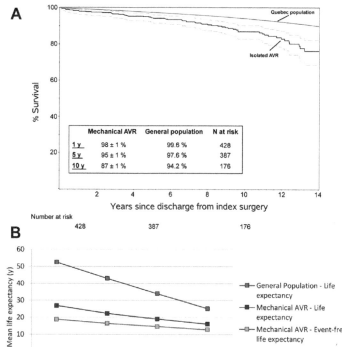

A

% Survival

Quebec population

Isolated AVR

	Mechanical AVR	General population	N at risk
1 y	98 ± 1 %	99.6 %	428
5 y	95 ± 1 %	97.6 %	387
10 y	87 ± 1 %	94.2 %	176

Years since discharge from index surgery

Number at risk
428   387   176

B

Mean life expectancy (y)

— General Population - Life expectancy

— Mechanical AVR - Life expectancy

— Mechanical AVR - Event-free life expectancy

Age at surgery (y)

Fig. 1. Excess mortality with mechanical AVR in non-elderly patients. (*From* Bouhout I, Stevens LM, Mazine A, Poirier N, Cartier R, Demers P, et al. Long-term outcomes after elective isolated mechanical aortic valve replacement in young adults. J Thorac Cardiovasc Surg. 2014;148(4):1341-6 e1 and Korteland NM, Etnel JRG, Arabkhani B, Mokhles MM, Mohamad A, Roos-Hesselink JW, et al. Mechanical aortic valve replacement in non-elderly adults: meta-analysis and microsimulation. Eur Heart J. 2017;38(45):3370-7; with permission.)

need for frequent laboratory testing, non-vitamin K antagonist oral anticoagulants (NOACs) were proposed as a potential alternative to warfarin in patients with mechanical valves. However, NOACs are currently contraindicated in these patients based on a single randomized study—the RE-ALIGN trial—in which a total of 252 patients were randomized to receive dabigatran versus warfarin immediately after mechanical AVR.[20] The trial was terminated early due to excess thromboembolic and bleeding events in the dabigatran group. One of the main limitations of the study was the fact that NOAC usage was initiated immediately after surgery. It is well established that the early postoperative period is characterized by intense inflammation and heightened thrombogenicity before neoendothelialization occurs, which is why bridging with warfarin for the first 3 postoperative months may be a more judicious approach. Despite the unfavorable results of the RE-ALIGN trial, the use of NOACs as an anticoagulation strategy in patients with mechanical valves remains an area of active research. The PROACT Xa trial, which will randomize patients to warfarin versus apixaban 3 months after mechanical AVR with the On-X valve (Cryolife Inc, Kennesaw, Georgia), should further address this question.

Another strategy, home international normalized ratio (INR) monitoring with point-of-care devices, has been thought to allow better INR control, lower rates of anticoagulation-related adverse events, and possibly improved survival in patients with mechanical valves who are taking warfarin.[21] However, there remains controversy surrounding the widespread applicability of home INR monitoring in a "real-world" setting, as well as the efficacy of this strategy. Indeed, the largest randomized controlled trial on this subject—the Home INR Study—did not demonstrate any advantage of weekly self-testing, as compared with monthly high-quality clinic testing, in delaying the time to a first stroke, major bleeding episode, or death.[22] Nevertheless, from a mere quality of life standpoint, home INR testing helps reduce the day-to-day burden of warfarin anticoagulation.

Finally, newer generations of mechanical prostheses may require less aggressive anticoagulation. The Prospective Randomized On-X Valve Anticoagulation Trial aimed to evaluate whether a lower INR target (1.5–2.0) was safe after implantation of the On-X bileaflet mechanical valve (Cryolife Inc, Kennesaw, Georgia) in patients at increased risk of thromboembolic events.[15] This multicenter study randomized 375 patients to either lower INR target (1.5–2.0) or standard INR target (2.0–

3.0). All patients concomitantly received aspirin, 80 mg, and were monitored using home INR testing. The main finding from this study was a significantly lower rate of the composite of major and minor bleeding, thromboembolism, and thrombosis events in the lower INR group, driven by lower bleeding rates with no significant increase in thromboembolic events. Although these data represent a major step forward in the management of patients following mechanical AVR, a closer look at the data reveals a more sobering picture. First, although not statistically significant, there was a 60% higher rate thromboembolic and thrombosis events in the lower INR group (2.96% per patient-year vs 1.85% per patient-year). Given that the trial was designed to demonstrate noninferiority of a composite endpoint of bleeding, thromboembolism, and thrombosis events, it is entirely possible that the lack of statistical significance may be related to insufficient statistical power. Furthering this point, it is noteworthy that when considering the composite endpoint while excluding minor events, there was no significant difference between the 2 study arms. Second—and perhaps most importantly— in this relatively young (mean age 55 years) and prospectively followed population with excellent INR monitoring, the linearized rate of major adverse events (ie, major bleeding, thromboembolism, or thrombosis) was 4.44% per patient-year in the lower INR group.[15] This suggests that even with lower INR targets, mechanical valves carry a significant thromboembolic and hemorrhagic burden. This has major implications, particularly for young patients with a long anticipated life expectancy.

In summary, mechanical AVR is associated with good overall durability—especially in young patients—but carries a significant clinical burden, both in terms of valve-related complications as well as lifestyle adjustment. Furthermore, even in low-risk elective patients, there is excess long-term mortality versus the age- and sex-matched general population.

BIOPROSTHETIC VALVES

The most frequently implanted stented bioprostheses are porcine xenografts or bovine pericardial tissue valves. Stentless bioprosthetic valves are also available, and the absence of stents improves hemodynamics. Unlike mechanical valves, bioprosthetic valves do not require anticoagulation. However, these valves are prone to structural deterioration—as well as other valve-related complications such as nonstructural valve dysfunction, endocarditis, patient-prosthesis

mismatch (PPM), and thromboembolism—which limits their durability, particularly in younger patient populations. Although porcine and pericardial valves have comparable durability,[23,24] their modes of failure tend to differ, with porcine valves most often failing due to leaflet tear, whereas pericardial valves failing due to calcification and thrombosis.

The most important determinant of reoperation for bioprosthetic valve degeneration is age at implantation. Bioprosthetic valves have excellent durability in elderly patients and are the valve substitute of choice in this patient population.[25] However, the use of bioprosthetic valves in young and middle-aged adults (<60 years) is more problematic. Numerous studies have shown that when implanted in young adults, bioprosthetic valves have poor durability,[25–30] which translates into excess mortality compared with the age- and sex-matched general population[28–30] (**Fig. 2**). In addition—similar to mechanical valves—this excess mortality is inversely proportional to patient age at surgery and is further compounded by the presence of PPM after surgery.[30,31] These findings are likely related to a higher functional demand in young patients, as well as a long period of exposure to valve-related complications. Using microsimulation, a 45-year-old patient undergoing bioprosthetic AVR has a life expectancy of 21 years (vs 33 years in the age- and sex-matched general population) and a lifetime risk of structural valve deterioration or reoperation of 71% and 78%, respectively.[32] Furthermore, although rates of reoperation are low in elderly patients who undergo bioprosthetic AVR, recent studies have demonstrated that subclinical hemodynamic valve deterioration is a common finding in this patient population.[33,34] This suggests that even in elderly patients, the durability of bioprosthetic valves may be overstated.

Despite these data, bioprosthetic valves are increasingly being implanted, including in young and middle-aged adults.[35] This trend is fueled— at least in part—by the promise of valve-in-valve transcatheter aortic valve implantation (TAVI). This approach is predicated on the erroneous notion that the poor outcomes observed with bioprosthetic AVR in non-elderly patients are mostly due to the mortality and morbidity of reoperation, which could be attenuated with percutaneous valve-in-valve technology. Rather, it is the obstructive nature of stented bioprostheses— and its deleterious impact on left ventricular health—that drives these outcomes. Indeed, clinically significant PPM occurs in an estimated 44% of patients who undergo prosthetic AVR[36] and is associated with increased rates of structural valve

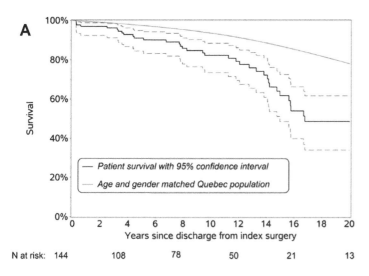

A

Survival

100%

80%

60%

40%

20%

0%

— Patient survival with 95% confidence interval

- - - Age and gender matched Quebec population

0 2 4 6 8 10 12 14 16 18 20

Years since discharge from index surgery

N at risk: 144   108   78   50   21   13

Fig. 2. Excess mortality with bio-prosthetic AVR in non-elderly patients. (*From* Forcillo J, El Hamamsy I, Stevens LM, Badrudin D, Pellerin M, Perrault LP, et al. The perimount valve in the aortic position: twenty-year experience with patients under 60 years old. Ann Thorac Surg. 2014;97(5):1526-32 and Bourguignon T, Bouquiaux-Stablo AL, Candolfi P, Mirza A, Loardi C, May MA, et al. Very long-term outcomes of the Carpentier-Edwards Perimount valve in aortic position. Ann Thorac Surg. 2015;99(3):831-7; with permission.)

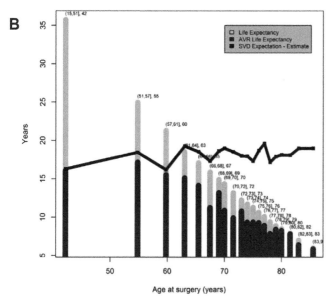

B

Years

Age at surgery (years)

deterioration,[37] increased mortality,[38] decreased left ventricular mass regression,[38] decreased quality of life,[38] and increased mortality after valve-in-valve TAVI.[39] Even in the current era, with heightened awareness about the importance of implanting large prostheses and avoiding PPM, the incidence remains significant. For instance, in the PARTNER III trial, despite the fact that 80% of surgically implanted valves were greater than or equal to 23 mm in size, rates of moderate-to-severe PPM were 56%.[40] It is worth emphasizing that this was no different than the rates observed in the TAVI arm (62% of moderate-to-severe PPM). In fact, at 1 year, the effective orifice area in the surgical group was higher than in the TAVI group (1.8 m² vs 1.7 cm²,

respectively). Finally, it is important to bear in mind that the estimated prevalence of PPM is derived from echocardiographic studies performed at rest, before hospital discharge. As a consequence, the true impact of PPM is probably understated in young, physically active patients who can generate large cardiac outputs with exercise through a fixed orifice. Furthermore, because bioprosthetic valves degenerate at a higher rates in young patients, this further exacerbates the impact of PPM and creates a vicious circle. This may explain why PPM has little impact on valve durability in elderly patients, but a significant impact in adults younger than 60 years.[37]

Stentless aortic bioprostheses have low rates of PPM and better hemodynamics compared with their stented counterparts.[41] However, stentless roots are also prone to structural valve degeneration and expose patients to challenging, higher-risk reoperations because of the extensive calcification of the xenograft root. To date, no studies comparing the long-term outcomes of stented versus stentless AVR in young and middle-aged adults have been performed.

In summary, bioprosthetic valves alleviate the need for lifelong anticoagulation but are associated with high rates of PPM and poor durability in young and middle-aged adults, which translates into loss in life expectancy compared with the age- and sex-matched general population. Nevertheless, the ease of implantation and the potential for future valve-in-valve procedures, combined for patient preference for avoiding anticoagulation, have resulted in an overall decrease in the age of implantation of bioprostheses in North America and Europe.

AORTIC HOMOGRAFTS

Aortic homografts represent another biological option for AVR. However, early calcification, limited availability, higher cost, comparable durability to bioprostheses, and increased complexity of reoperations have restricted their use.[42–44] Today, their use is primarily reserved for cases of severe active endocarditis with aortic root abscess in the aortic-mitral continuity, affecting the anterior leaflet of the mitral valve.[45,46]

THE ROSS PROCEDURE (PULMONARY AUTOGRAFT)

The Ross procedure consists in the replacement of the aortic valve with the patient's own pulmonary root (ie, pulmonary autograft) and subsequent implantation of a homograft in the pulmonary position. This operation has several advantages over prosthetic and homograft valve replacement. The Ross procedure is the only operation that allows replacement of the diseased aortic valve with a living substitute, thus allowing adaptive remodeling,[47] normal hemodynamics at rest and with exercise,[48,49] and long-term viability of the aortic valve substitute.[50] Importantly, the Ross procedure is the only operation that has resulted in restored life expectancy in young and middle-aged adults undergoing AVR (**Fig. 3**). Indeed, several contemporary series reporting long-term outcomes (≥15 years) of the Ross procedure in adults have demonstrated a survival equivalent to that of the age- and sex-matched general population.[43,51–56] Furthermore, because of the absence of anticoagulation and use of autologous material, the

Ross procedure is associated with very low rates of valve-related complications, namely thromboembolic events or endocarditis.[57]

In addition to long-term survival and valve-related complications, quality of life is a particularly important consideration for young and middle-aged adults who undergo AVR. Owing to excellent hemodynamic performance and avoidance of anticoagulation, patients who undergo the Ross procedure enjoy enhanced quality of life compared with those who undergo mechanical AVR.[58–60]

Despite these excellent outcomes, the Ross procedure has largely been abandoned in adults and its use remains limited to a handful of experienced centers worldwide.[61] Barriers to widespread adoption are multifold. The Ross procedure is a more technically complex operation than conventional AVR, raising concerns about a potentially increased operative risk. Although several high-volume centers have reported an operative mortality ranging from 0.3% to 1.1%[54,55,62,63]—similar to that of conventional prosthetic AVR—a propensity-matched study demonstrated a 3-fold increase in perioperative mortality with the Ross procedure compared with prosthetic AVR across the Society of Thoracic Surgeons database.[61] It is noteworthy, however, that the median annual number of Ross procedures performed per center was less than 1, and only 6 of 231 centers performed greater than or equal to 5 Ross procedures annually.[61] Given the well-established inverse relationship between surgical volumes and outcomes following aortic root surgery,[64] it is likely that the variability observed in operative outcomes of the Ross procedure are related to surgeon expertise. The Ross operation should not be carried out sporadically nor by surgeons who are not facile in aortic root procedures.

The potential long-term failure of 2 valves in a patient initially presenting with single valve disease has long been considered the Achilles heel of the Ross procedure. The Rotterdam group reported very high rates of autograft dilatation requiring reoperation (47% at 13 years), leading them and others to abandon the Ross procedure in adults.[65] Importantly, studies from the same group have demonstrated that in patients who developed autograft dilatation leading to reoperation, most of the increase in neoaortic root diameter had been reached during the perioperative period, highlighting the importance of surgical technique.[66] Advocates of the Ross operation have argued that the risk of late failure requiring reintervention can be mitigated by minute technical refinements and strict blood pressure control for the first 6 to 12 months after surgery to avoid early

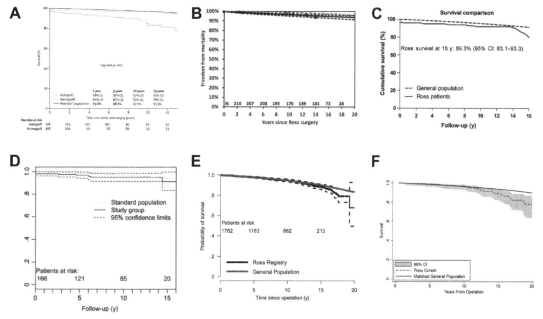

Fig. 3. Long-term survival after the Ross procedure compared with the age- and sex-matched general population. ([A] *Reprinted with permission from* Elsevier [El-Hamamsy I, Eryigit Z, Stevens LM, Sarang Z, George R, Clark L, et al. Long-term outcomes after autograft versus homograft aortic root replacement in adults with aortic valve disease: a randomised controlled trial. Lancet 2010;376(9740):524-31]; and [B-F] *From* Refs.[51–53,55,71]; with permission.)

autograft dilatation and instead promote autograft adaptation.[67] Supporting this notion, several contemporary cohorts have reported rates of reintervention (for the pulmonary autograft and/or homograft) ranging between 0.5% and 1.5% per patient-year, yielding a freedom from reintervention of 85% to 95% at 10 years.[43,51–57,68] Importantly, all these series have included a significant proportion of patients with pure aortic insufficiency, ranging from 20% to 50%. Thus, although preoperative aortic insufficiency is a known predictor of late failure of the pulmonary autograft, these data demonstrate that a tailored Ross procedure can still be carried out with good durability in young adults with nonrepairable aortic insufficiency and may still represent the best option in this patient population.[67,69]

Despite the aforementioned technical refinements, a small subset of patients who undergo the Ross procedure will require reoperation. Reoperative surgery after the Ross procedure is more complex than after standard AVR. In a series of 56 patients who underwent reoperation after a failed Ross, the Mayo Clinic group reported 1 in-hospital mortality (1.8%) and 4 additional deaths (7.1%) within a median follow-up of 8 months.[70] In contrast, other centers with larger Ross experiences reported better results, with mortality rates at reoperation ranging from 0% to 2.9%.[55,63,71]

Furthermore, in most cases, the pulmonary autograft valve can be salvaged at the time of reintervention, thus retaining its benefits as a living valve substitute.[71,72] This can be achieved through valve repair,[73] valve-sparing root replacement,[74,75] or by placing the pulmonary autograft back in the native pulmonary position.[76]

In summary, when performed in high-volume centers by experienced surgeons, the Ross procedure results in restored survival, normal hemodynamics with absence of PPM,[67] low rates of valve-related complications, and excellent quality of life in non-elderly patients undergoing AVR. When homografts are not available for right ventricular reconstruction during the Ross procedure, viable alternatives include stentless bioprostheses[77] as well as a variety of other xenografts.[78]

COMPARATIVE STUDIES
Mechanical Versus Bioprosthetic Valves

The 2017 American Heart Association/American College of Cardiology guidelines on valvular heart disease recommend the use of mechanical valves in patients younger than 50 years and bioprosthetic valves in patients older than 70 years.[79] For patients aged between 50 and 70 years, both options are reasonable and the choice should be individualized based on patient factors and preferences. The previous iteration of these American guidelines, published in 2014, recommended mechanical valves for patients younger than 60 years.[80] Meanwhile, the 2017 European Society of Cardiology guidelines on valvular heart disease recommend the use of a mechanical prosthesis in patients younger than 60 years and bioprosthetic valves in patients older than 65 years.[81] The discrepancy between American and European guidelines published the same year—as well as the fact that the age cut-off for mechanical valves was lowered in the American guidelines—reflects the persistent uncertainty surrounding the choice of an aortic valve substitute in non-elderly patients.

These guideline recommendations are based on 2 historical randomized controlled trials conducted in the 1970s and 1980s,[14,82] a more recent randomized trial comparing second-generation devices[16] and several observational studies comparing newer generation devices. No randomized controlled trial has been conducted with contemporary valves. A recent systematic review listed all observational studies comparing long-term survival between mechanical and bioprosthetic valves in non-elderly patients, focusing on studies that applied propensity matching or performed multivariable analysis to account for baseline differences.[36] Results were conflicting, with some studies showing enhanced survival with mechanical valves, whereas others demonstrated no difference.[83,84] However, it should be noted that none of the studies reported improved survival rates with bioprosthetic over mechanical valves.[36] Simultaneously, a large California-wide cohort study comparing long-term outcomes of mechanical and bioprosthetic valves in ~10,000 patients undergoing isolated AVR showed similar 15-year survival for patients aged 55 to 64 years, but increased mortality at 15 years with bioprosthetic AVR compared with mechanical AVR in patients aged 45 to 54 years.[85] Similarly, in a study reporting outcomes of all patients aged 50 to 69 years who underwent primary isolated AVR in Sweden from 1997 through 2013, patients who received mechanical valves had better long-term survival after AVR compared with those who received bioprostheses.[86]

Despite these findings—and the aforementioned guideline recommendations—the use of bioprosthetic valves has significantly increased in the last 2 decades.[35] This increase was observed across all age groups—including young adults—and was most pronounced in patients aged 55 to 64 years. The promise of valve-in-valve TAVI has undoubtedly contributed to the increased use of bioprosthetic valves in non-elderly patients,

although this trend preceded the introduction of TAVI. Although valve-in-valve TAVI represents a promising avenue to treat bioprosthetic valve failure, the impact of this approach on long-term survival and valve-related complications in non-elderly adults has yet to be determined.[87]

Ross Versus Homograft

In a single-center randomized controlled trial—conducted by Sir Magdi Yacoub—comparing the Ross procedure with aortic homograft replacement in 216 young adults (mean age 39 years, mean follow-up 11 years, completeness of follow-up 97%), survival at 13 years was significantly higher in the Ross group (95% vs 78%, $P = .006$).[43] Furthermore, 13-year survival following the Ross procedure was identical to the age- and sex-matched general population of UK. These findings are all the more impressive considering this cohort was composed of "all comers," including 42% of patients who had undergone previous cardiac surgery and 8% who were operated for active endocarditis. Although nowadays, homografts are no longer considered a surgical option for elective AVR, this study was important in that it highlighted for the first time the possibility of restoring late survival after aortic valve surgery in young adults with aortic stenosis.

Ross Versus Mechanical Valves

There is a relative paucity of studies comparing long-term outcomes of the Ross procedure versus prosthetic AVR (**Fig. 4**) and no large-scale RCT has been conducted to date. A recently published systematic review and meta-analysis, which identified 18 comparative studies, demonstrated a 46% lower all-cause mortality in patients undergoing the Ross procedure compared with mechanical AVR (incidence rate ratio 0.54, $P = .004$).[88] The Ross procedure was also associated with lower rates of stroke (incidence rate ratio 0.26, $P = .02$) and major bleeding (incidence rate ratio 0.17, $P<.001$) but higher rates of reintervention (incidence rate ratio 1.76, $P = .007$). Most of the studies included, however, had limited follow-up (median average follow-up 5.8 years).

The longest available longitudinal study comparing the Ross with mechanical AVR is a propensity-matched cohort study, which included 208 pairs of patients (mean age 37 years, mean follow-up 14 years, completeness of follow-up 98%).[63] Although this study demonstrated equivalent early outcomes and overall survival between the 2 groups, patients in the Ross group had significantly lower rates of cardiac- and valve-related mortality (hazard ratio 0.22, $P = .03$) and

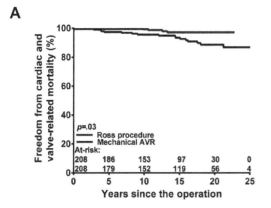

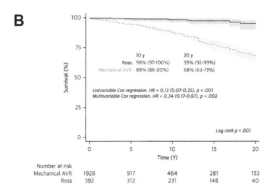

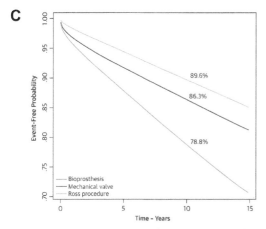

Fig. 4. Long-term outcomes of the Ross procedure versus prosthetic AVR. (*From* Refs.[63,89,97]; with permission.)

thrombohemorrhagic complications (hazard ratio 0.09, *P*<.001). Interestingly, long-term freedom from any reintervention was similar between the groups (87% in the Ross groups vs 94% in the mechanical AVR group at 20 years, *P* = .19) despite the fact that reintervention in the Ross group included any surgical or percutaneous reintervention on the aortic and/or pulmonary position.

In a similar study, Buratto and colleagues[89] reported outcomes of 275 propensity-matched pairs

of patients undergoing the Ross procedure or mechanical AVR (mean age 44 years, mean follow-up 10 years). Early mortality was similar, but patients in the Ross group had superior survival at 20 years (94% vs 84%, *P* = .018). This study is the first large-scale propensity-matched analysis to demonstrate a survival benefit of the Ross procedure over mechanical AVR.

WHAT ABOUT THE GUIDELINES?

Despite a growing body of evidence demonstrating superior outcomes of the Ross procedure versus prosthetic AVR in young and middle-aged adults, current American guidelines give the Ross operation a class IIb recommendation,[79] whereas the European guidelines fail to mention the Ross procedure as a surgical option altogether,[81] in spite of numerous series showing excellent outcomes into the second decade and a randomized controlled trial. Since these guidelines were drafted, a further 2 propensity-matched studies[63,89] and a meta-analysis of comparative studies have been published.[88] The authors believe that future iterations of the guidelines should take this additional evidence into account and propose a more central role for the Ross procedure in the treatment of aortic valve disease in non-elderly patients (**Fig. 5**), provided that the operation is carried out in centers of excellence where high volumes of aortic root surgery are performed.[90–92]

PATIENT SELECTION

Bioprosthetic valves are the substitute of choice in elderly patients undergoing AVR. Bioprostheses have excellent durability in this age group and will last the entirety of the patient's lifespan in most of the cases. In contrast, bioprosthetic valves should be avoided in young and middle-aged adults with aortic valve disease, unless there are other concomitant conditions that limit the patient's life expectancy (eg, end-stage renal disease, malignancy, etc.). Although valve-in-valve TAVI represents a promising avenue, the best available evidence does not currently support a prospective strategy in which a young patient is advised to undergo bioprosthetic AVR with the hope of performing valve-in-valve TAVI if the first valve fails.

In the absence of contraindications (eg, familial aortopathy, connective tissue disorder, autoimmune disease),[57,93] the authors believe the Ross procedure is the best operation to treat nonrepairable aortic valve disease in young and middle-aged adults,[94] provided it can be performed by

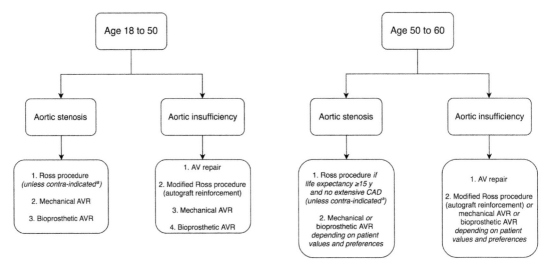

Fig. 5. Proposed algorithm for the management of aortic valve disease in non-elderly adults. [a] Contraindications to the Ross procedure: familial aortopathy, connective tissue disorder, autoimmune disorder, or any condition that limits life expectancy to less than 15 years.

dedicated teams in high-volume centers. It is a particularly desirable option for patients with aortic stenosis who present high levels of physical activity, patients with aortic annular diameter of 23 mm or less, as well as women contemplating pregnancy. Despite the generalized negative bias toward anticoagulation, evidence suggests that mechanical valves may still represent the alternative of choice for young patients who are not candidates for the Ross procedure and have no contraindication for anticoagulation. However, these data must be weighed against patients' preferences and values regarding the burden of anticoagulation versus the prospect of reoperation. Finally, aortic homografts remain useful in the setting of extensive aortic endocarditis with root abscess.

SUMMARY

The management of aortic valve disease in non-elderly adults has evolved rapidly over the last 2 decades. Several factors have contributed to this evolution: the development of transcatheter approaches, wider availability of home anticoagulation monitoring, and improved design of tissue and mechanical prostheses. However, the most significant factor is the increasing number of studies with a specific focus on this patient population. As a result, it is now clearly apparent that, counter to intuition, the younger the patients are, the bigger the loss in life expectancy after prosthetic AVR. In contrast, having a living valve substitute in the aortic position (Ross procedure) translates into improvements in clinically relevant

outcomes, including long-term survival. Nevertheless, it is important to tailor the surgery to the specific patient, through clear information while respecting their values and preferences. A patient-centered heart team approach is the optimal means of achieving this purpose. Continued research focused on this specific patient population will continue to yield new information and there is little doubt that, a decade from now, the field will have evolved even further. In the meantime, continued research is required to achieve the next quantum step in the surgical treatment of aortic valve disease: a tissue-engineered "off-the-shelf" living heart valve.[95]

DISCLOSURES

The authors have nothing to disclose.

REFERENCES

1. Nkomo VT, Gardin JM, Skelton TN, et al. Burden of valvular heart diseases: a population-based study. Lancet 2006;368(9540):1005–11.
2. Iung B, Baron G, Butchart EG, et al. A prospective survey of patients with valvular heart disease in Europe: the Euro heart Survey on valvular heart disease. Eur Heart J 2003;24(13):1231–43.
3. Carabello BA, Paulus WJ. Aortic stenosis. Lancet 2009;373(9667):956–66.
4. Cowell SJ, Newby DE, Prescott RJ, et al. A randomized trial of intensive lipid-lowering therapy in calcific aortic stenosis. N Engl J Med 2005;352(23):2389–97.
5. Yang LT, Michelena HI, Scott CG, et al. Outcomes in chronic hemodynamically significant aortic

regurgitation and limitations of current guidelines. J Am Coll Cardiol 2019;73(14):1741–52.

6. Dagum P, Green GR, Nistal FJ, et al. Deformational dynamics of the aortic root: modes and physiologic determinants. Circulation 1999;100(19 Suppl):II54–62.

7. DeWall RA, Qasim N, Carr L. Evolution of mechanical heart valves. Ann Thorac Surg 2000;69(5):1612–21.

8. Ikonomidis JS, Kratz JM, Crumbley AJ 3rd, et al. Twenty-year experience with the St Jude Medical mechanical valve prosthesis. J Thorac Cardiovasc Surg 2003;126(6):2022–31.

9. Van Nooten GJ, Caes F, Francois K, et al. Twenty years' single-center experience with mechanical heart valves: a critical review of anticoagulation policy. J Heart Valve Dis 2012;21(1):88–98.

10. Steinberg ZL, Dominguez-Islas CP, Otto CM, et al. Maternal and fetal outcomes of anticoagulation in pregnant women with mechanical heart valves. J Am Coll Cardiol 2017;69(22):2681–91.

11. D'Souza R, Ostro J, Shah PS, et al. Anticoagulation for pregnant women with mechanical heart valves: a systematic review and meta-analysis. Eur Heart J 2017;38(19):1509–16.

12. Bouhout I, Poirier N, Mazine A, et al. Cardiac, obstetric, and fetal outcomes during pregnancy after biological or mechanical aortic valve replacement. Can J Cardiol 2014;30(7):801–7.

13. Batra J, Itagaki S, Egorova NN, et al. Outcomes and long-term effects of pregnancy in women with biologic and mechanical valve prostheses. Am J Cardiol 2018;122(10):1738–44.

14. Hammermeister K, Sethi GK, Henderson WG, et al. Outcomes 15 years after valve replacement with a mechanical versus a bioprosthetic valve: final report of the Veterans Affairs randomized trial. J Am Coll Cardiol 2000;36(4):1152–8.

15. Puskas J, Gerdisch M, Nichols D, et al. Reduced anticoagulation after mechanical aortic valve replacement: interim results from the prospective randomized on-X valve anticoagulation clinical trial randomized Food and Drug Administration investigational device exemption trial. J Thorac Cardiovasc Surg 2014;147(4):1202–10 [discussion: 10–1].

16. Stassano P, Di Tommaso L, Monaco M, et al. Aortic valve replacement: a prospective randomized evaluation of mechanical versus biological valves in patients ages 55 to 70 years. J Am Coll Cardiol 2009;54(20):1862–8.

17. Bouhout I, Stevens LM, Mazine A, et al. Long-term outcomes after elective isolated mechanical aortic valve replacement in young adults. J Thorac Cardiovasc Surg 2014;148(4):1341–6.e1.

18. Kvidal P, Bergstrom R, Horte LG, et al. Observed and relative survival after aortic valve replacement. J Am Coll Cardiol 2000;35(3):747–56.

19. Korteland NM, Etnel JRG, Arabkhani B, et al. Mechanical aortic valve replacement in non-elderly adults: meta-analysis and microsimulation. Eur Heart J 2017;38(45):3370–7.

20. Eikelboom JW, Connolly SJ, Brueckmann M, et al. Dabigatran versus warfarin in patients with mechanical heart valves. N Engl J Med 2013;369(13):1206–14.

21. Heneghan C, Ward A, Perera R, et al. Self-monitoring of oral anticoagulation: systematic review and meta-analysis of individual patient data. Lancet 2012;379(9813):322–34.

22. Matchar DB, Jacobson A, Dolor R, et al. Effect of home testing of international normalized ratio on clinical events. N Engl J Med 2010;363(17):1608–20.

23. Grunkemeier GL, Furnary AP, Wu Y, et al. Durability of pericardial versus porcine bioprosthetic heart valves. J Thorac Cardiovasc Surg 2012;144(6):1381–6.

24. Hickey GL, Grant SW, Bridgewater B, et al. A comparison of outcomes between bovine pericardial and porcine valves in 38,040 patients in England and Wales over 10 years. Eur J Cardiothorac Surg 2015;47(6):1067–74.

25. David TE, Armstrong S, Maganti M. Hancock II bioprosthesis for aortic valve replacement: the gold standard of bioprosthetic valves durability? Ann Thorac Surg 2010;90(3):775–81.

26. Myken PS, Bech-Hansen O. A 20-year experience of 1712 patients with the Biocor porcine bioprosthesis. J Thorac Cardiovasc Surg 2009;137(1):76–81.

27. Jamieson WR, Burr LH, Miyagishima RT, et al. Carpentier-Edwards supra-annular aortic porcine bioprosthesis: clinical performance over 20 years. J Thorac Cardiovasc Surg 2005;130(4):994–1000.

28. Bourguignon T, Lhommet P, El Khoury R, et al. Very long-term outcomes of the Carpentier-Edwards Perimount aortic valve in patients aged 50-65 years. Eur J Cardiothorac Surg 2016;49(5):1462–8.

29. Forcillo J, El Hamamsy I, Stevens LM, et al. The perimount valve in the aortic position: twenty-year experience with patients under 60 years old. Ann Thorac Surg 2014;97(5):1526–32.

30. Mihaljevic T, Nowicki ER, Rajeswaran J, et al. Survival after valve replacement for aortic stenosis: implications for decision making. J Thorac Cardiovasc Surg 2008;135(6):1270–8 [discussion: 8–9].

31. Bourguignon T, Bouquiaux-Stablo AL, Candolfi P, et al. Very long-term outcomes of the Carpentier-Edwards Perimount valve in aortic position. Ann Thorac Surg 2015;99(3):831–7.

32. Etnel JRG, Huygens SA, Grashuis P, et al. Bioprosthetic aortic valve replacement in nonelderly adults: a systematic review, meta-analysis, Microsimulation. Circ Cardiovasc Qual Outcomes 2019;12(2):e005481.

33. Salaun E, Mahjoub H, Girerd N, et al. Rate, timing, correlates, and outcomes of hemodynamic valve deterioration after bioprosthetic surgical aortic valve replacement. Circulation 2018;138(10):971–85.

34. Salaun E, Mahjoub H, Dahou A, et al. Hemodynamic deterioration of surgically implanted bioprosthetic aortic valves. J Am Coll Cardiol 2018;72(3):241–51.

35. Isaacs AJ, Shuhaiber J, Salemi A, et al. National trends in utilization and in-hospital outcomes of mechanical versus bioprosthetic aortic valve replacements. J Thorac Cardiovasc Surg 2015;149(5):1262–9.e3.

36. Head SJ, Celik M, Kappetein AP. Mechanical versus bioprosthetic aortic valve replacement. Eur Heart J 2017;38(28):2183–91.

37. Johnston DR, Soltesz EG, Vakil N, et al. Long-term durability of bioprosthetic aortic valves: implications from 12,569 implants. Ann Thorac Surg 2015;99(4):1239–47.

38. Bilkhu R, Jahangiri M, Otto CM. Patient-prosthesis mismatch following aortic valve replacement. Heart 2019;105(Suppl 2):s28–33.

39. Pibarot P, Simonato M, Barbanti M, et al. Impact of pre-existing prosthesis-patient mismatch on survival following aortic valve-in-valve procedures. JACC Cardiovasc Interv 2018;11(2):133–41.

40. Mack MJ, Leon MB, Thourani VH, et al. Transcatheter aortic-valve replacement with a balloon-expandable valve in low-risk patients. N Engl J Med 2019;380(18):1695–705.

41. Ghoneim A, Bouhout I, Demers P, et al. Management of small aortic annulus in the era of sutureless valves: a comparative study among different biological options. J Thorac Cardiovasc Surg 2016;152(4):1019–28.

42. El-Hamamsy I, Clark L, Stevens LM, et al. Late outcomes following freestyle versus homograft aortic root replacement: results from a prospective randomized trial. J Am Coll Cardiol 2010;55(4):368–76.

43. El-Hamamsy I, Eryigit Z, Stevens LM, et al. Long-term outcomes after autograft versus homograft aortic root replacement in adults with aortic valve disease: a randomised controlled trial. Lancet 2010;376(9740):524–31.

44. El-Hamamsy I, Zaki M, Stevens LM, et al. Rate of progression and functional significance of aortic root calcification after homograft versus freestyle aortic root replacement. Circulation 2009;120(11 Suppl):S269–75.

45. Solari S, Mastrobuoni S, De Kerchove L, et al. Over 20 years experience with aortic homograft in aortic valve replacement during acute infective endocarditis. Eur J Cardiothorac Surg 2016;50(6):1158–64.

46. Sabik JF, Lytle BW, Blackstone EH, et al. Aortic root replacement with cryopreserved allograft for prosthetic valve endocarditis. Ann Thorac Surg 2002;74(3):650–9 [discussion: 9].

47. Rabkin-Aikawa E, Aikawa M, Farber M, et al. Clinical pulmonary autograft valves: pathologic evidence of adaptive remodeling in the aortic site. J Thorac Cardiovasc Surg 2004;128(4):552–61.

48. Laforest I, Dumesnil JG, Briand M, et al. Hemodynamic performance at rest and during exercise after aortic valve replacement: comparison of pulmonary autografts versus aortic homografts. Circulation 2002;106(12 Suppl 1):I57–62.

49. Torii R, El-Hamamsy I, Donya M, et al. Integrated morphologic and functional assessment of the aortic root after different tissue valve root replacement procedures. J Thorac Cardiovasc Surg 2012;143(6):1422–8.

50. Hon JK, Melina G, Wray J, et al. Insights from 36 years' follow up of a patient with the Ross operation. J Heart Valve Dis 2003;12(5):561–5.

51. David TE, David C, Woo A, et al. The Ross procedure: outcomes at 20 years. J Thorac Cardiovasc Surg 2014;147(1):85–93.

52. da Costa FD, Takkenberg JJ, Fornazari D, et al. Long-term results of the Ross operation: an 18-year single institutional experience. Eur J Cardiothorac Surg 2014;46(3):415–22 [discussion: 22].

53. Andreas M, Seebacher G, Reida E, et al. A single-center experience with the ross procedure over 20 years. Ann Thorac Surg 2014;97(1):182–8.

54. Skillington PD, Mokhles MM, Takkenberg JJ, et al. The Ross procedure using autologous support of the pulmonary autograft: techniques and late results. J Thorac Cardiovasc Surg 2015;149(2 Suppl):S46–52.

55. Sievers HH, Stierle U, Charitos EI, et al. A multicentre evaluation of the autograft procedure for young patients undergoing aortic valve replacement: update on the German Ross Registrydagger. Eur J Cardiothorac Surg 2016;49(1):212–8.

56. Sievers HH, Stierle U, Petersen M, et al. Valve performance classification in 630 subcoronary Ross patients over 22 years. J Thorac Cardiovasc Surg 2018;156(1):79–86.e2.

57. Mazine A, El-Hamamsy I, Verma S, et al. Ross procedure in adults for cardiologists and cardiac surgeons: JACC state-of-the-art review. J Am Coll Cardiol 2018;72(22):2761–77.

58. Aicher D, Holz A, Feldner S, et al. Quality of life after aortic valve surgery: replacement versus reconstruction. J Thorac Cardiovasc Surg 2011;142(2):e19–24.

59. Notzold A, Huppe M, Schmidtke C, et al. Quality of life in aortic valve replacement: pulmonary autografts versus mechanical prostheses. J Am Coll Cardiol 2001;37(7):1963–6.

60. Zacek P, Holubec T, Vobornik M, et al. Quality of life after aortic valve repair is similar to Ross patients and superior to mechanical valve replacement: a

cross-sectional study. BMC Cardiovasc Disord 2016;16:63.

61. Reece TB, Welke KF, O'Brien S, et al. Rethinking the ross procedure in adults. Ann Thorac Surg 2014; 97(1):175–81.

62. Bouhout I, Noly PE, Ghoneim A, et al. Is the Ross procedure a riskier operation? Perioperative outcome comparison with mechanical aortic valve replacement in a propensity-matched cohort. Interact Cardiovasc Thorac Surg 2017;24(1):41–7.

63. Mazine A, David TE, Rao V, et al. Long-term outcomes of the ross procedure versus mechanical aortic valve replacement: propensity-matched cohort study. Circulation 2016;134(8):576–85.

64. Hughes GC, Zhao Y, Rankin JS, et al. Effects of institutional volumes on operative outcomes for aortic root replacement in North America. J Thorac Cardiovasc Surg 2013;145(1):166–70.

65. Klieverik LM, Takkenberg JJ, Bekkers JA, et al. The Ross operation: a Trojan horse? Eur Heart J 2007; 28(16):1993–2000.

66. Hokken RB, Takkenberg JJ, van Herwerden LA, et al. Excessive pulmonary autograft dilatation causes important aortic regurgitation. Heart 2003;89(8): 933–4.

67. Bouhout I, Ghoneim A, Tousch M, et al. Impact of a tailored surgical approach on autograft root dimensions in patients undergoing the Ross procedure for aortic regurgitationdagger. Eur J Cardiothorac Surg 2019. https://doi.org/10.1093/ejcts/ezz105.

68. Martin E, Mohammadi S, Jacques F, et al. Clinical outcomes following the ross procedure in adults: a 25-year longitudinal study. J Am Coll Cardiol 2017; 70(15):1890–9.

69. Poh CL, Buratto E, Larobina M, et al. The Ross procedure in adults presenting with bicuspid aortic valve and pure aortic regurgitation: 85% freedom from reoperation at 20 years. Eur J Cardiothorac Surg 2018;54(3):420–6.

70. Stulak JM, Burkhart HM, Sundt TM 3rd, et al. Spectrum and outcome of reoperations after the Ross procedure. Circulation 2010;122(12):1153–8.

71. Mastrobuoni S, de Kerchove L, Solari S, et al. The Ross procedure in young adults: over 20 years of experience in our Institution. Eur J Cardiothorac Surg 2016;49(2):507–12 [discussion: 12–3].

72. Kumar SR, Bansal N, Wells WJ, et al. Outcomes of reintervention on the autograft after ross procedure. Ann Thorac Surg 2016;102(5):1517–21.

73. Luciani GB, Lucchese G, De Rita F, et al. Reparative surgery of the pulmonary autograft: experience with Ross reoperations. Eur J Cardiothorac Surg 2012; 41(6):1309–14 [discussion: 14–5].

74. Liebrich M, Weimar T, Tzanavaros I, et al. The David procedure for salvage of a failing autograft after the Ross operation. Ann Thorac Surg 2014;98(6): 2046–52.

75. Mookhoek A, de Kerchove L, El Khoury G, et al. European multicenter experience with valve-sparing reoperations after the Ross procedure. J Thorac Cardiovasc Surg 2015;150(5):1132–7.

76. Hussain ST, Majdalany DS, Dunn A, et al. Early and mid-term results of autograft rescue by Ross reversal: a one-valve disease need not become a two-valve disease. J Thorac Cardiovasc Surg 2018;155(2):562–72.

77. Marathe SP, Bell D, Betts K, et al. Homografts versus stentless bioprosthetic valves in the pulmonary position: a multicentre propensity-matched comparison in patients younger than 20 years. Eur J Cardiothorac Surg 2019. https://doi.org/10.1093/ejcts/ezz021.

78. Karaskov A, Sharifulin R, Zheleznev S, et al. Results of the Ross procedure in adults: a single-centre experience of 741 operations. Eur J Cardiothorac Surg 2016;49(5):e97–104.

79. Nishimura RA, Otto CM, Bonow RO, et al. 2017 AHA/ACC focused update of the 2014 AHA/ACC guideline for the management of patients with valvular heart disease: a report of the American College of Cardiology/American Heart Association Task Force on clinical practice guidelines. J Am Coll Cardiol 2017;70(2):252–89.

80. Nishimura RA, Otto CM, Bonow RO, et al. 2014 AHA/ACC guideline for the management of patients with valvular heart disease: a report of the American College of Cardiology/American Heart Association task force on practice guidelines. J Am Coll Cardiol 2014; 63(22):e57–185.

81. Baumgartner H, Falk V, Bax JJ, et al. 2017 ESC/EACTS guidelines for the management of valvular heart disease. Eur Heart J 2017;38(36):2739–91.

82. Oxenham H, Bloomfield P, Wheatley DJ, et al. Twenty year comparison of a Bjork-Shiley mechanical heart valve with porcine bioprostheses. Heart 2003;89(7):715–21.

83. Ruel M, Chan V, Bedard P, et al. Very long-term survival implications of heart valve replacement with tissue versus mechanical prostheses in adults <60 years of age. Circulation 2007;116(11 Suppl):I294–300.

84. Glaser N, Persson M, Jackson V, et al. Loss in life expectancy after surgical aortic valve replacement: SWEDEHEART Study. J Am Coll Cardiol 2019; 74(1):26–33.

85. Goldstone AB, Chiu P, Baiocchi M, et al. Mechanical or biologic prostheses for aortic-valve and mitral-valve replacement. N Engl J Med 2017;377(19): 1847–57.

86. Glaser N, Jackson V, Holzmann MJ, et al. Aortic valve replacement with mechanical vs. biological prostheses in patients aged 50-69 years. Eur Heart J 2016;37(34):2658–67.

87. Carabello BA. Valve-in-Valve TAVR: insights into the pathophysiology of aortic stenosis. J Am Coll Cardiol 2017;69(18):2263–5.

88. Mazine A, Rocha RV, El-Hamamsy I, et al. Ross procedure vs mechanical aortic valve replacement in adults: a systematic review and meta-analysis. JAMA Cardiol 2018;3(10):978–87.

89. Buratto E, Shi WY, Wynne R, et al. Improved survival after the ross procedure compared with mechanical aortic valve replacement. J Am Coll Cardiol 2018; 71(12):1337–44.

90. El-Hamamsy I, Bouhout I. The Ross procedure: time for a hard look at current practices and a reexamination of the guidelines. Ann Transl Med 2017;5(6): 142.

91. Misfeld M, Borger MA. The Ross procedure: time to reevaluate the guidelines. J Thorac Cardiovasc Surg 2019;157(1):211–2.

92. Pettersson GB, Blackstone EH. Is it time to reconsider use of the ross procedure for adults? J Am Coll Cardiol 2018;71(12):1345–6.

93. Mazine A, El-Hamamsy I, Ouzounian M. The Ross procedure in adults: which patients, which disease? Curr Opin Cardiol 2017;32(6):663–71.

94. Ouzounian M, Mazine A, David TE. The Ross procedure is the best operation to treat aortic stenosis in young and middle-aged adults. J Thorac Cardiovasc Surg 2017;154(3):778–82.

95. Yacoub MH, Takkenberg JJ. Will heart valve tissue engineering change the world? Nat Clin Pract Cardiovasc Med 2005;2(2):60–1.

96. Schnittman SR, Adams DH, Itagaki S, et al. Bioprosthetic aortic valve replacement: revisiting prosthesis choice in patients younger than 50 years old. J Thorac Cardiovasc Surg 2018;155(2):539–47.e9.

97. Sharabiani MT, Dorobantu DM, Mahani AS, et al. Aortic valve replacement and the ross operation in children and young adults. J Am Coll Cardiol 2016; 67(24):2858–70.

Planning for Success
Pre-procedural Evaluation for Transcatheter Aortic Valve Replacement

Vivian G. Ng, MD, Rebecca T. Hahn, MD, Tamim M. Nazif, MD*

KEYWORDS

- Transcatheter Aortic Valve Replacement • TAVR • TAVI • Multi-modality Imaging
- Echocardiography • MSCT

KEY POINTS

- While TAVR devices and techniques have matured, comprehensive multi-modality imaging has remained vital to performing the procedure safely and effectively.
- Pre-procedural echocardiography and MSCT facilitate procedure planning, choice of the appropriate transcatheter valve type and size, and prediction of potential complications.
- Intra-procedure echocardiography can be used to provide additional real-time procedure guidance.

INTRODUCTION

Since its inception in 2002, the use of transcatheter aortic valve replacement (TAVR) has rapidly increased over the last 17 years.[1,2] Many of the challenges encountered in the early phases of TAVR adoption have been overcome with technological improvements in both the transcatheter valves and delivery systems.[3,4] Nonetheless, as TAVR indications broaden to include lower-risk populations,[5,6] detailed pre-procedural planning is crucial to maintain the safety and efficacy of this therapy. The 2017 American College of Cardiology (ACC) Expert Consensus Decision Pathway for Transcatheter Aortic Valve Replacement suggested a decision pathway for clinicians caring for patients with aortic stenosis (AS).[7] This pathway starts at the point where a patient with severe AS is being considered for TAVR based on the indication for aortic valve (AV) intervention and choice of valve type indicated in the ACC guidelines.[8] The shared decision-making by the Heart Valve Team is based on a comprehensive understanding of the patient-specific anatomy,

best defined by multi-modality imaging. In this review, we discuss the key elements of the pre-procedural evaluations in patients referred to a multi-disciplinary, collaborative Heart Valve Team with possible severe, symptomatic AS.[7]

PRE-PROCEDURAL ECHOCARDIOGRAPHIC EVALUATION

The 2014 ACC/American Heart Association valvular heart disease guidelines[9] divide specific valvular diseases into stages, with stage D including symptomatic patients with severe disease. Class I indications for TAVR include patients with severe symptomatic high-gradient AS (stage D1) with prohibitive or high surgical risk and asymptomatic patients with high gradients and left ventricular ejection fraction <50% (stage C2). In addition, there are class IIa indications for AV replacement in patients with severe low-flow low-gradient with reduced ejection fraction (stage D2) and paradoxic low-flow low-gradient AS (stage D3), and the 2017 focused update[8] included a class IIa indication for high-gradient patients with

Division of Cardiology, Columbia University Medical Center, NewYork-Presbyterian Hospital, 177 Fort Washington Avenue, 5th Floor, Room 5C-501, New York, NY 10032, USA
* Corresponding author. 177 Fort Washington Avenue, 5th Floor, Room 5C-501, New York, NY 10032.
E-mail address: tmn31@columbia.edu

Cardiol Clin 38 (2020) 103–113
https://doi.org/10.1016/j.ccl.2019.09.013
0733-8651/20/© 2019 Elsevier Inc. All rights reserved.

intermediate surgical risk. The identification of the D2 and D3 stages of disease is thus an essential task for the Heart Valve Team (see Julien Ternacle and Marie-Annick Clavel's article, "Assessment of Aortic Stenosis Severity: A Multimodality Approach," in this issue).

Another aspect to consider when choosing the AV intervention and valve may be avoidance of prosthesis-patient mismatch (PPM).[10] PPM is considered not clinically significant, moderate, or severe when the indexed effective orifice area (EOA) is >0.85 cm^2/m^2, between 0.85 and 0.65 cm^2/m^2, and less than 0.65 cm^2/m^2, respectively. However, the indexed EOA may overestimate the severity of PPM in obese patients (body mass index $\geq$ 30 kg/m^2), and the European Association of Cardiovascular Imaging and Valve Academic Research Consortium 2 therefore recommend using lower cut-points of indexed EOA in obese patients: that is, less than 0.70 cm^2/m^2 for moderate PPM and less than 0.55 cm^2/m^2 for severe PPM.[11] Following TAVR, the incidence of outcomes related to PPM for different valve types have been discordant.[12,13] The most recent report from the From the Society of Thoracic Surgeons/ACC Transcatheter Valve Therapy Registry reported the incidence of severe PPM in 12% of patients. At 1 year, mortality (17.2% vs 15.9%, P = .02) and heart failure rehospitalization (14.7% vs 11.9%, $P<$.0001) were more frequent in severe than in no PPM patients. To predict possible PPM following TAVR, the expected indexed aortic valve area (AVA) of the balloon expandable and self-expanding transcatheter AVs based on native annular measurements can be found in the tables published by Hahn and colleagues.[14] The expected valve area is then divided by the patient's body surface area to determine the indexed AVA.

Although avoiding PPM is reasonable, PPM likely has less impact on outcomes than paravalvular regurgitation (PVR). Hence, in general, the largest possible valve size with appropriate degrees of over-sizing is used to minimize the risk of PPM and PVL.

COMPUTED TOMOGRAPHY ANGIOGRAPHY EVALUATION
Vascular Access Assessment

Vascular complications are one of the more frequent complications of TAVR (2%–30%) and are associated with significant morbidity and mortality.[15–19] Although TAVR vascular complication have clearly decreased over time, TAVR procedures continue to require large-bore arterial sheaths. Planning for a TAVR procedure therefore involves a comprehensive assessment of vascular anatomy and pathology to determine the most appropriate access route. This is most commonly achieved using contrast-enhanced multi-slice computed tomography (MSCT) of the aorta and peripheral vessels. Consensus guidelines have been created to facilitate appropriate preprocedural TAVR imaging.[20] Although contrast-enhanced imaging provides the most comprehensive vascular assessment, low-contrast CT or a hybrid approach using non-contrast CT and magnetic resonance imaging can provide significant amounts of information in patients with prohibitive renal dysfunction or untreatable contrast allergy. This can be paired with iliofemoral arterial intravascular ultrasound for 3-dimensional vascular imaging in borderline cases.[21]

The vascular access assessment should include evaluation of the aorta, common iliac, external iliac, and femoral arteries. Small vessel diameter, severe calcification, vessel tortuosity, and peripheral arterial disease have all been described as risk factors for vascular complications during transfemoral TAVR procedures.[17,22] A sheath to femoral artery size ratio of 1.10 can be used when there is no vascular calcification, but a ratio of 1.00 may be more appropriate when there is significant vascular calcification.[23] Relative contraindications to a transfemoral approach to TAVR with currently available systems generally include iliofemoral vessel diameter less than 5.0 mm, severe calcification (especially if circumferential and at the puncture site), significant tortuosity, previous aorto-femoral bypass, aortic dissection, aortic thrombus protruding into the lumen, and significant atherosclerotic disease. Notably, these vessel characteristics must be taken into consideration together. For example, iliac and femoral arteries with substantial calcification may provide appropriate TAVR access if the vessels have adequate diameters and no significant tortuosity. Similarly, tortuous vessels that have adequate diameters and no significant calcification are frequently compliant and may straighten with a stiff wire and sheath. Of note, each transcatheter heart valve system requires a minimum vessel diameter, which should be carefully observed (**Table 1**).

Although transfemoral access is by far the most common method of performing TAVR, accounting for more than 85% of all procedures in the United States by 2015,[2] there remain challenging cases. In these situations, potential alternative access routes include transsubclavian,[24] transaxillary,[25] transcarotid,[26,27] suprasternal,[28] transcaval,[29,30] and direct aortic access.[31,32] With increasing experience with these various other alternative

Table 1
Minimum vessel diameters required for valve delivery systems

Transcatheter Valve Type	Minimum Vessel Diameter Required (mm)
Edwards Sapien 3 valve	
20 mm, 23 mm, 26 mm	5.5
29 mm	6.0
Medtronic Evolut-R	
23 mm, 26 mm, 29 mm	5.0
34 mm	5.5
Medtronic Evolut-Pro	
23 mm, 26 mm, 29 mm	5.5

access routes, transapical access[33] has become infrequently used for TAVR, but remains a potential option in selected cases. Contrast-enhanced CT remains the mainstay of assessment for alternative access.

Transcatheter Aortic Valve Sizing and Risk Assessment

Unlike in surgical AV replacement, direct visualization of the AV for sizing is not possible during TAVR. Pre-procedural MSCT, transesophageal echocardiography (TEE), or cardiac MRI is therefore required to assess the aortic valvar anatomic suitability for TAVR and to measure the AV annulus.[34,35] Three-dimensional imaging is essential to obtain detailed anatomic information including: left ventricular outflow tract, AV annulus and aortic dimensions, the location and burden of calcification, and the relationship to surrounding structures including the coronary artery ostia. Contrast-enhanced MSCT is the preferred method of evaluation and it must be performed with either retrospective or prospective electrocardiogram triggering (gated) and during suspended respirations to decrease motion artifact.[36]

Measurement of the AV annulus should generally be performed in systole because the annulus is usually slightly larger in systole.[20] The aortic annulus is not a fibrous structure, but rather a virtual ring that connects the 3 lowest points of the AV cusps (leaflet hinge points) and is usually the smallest part of the aortic root.[34] This virtual ring is orthogonal to the central axis of the left ventricular outflow tract and is the reference structure for TAVR device sizing. The perimeter or area of the

annulus is calculated in the axial plane to determine the most appropriate transcatheter heart valve size for the individual anatomy (**Tables 2 and 3**). The annulus area is generally used for sizing balloon expandable or mechanically expandable transcatheter valves, whereas the perimeter is favored for self-expanding. The appropriate degree of transcatheter heart valve over-sizing ([transcatheter valve nominal diameter/annular diameter – 1] $\times$ 100) varies depending on the specific TAVR system used and whether diameter, perimeter or area measurements are employed in the calculation. If the implanted prosthesis is too large for the annulus or the surrounding structures, annular rupture or root injury (aortic dissection or hematoma) can occur, which are potentially fatal complications.[37,38] In addition, prosthesis over-sizing may limit the durability of the valve[39] and increase the risk of conduction disturbances.[40] The presence of severe aortic root calcification, left ventricular outflow tract calcification, and valve over-sizing can also lead to aortic root injury.[38,41] The acceptable degree of oversizing therefore depends not just on the transcatheter heart valve system used, but on anatomy of the individual aortic valvar complex.

Severe TAVR under-sizing can lead to device instability or even embolization,[42] while lesser degrees of under-sizing are associated with increased PVR and PPM, which are associated with worse clinical outcomes over time.[43–45] Adoption of routine CT-based annular sizing has been shown to reduce the risk of PVR.[42,46] It remains controversial whether leaflet calcification severity and location impact PVR.[47–51] Qualitatively, patients with annular calcification that protrudes into the lumen or calcifications located in the left ventricular outflow tract may be at higher risk of having PVR.[47,50]

In addition to annular sizing, measurements such as the height of the coronary ostia above the aortic annulus, AV leaflet length, aortic sinus width, left ventricular outflow tract diameter, and sinotubular junction diameter are also necessary.[20,52–54] Because the AV leaflets are pushed open into the sinuses by the TAVR prosthesis,

Table 2
Sizing chart for Edwards Sapien 3 valve

	20 mm	23 mm	26 mm	29 mm
Annulus area (mm²)	273–345	338–430	430–546	540–680
Expanded length (mm)	15.5	18	20	22.5

Table 3
Sizing chart for Medtronic Evolut valves

Valve Size	Evolut-R and Pro			Evolut-R
	23 mm	26 mm	29 mm	34 mm
Annulus				
Diameter (mm)	18–20	20–23	23–26	26–30
Perimeter (mm)	56.5–62.8	62.8–72.3	72.3–81.7	81.7–94.2
Sinus of Valsalva				
Diameter (mm)	≥25	≥27	≥29	≥31
Height (mm)	≥15	≥15	≥15	≥16

the leaflets can be displaced over the coronary ostia in certain anatomies causing coronary obstruction.[15] Although the rate of coronary occlusion is low at 0.1% to 1.2% in randomized clinical trials,[55–57] this is a potentially life-threatening complication that is associated with a high mortality rate.[58-60] The risk of coronary occlusion increases with low height of the coronary ostia (≤10 mm), increased coronary leaflet length, leaflet tip calcification, and narrow sinus of Valsalva.[52,59-61] However, approximately 25% of cases with coronary obstruction had a coronary height greater than 12 mm, highlighting the importance of additional anatomic features.[59]

Bicuspid Aortic Valve Considerations

Patients with bicuspid AV disease were excluded from the pivotal TAVR trials.[16,62,63] Compared with patients with senile, degenerative AS, those with bicuspid AV disease tend to be younger with lower surgical risk. Anatomically, these patients have not been considered ideal for TAVR because of concerns about TAVR sizing, positioning, and expansion, and risks of PVR, aortic rupture,[64,65] and coronary obstruction from longer fused leaflets.[66,67] Furthermore, bicuspid AV disease is frequently associated with aortopathy.[68–70] Thus, surgery remains the gold standard treatment for AS due to bicuspid AV disease. Nevertheless, recent registries have demonstrated that TAVR with newer-generation transcatheter heart valve systems can be an acceptable alternative in selected patients at elevated risk for surgery.[66,67,71,72] The presence of a bicuspid valve may impact the selection and sizing of the transcatheter valve. The Sievers and Schmidtke classification (**Fig. 1**) should also be used on preprocedural imaging using MSCT and echocardiography.[73] The type of bicuspid valve may impact TAVR procedural risk; type 1 valves have more leaflet asymmetry, which may lead to incomplete

transcatheter valve expansion[66] and have been associated with higher rates of PVR than Sievers type 0 valves.[66] Other anatomic features related to bicuspid AV should be considered: the aortic annulus is less elliptical[72,74] and tends to be larger with asymmetric calcification,[74] and the presence of dilated horizontal ascending aortas and effaced sinuses.[74] Balloon aortic valvuloplasty can be helpful before TAVR for bicuspid AV to confirm sizing and coronary obstruction risk. Recent data suggest that newer-generation transcatheter and self-expandable valves may have an advantage in this patient population,[75] but additional studies are required.

PROCEDURAL PLANNING
Fluoroscopic C-arm Position

Transcatheter valve deployment is typically performed in a fluoroscopic projection that is orthogonal to the aortic annular plane, which can be predicted before the procedure using CT angiography.[76,77] Once the aortic annular plane has been identified by the selecting the lowest point of each aortic cusp, CT imaging processing programs can determine the corresponding fluoroscopic C-arm position as the "implanter's view." Additional fine adjustments are usually required at the time of the procedure because the patient may not be in exactly the same body position as during the CT scan. Recent use of echo-fluoro fusion imaging has also been used to intraprocedurally determine and confirm co-planar imaging views.[78]

Anesthetic Choice

The early procedures in inoperable or high surgical risk patients were modeled after cardiac surgery and performed under general anesthesia and guided by TEE. However, TAVR technology and experience have greatly improved and TAVR indications are now expanding to include lower-risk

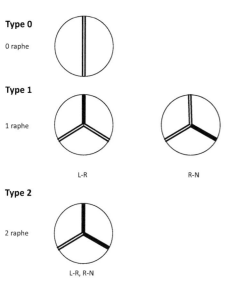

Type 0

0 raphe

Type 1

1 raphe

L-R   R-N   N-L

Type 2

2 raphe

L-R, R-N

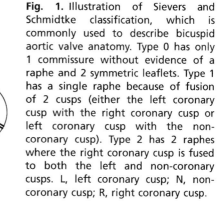

Fig. 1. Illustration of Sievers and Schmidtke classification, which is commonly used to describe bicuspid aortic valve anatomy. Type 0 has only 1 commissure without evidence of a raphe and 2 symmetric leaflets. Type 1 has a single raphe because of fusion of 2 cusps (either the left coronary cusp with the right coronary cusp or left coronary cusp with the non-coronary cusp). Type 2 has 2 raphes where the right coronary cusp is fused to both the left and non-coronary cusps. L, left coronary cusp; N, non-coronary cusp; R, right coronary cusp.

populations. Hence, TAVR procedures have been simplified by adopting a minimalist approach, which includes local anesthesia and monitored anesthesia care or conscious sedation.[79] Avoidance of general anesthesia may reduce procedural times, pulmonary complications, delirium, and duration of hospital stay,[80–82] and seemed to be at least as safe as general anesthesia for TAVR.[82–84]

In the current era, anesthetic choice should ideally be tailored to each individual patient considering clinical risk factors (e.g., left ventricular systolic dysfunction, concomitant coronary artery disease [CAD], multi-valvular disease, lung disease, or neurologic disease) and anatomic risk factors (e.g., high-risk vascular access, alternative access, high risk of coronary occlusion, annulus disruption, or PVR). For example, a patient who is at high risk of coronary occlusion or annular disruption may benefit from general anesthesia and TEE imaging during the procedure for immediate identification and management of complications.

Embolic Protection

Although 30-day rates of stroke after surgical AV replacement have been reported to be between 0.7% and 6.5%, 30-day rates of stroke have been reported to be approximately 3% to 6% after TAVR.[16,57,85] Most neurologic events occur in the peri-procedural period[86,87] and are thought to be related to cerebral embolization and hypoperfusion.[88] Despite improvements in TAVR device technology, rates of neurologic events seem to be relatively consistent over time and not related

to site experience.[89,90] The Sentinel Cerebral Protection System is currently the only US Food and Drug Administration-approved device for neuroprotection during TAVR. The device is inserted via the right radial artery (6Fr) and consists of 2 interconnected filters. One filter is deployed in the proximal right brachiocephalic artery and the second filter is deployed in the proximal left common carotid artery. The anatomy and diameters of the brachiocephalic and left common carotid arteries should be evaluated on the pre-procedural CT. A meta-analysis of 4 studies evaluating 606 patients receiving embolic protection with the Sentinel device during TAVR compared with 724 patients who did not receive embolic protection found that embolic protection was associated with lower rates of symptomatic stroke at 30 days.[91] This device is currently also being studied in the PROTECT-TAVI European multicenter trial.

Management of Coronary Artery Disease

There is a high burden (>50%) of concomitant CAD in patients with AS undergoing evaluation for TAVR.[92] As a result, TAVR patients routinely receive coronary angiography; although, there is emerging data that suggest that coronary CT angiography is an acceptable alternative to evaluate for significant CAD before TAVR.[93] Because TAVR trials have required revascularization of significant CAD, it is generally recommended in clinical practice to perform coronary angiography and pursue revascularization through percutaneous coronary intervention (PCI) on patients with AS and significant proximal CAD.[94,95]

However, it is unclear whether routine PCI before TAVR is actually associated with any clinical advantage.[92] In addition, if PCI is planned, it remains unclear whether it should be performed at the time of TAVR or as a staged procedure before or after TAVR.[96–98] Additional studies are necessary to determine which TAVR patients would benefit most from routine angiography and PCI, as well as the optimal timing for PCI relative to the TAVR procedure.

INTRA-PROCEDURAL CONSIDERATIONS
Balloon Aortic Valvuloplasty Sizing

At times, balloon aortic valvuloplasty (BAV) sizing may be helpful for selecting the optimal transcatheter heart valve size,[99,100] and in assessing if the risk ofr coronary artery ostial occlusion when pre-procedural imaging cannot be performed is inadequate or there are conflicting or borderline measurements. The balloon should be matched in size to the smaller TAVR size being considered. The BAV is then performed under rapid pacing with contrast injection at the level of the aortic root or ascending aorta after full balloon inflation. Signs of correct sizing include a lack of balloon movement within the AV, a waist on the balloon at the level of the aortic annulus, and a lack of contrast regurgitation into the left ventricle. TEE imaging during BAV may also be useful not only for sizing but also to assess the displacement of calcium and risk of complications, such as annular or aortic root rupture and coronary artery occlusion.[101]

Coronary Occlusion Risk Management

As discussed above, coronary artery occlusion is a potentially devastating complication of TAVR. Most cases present immediately after valve deployment, but late presentations (≥48 hours) have been reported.[62] In addition to CT parameters, the risk of coronary occlusion can be further evaluated during the TAVR procedure by performing BAV with concomitant aortography. The absence of coronary opacification during the BAV confirms high risk of coronary occlusion after TAVR deployment. When pre-procedural imaging suggests a high risk of coronary occlusion, a guidewire and undeployed stent may be positioned in the threatened coronary artery to maintain an access after valve deployment. A guide catheter with side holes is helpful in these situations because the guide catheter can be pulled away from the coronary ostium during valve deployment and used for the aortogram instead of a pigtail catheter. A guide extension may also be useful to facilitate positioning or removal of the coronary stent after TAVR deployment. After valve deployment, if the coronary ostium is indeed occluded by the native leaflet, the undeployed stent can be pulled back and deployed rapidly. The proximal edge of the stent should extend above the level of the native valve leaflet and to the edge of the TAVR stent frame in a "snorkel" or "chimney" fashion, to ensure coronary perfusion. In addition, the laceration of the AV leaflets (native or failed prosthetic) may be performed before TAVR implantation using the BASILICA (Bioprosthetic or native Aortic Scallop Intentional Laceration to prevent Iatrogenic Coronary Artery obstruction during TAVR) technique.[102,103]

Confirmation of Aortic Root Anatomy

If pre-procedural CT or other imaging is inadequate for annular sizing or confirmation of sizing is indicated, intra-procedural TEE may be appropriate. Three-dimensional TEE using multiplanar reconstruction overcomes the limitations of 2D by allowing measurements of the annular area and perimeter, and has demonstrated comparable results with MSCT, at the same time avoiding the risks associated with exposure to radiation and contrast dye.[104–106] In addition, other measurements of the aortic valvular complex should be performed, including the size of the sinuses of Valsalva, diameter of the sinotubular junction, and the height of the coronary arteries ostia above the annulus.[107] These measurements should be used in concert with a three-dimensional assessment of the anatomic relationships and calcium location and burden to perform transcatheter valve sizing and risk assessment.

SUMMARY

Advancements in transcatheter heart valve technology have greatly improved the ease and safety of the TAVR procedure. Nevertheless, comprehensive multi-modality imaging remains vital to performing these procedures safely and effectively. Echocardiography and MSCT should be used for pre-procedural planning to choose the appropriate valve type/size and to anticipate potential complications. Furthermore, echocardiography can be used to provide additional real-time guidance intra-procedurally.

DISCLOSURE

R.T. Hahn reports speaker fees from Boston Scientific Corporation and Baylis Medical; consulting for Abbott Structural, Edwards Lifesciences, Gore & Associates, Medtronic, Navigate, Philips Healthcare, and Siemens Healthcare; non-financial support from 3mensio and GE Healthcare; is Chief Scientific Officer for the Echocardiography Core Laboratory at the Cardiovascular Research Foundation for multiple industry-sponsored trials, for which she receives no direct industry compensation. T.M. Nazif reports consulting or honoraria for Edwards Lifesciences, Medtronic, Boston Scientific, Baylis Medical, and BioTrace Medical.

REFERENCES

1. Cribier A, Eltchaninoff H, Tron C, et al. Early experience with percutaneous transcatheter implantation of heart valve prosthesis for the treatment of end-stage inoperable patients with calcific aortic stenosis. J Am Coll Cardiol 2004;43(4):698–703.

2. Grover FL, Vemulapalli S, Carroll JD, et al. 2016 annual report of the Society of Thoracic Surgeons/American College of Cardiology transcatheter valve therapy registry. J Am Coll Cardiol 2017;69(10):1215–30.

3. Forrest JK, Mangi AA, Popma JJ, et al. Early outcomes with the Evolut PRO repositionable self-expanding transcatheter aortic valve with pericardial wrap. JACC Cardiovasc Interv 2018;11(2):160–8.

4. Thourani VH, Kodali S, Makkar RR, et al. Transcatheter aortic valve replacement versus surgical valve replacement in intermediate-risk patients: a propensity score analysis. Lancet 2016;387(10034):2218–25.

5. Mack MJ, Leon MB, Thourani VH, et al. Transcatheter aortic-valve replacement with a balloon-expandable valve in low-risk patients. N Engl J Med 2019;380(18):1695–705.

6. Popma JJ, Deeb GM, Yakubov SJ, et al. Transcatheter aortic-valve replacement with a self-expanding valve in low-risk patients. N Engl J Med 2019;380(18):1706–15.

7. Otto CM, Kumbhani DJ, Alexander KP, et al. 2017 ACC expert consensus decision pathway for transcatheter aortic valve replacement in the management of adults with aortic stenosis: a report of the American College of Cardiology task force on clinical expert consensus documents. J Am Coll Cardiol 2017;69(10):1313–46.

8. Nishimura RA, Otto CM, Bonow RO, et al. 2017 AHA/ACC focused update of the 2014 AHA/ACC guideline for the management of patients with valvular heart disease: a report of the American College of Cardiology/American Heart Association Task Force on clinical practice guidelines. Circulation 2017;135(25):e1159–95.

9. Nishimura RA, Otto CM, Bonow RO, et al. 2014 AHA/ACC guideline for the management of patients with valvular heart disease: executive summary. A report of the American College of Cardiology/American Heart Association Task Force on Practice Guidelines. J Am Coll Cardiol 2014;63(22):2438–88.

10. Pibarot P, Dumesnil JG. Prosthesis-patient mismatch: definition, clinical impact, and prevention. Heart 2006;92(8):1022–9.

11. Kappetein AP, Head SJ, Genereux P, et al. Updated standardized endpoint definitions for transcatheter aortic valve implantation: the Valve Academic Research Consortium-2 consensus document. J Am Coll Cardiol 2012;60(15):1438–54.

12. Zorn GL 3rd, Little SH, Tadros P, et al. Prosthesis-patient mismatch in high-risk patients with severe aortic stenosis: a randomized trial of a self-expanding prosthesis. J Thorac Cardiovasc Surg 2016;151(4):1014–1023 e1013.

13. Pibarot P, Weissman NJ, Stewart WJ, et al. Incidence and sequelae of prosthesis-patient mismatch in transcatheter versus surgical valve replacement in high-risk patients with severe aortic stenosis: a PARTNER trial cohort-A analysis. J Am Coll Cardiol 2014;64(13):1323–34.

14. Hahn RT, Leipsic J, Douglas PS, et al. Comprehensive echocardiographic assessment of normal transcatheter valve function. JACC Cardiovasc Imaging 2019;12(1):25–34.

15. Genereux P, Head SJ, Van Mieghem NM, et al. Clinical outcomes after transcatheter aortic valve replacement using valve academic research consortium definitions: a weighted meta-analysis of 3,519 patients from 16 studies. J Am Coll Cardiol 2012;59(25):2317–26.

16. Leon MB, Smith CR, Mack M, et al. Transcatheter aortic-valve implantation for aortic stenosis in patients who cannot undergo surgery. N Engl J Med 2010;363(17):1597–607.

17. Hayashida K, Lefevre T, Chevalier B, et al. Transfemoral aortic valve implantation new criteria to predict vascular complications. JACC Cardiovasc Interv 2011;4(8):851–8.

18. Tchetche D, Dumonteil N, Sauguet A, et al. Thirty-day outcome and vascular complications after transarterial aortic valve implantation using both Edwards Sapien and Medtronic CoreValve bioprostheses in a mixed population. EuroIntervention 2010;5(6):659–65.

19. Van Mieghem NM, Nuis RJ, Piazza N, et al. Vascular complications with transcatheter aortic valve implantation using the 18 Fr Medtronic CoreValve System: the Rotterdam experience. EuroIntervention 2010;5(6):673–9.

20. Achenbach S, Delgado V, Hausleiter J, et al. SCCT expert consensus document on computed tomography imaging before transcatheter aortic valve implantation (TAVI)/transcatheter aortic valve replacement (TAVR). J Cardiovasc Comput Tomogr 2012;6(6):366–80.

21. Essa E, Makki N, Bittenbender P, et al. Vascular assessment for transcatheter aortic valve replacement: intravascular ultrasound compared with computed tomography. J Invasive Cardiol 2016; 28(12):E172–8.

22. Toggweiler S, Gurvitch R, Leipsic J, et al. Percutaneous aortic valve replacement: vascular outcomes with a fully percutaneous procedure. J Am Coll Cardiol 2012;59(2):113–8.

23. Piazza N, Lange R, Martucci G, et al. Patient selection for transcatheter aortic valve implantation: patient risk profile and anatomical selection criteria. Arch Cardiovasc Dis 2012;105(3):165–73.

24. Petronio AS, De Carlo M, Bedogni F, et al. Safety and efficacy of the subclavian approach for transcatheter aortic valve implantation with the CoreValve revalving system. Circ Cardiovasc Interv 2010;3(4):359–66.

25. Dahle TG, Kaneko T, McCabe JM. Outcomes following subclavian and axillary artery access for transcatheter aortic valve replacement: Society of the Thoracic Surgeons/American College of Cardiology TVT registry report. JACC Cardiovasc Interv 2019;12(7):662–9.

26. Mylotte D, Sudre A, Teiger E, et al. Transcarotid transcatheter aortic valve replacement: feasibility and safety. JACC Cardiovasc Interv 2016;9(5): 472–80.

27. Thourani VH, Li C, Devireddy C, et al. High-risk patients with inoperative aortic stenosis: use of transapical, transaortic, and transcarotid techniques. Ann Thorac Surg 2015;99(3):817–23 [discussion: 823–5].

28. Codner P, Pugliese D, Kouz R, et al. Transcatheter aortic valve replacement by a novel suprasternal approach. Ann Thorac Surg 2018;105(4):1215–22.

29. Greenbaum AB, O'Neill WW, Paone G, et al. Cavalaortic access to allow transcatheter aortic valve replacement in otherwise ineligible patients: initial human experience. J Am Coll Cardiol 2014;63(25 Pt A):2795–804.

30. Lederman RJ, Babaliaros VC, Rogers T, et al. The fate of transcaval access tracts: 12-month results of the prospective NHLBI transcaval transcatheter aortic valve replacement study. JACC Cardiovasc Interv 2019;12(5):448–56.

31. Bruschi G, de Marco F, Botta L, et al. Direct aortic access for transcatheter self-expanding aortic bioprosthetic valves implantation. Ann Thorac Surg 2012;94(2):497–503.

32. Etienne PY, Papadatos S, El Khoury E, et al. Transaortic transcatheter aortic valve implantation with the Edwards SAPIEN valve: feasibility, technical considerations, and clinical advantages. Ann Thorac Surg 2011;92(2):746–8.

33. Kempfert J, Rastan A, Holzhey D, et al. Transapical aortic valve implantation: analysis of risk factors and learning experience in 299 patients. Circulation 2011;124(11 Suppl):S124–9.

34. Piazza N, de Jaegere P, Schultz C, et al. Anatomy of the aortic valvar complex and its implications for transcatheter implantation of the aortic valve. Circ Cardiovasc Interv 2008;1(1):74–81.

35. Kasel AM, Cassese S, Bleiziffer S, et al. Standardized imaging for aortic annular sizing: implications for transcatheter valve selection. JACC Cardiovasc Imaging 2013;6(2):249–62.

36. Schultz C, Moelker A, Tzikas A, et al. The use of MSCT for the evaluation of the aortic root before transcutaneous aortic valve implantation: the Rotterdam approach. EuroIntervention 2010;6(4): 505–11.

37. Blanke P, Reinohl J, Schlensak C, et al. Prosthesis oversizing in balloon-expandable transcatheter aortic valve implantation is associated with contained rupture of the aortic root. Circ Cardiovasc Interv 2012;5(4):540–8.

38. Barbanti M, Yang TH, Rodes Cabau J, et al. Anatomical and procedural features associated with aortic root rupture during balloon-expandable transcatheter aortic valve replacement. Circulation 2013;128(3):244–53.

39. Stanova V, Zenses A-S, Rieu R, et al. Effect of valve oversizing on leaflet bending stress in the corevalve: an in vitro study. J Am Coll Cardiol 2017; 69:1044.

40. Nazif TM, Dizon JM, Hahn RT, et al. Predictors and clinical outcomes of permanent pacemaker implantation after transcatheter aortic valve replacement: the PARTNER (Placement of AoRtic TraNscathetER Valves) trial and registry. JACC Cardiovasc Interv 2015;8(1 Pt A):60–9.

41. Hansson NC, Norgaard BL, Barbanti M, et al. The impact of calcium volume and distribution in aortic root injury related to balloon-expandable transcatheter aortic valve replacement. J Cardiovasc Comput Tomogr 2015;9(5):382–92.

42. Tay EL, Gurvitch R, Wijeysinghe N, et al. Outcome of patients after transcatheter aortic valve embolization. JACC Cardiovasc Interv 2011;4(2):228–34.

43. Detaint D, Lepage L, Himbert D, et al. Determinants of significant paravalvular regurgitation after transcatheter aortic valve: implantation impact of device and annulus discongruence. JACC Cardiovasc Interv 2009;2(9):821–7.

44. Kodali SK, Williams MR, Smith CR, et al. Two-year outcomes after transcatheter or surgical aortic-valve replacement. N Engl J Med 2012;366(18): 1686–95.

45. Sinning JM, Hammerstingl C, Vasa-Nicotera M, et al. Aortic regurgitation index defines severity of peri-prosthetic regurgitation and predicts outcome in patients after transcatheter aortic valve implantation. J Am Coll Cardiol 2012;59(13):1134–41.

46. Binder RK, Webb JG, Willson AB, et al. The impact of integration of a multidetector computed tomography annulus area sizing algorithm on outcomes of transcatheter aortic valve replacement: a prospective, multicenter, controlled trial. J Am Coll Cardiol 2013;62(5):431–8.

47. Feuchtner G, Plank F, Bartel T, et al. Prediction of paravalvular regurgitation after transcatheter aortic valve implantation by computed tomography: value of aortic valve and annular calcification. Ann Thorac Surg 2013;96(5):1574–80.

48. Ewe SH, Ng AC, Schuijf JD, et al. Location and severity of aortic valve calcium and implications for aortic regurgitation after transcatheter aortic valve implantation. Am J Cardiol 2011;108(10): 1470–7.

49. John D, Buellesfeld L, Yuecel S, et al. Correlation of device landing zone calcification and acute procedural success in patients undergoing transcatheter aortic valve implantations with the self-expanding CoreValve prosthesis. JACC Cardiovasc Interv 2010;3(2):233–43.

50. Hansson NC, Leipsic J, Pugliese F, et al. Aortic valve and left ventricular outflow tract calcium volume and distribution in transcatheter aortic valve replacement: influence on the risk of significant paravalvular regurgitation. J Cardiovasc Comput Tomogr 2018;12(4):290–7.

51. Khalique OK, Hahn RT, Gada H, et al. Quantity and location of aortic valve complex calcification predicts severity and location of paravalvular regurgitation and frequency of post-dilation after balloon-expandable transcatheter aortic valve replacement. JACC Cardiovasc Interv 2014;7(8): 885–94.

52. Tops LF, Wood DA, Delgado V, et al. Noninvasive evaluation of the aortic root with multislice computed tomography implications for transcatheter aortic valve replacement. JACC Cardiovasc Imaging 2008;1(3):321–30.

53. Schoenhagen P, Tuzcu EM, Kapadia SR, et al. Three-dimensional imaging of the aortic valve and aortic root with computed tomography: new standards in an era of transcatheter valve repair/implantation. Eur Heart J 2009;30(17):2079–86.

54. Schoenhagen P, Numburi U, Halliburton SS, et al. Three-dimensional imaging in the context of minimally invasive and transcatheter cardiovascular interventions using multi-detector computed tomography: from pre-operative planning to intraoperative guidance. Eur Heart J 2010;31(22): 2727–40.

55. Smith CR, Leon MB, Mack MJ, et al. Transcatheter versus surgical aortic-valve replacement in high-risk patients. N Engl J Med 2011;364(23):2187–98.

56. Eltchaninoff H, Prat A, Gilard M, et al. Transcatheter aortic valve implantation: early results of the FRANCE (FRench Aortic National CoreValve and Edwards) registry. Eur Heart J 2011;32(2):191–7.

57. Rodes-Cabau J, Webb JG, Cheung A, et al. Transcatheter aortic valve implantation for the treatment of severe symptomatic aortic stenosis in patients at very high or prohibitive surgical risk: acute and late outcomes of the multicenter Canadian experience. J Am Coll Cardiol 2010;55(11):1080–90.

58. Ribeiro HB, Nombela-Franco L, Urena M, et al. Coronary obstruction following transcatheter aortic valve implantation: a systematic review. JACC Cardiovasc Interv 2013;6(5):452–61.

59. Ribeiro HB, Webb JG, Makkar RR, et al. Predictive factors, management, and clinical outcomes of coronary obstruction following transcatheter aortic valve implantation: insights from a large multicenter registry. J Am Coll Cardiol 2013;62(17):1552–62.

60. Jabbour RJ, Tanaka A, Finkelstein A, et al. Delayed coronary obstruction after transcatheter aortic valve replacement. J Am Coll Cardiol 2018; 71(14):1513–24.

61. Tamborini G, Fusini L, Gripari P, et al. Feasibility and accuracy of 3DTEE versus CT for the evaluation of aortic valve annulus to left main ostium distance before transcatheter aortic valve implantation. JACC Cardiovasc Imaging 2012; 5(6):579–88.

62. Leon MB, Smith CR, Mack MJ, et al. Transcatheter or surgical aortic-valve replacement in intermediate-risk patients. N Engl J Med 2016; 374(17):1609–20.

63. Adams DH, Popma JJ, Reardon MJ, et al. Transcatheter aortic-valve replacement with a self-expanding prosthesis. N Engl J Med 2014;370(19): 1790–8.

64. Mylotte D, Lefevre T, Sondergaard L, et al. Transcatheter aortic valve replacement in bicuspid aortic valve disease. J Am Coll Cardiol 2014;64(22): 2330–9.

65. Bauer T, Linke A, Sievert H, et al. Comparison of the effectiveness of transcatheter aortic valve implantation in patients with stenotic bicuspid versus tricuspid aortic valves (from the German TAVI Registry). Am J Cardiol 2014;113(3):518–21.

66. Al Emam AR, Chamsi-Pasha M, Pavlides G. Ostial coronary occlusion during TAVR in bicuspid aortic valve, should we redefine what is a safe ostial height? Int J Cardiol 2016;212:288–9.

67. Frangieh AH, Kasel AM. TAVI in bicuspid aortic valves 'made easy'. Eur Heart J 2017;38(16): 1177–81.

68. Nkomo VT, Enriquez-Sarano M, Ammash NM, et al. Bicuspid aortic valve associated with aortic dilatation: a community-based study. Arterioscler Thromb Vasc Biol 2003;23(2):351–6.

69. Keane MG, Wiegers SE, Plappert T, et al. Bicuspid aortic valves are associated with aortic dilatation

out of proportion to coexistent valvular lesions. Circulation 2000;102(19 Suppl 3):Iii35–9.

70. Pachulski RT, Weinberg AL, Chan KL. Aortic aneurysm in patients with functionally normal or minimally stenotic bicuspid aortic valve. Am J Cardiol 1991;67(8):781–2.

71. Himbert D, Pontnau F, Messika-Zeitoun D, et al. Feasibility and outcomes of transcatheter aortic valve implantation in high-risk patients with stenotic bicuspid aortic valves. Am J Cardiol 2012;110(6):877–83.

72. Hayashida K, Bouvier E, Lefevre T, et al. Transcatheter aortic valve implantation for patients with severe bicuspid aortic valve stenosis. Circ Cardiovasc Interv 2013;6(3):284–91.

73. Sievers HH, Schmidtke C. A classification system for the bicuspid aortic valve from 304 surgical specimens. J Thorac Cardiovasc Surg 2007;133(5):1226–33.

74. Philip F, Faza NN, Schoenhagen P, et al. Aortic annulus and root characteristics in severe aortic stenosis due to bicuspid aortic valve and tricuspid aortic valves: implications for transcatheter aortic valve therapies. Catheter Cardiovasc Interv 2015;86(2):E88–98.

75. Yoon SH, Lefevre T, Ahn JM, et al. Transcatheter aortic valve replacement with early- and new-generation devices in bicuspid aortic valve stenosis. J Am Coll Cardiol 2016;68(11):1195–205.

76. Gurvitch R, Wood DA, Leipsic J, et al. Multislice computed tomography for prediction of optimal angiographic deployment projections during transcatheter aortic valve implantation. JACC Cardiovasc Interv 2010;3(11):1157–65.

77. Kurra V, Kapadia SR, Tuzcu EM, et al. Pre-procedural imaging of aortic root orientation and dimensions: comparison between X-ray angiographic planar imaging and 3-dimensional multidetector row computed tomography. JACC Cardiovasc Interv 2010;3(1):105–13.

78. Kim MS, Bracken J, Nijhof N, et al. Integrated 3D echo-X-ray navigation to predict optimal angiographic deployment projections for TAVR. JACC Cardiovasc Imaging 2014;7(8):847–8.

79. Bufton KA, Augoustides JG, Cobey FC. Anesthesia for transfemoral aortic valve replacement in North America and Europe. J Cardiothorac Vasc Anesth 2013;27(1):46–9.

80. Aitkenhead AR. Injuries associated with anaesthesia. A global perspective. Br J Anaesth 2005;95(1):95–109.

81. Guarracino F, Landoni G. Con: transcatheter aortic valve implantation should not be performed under general anesthesia. J Cardiothorac Vasc Anesth 2012;26(4):736–9.

82. Husser O, Fujita B, Hengstenberg C, et al. Conscious sedation versus general anesthesia in transcatheter aortic valve replacement: the German aortic valve registry. JACC Cardiovasc Interv 2018;11(6):567–78.

83. Ehret C, Rossaint R, Foldenauer AC, et al. Is local anaesthesia a favourable approach for transcatheter aortic valve implantation? A systematic review and meta-analysis comparing local and general anaesthesia. BMJ open 2017;7(9):e016321.

84. Hyman MC, Vemulapalli S, Szeto WY, et al. Conscious sedation versus general anesthesia for transcatheter aortic valve replacement: insights from the National Cardiovascular Data Registry Society of Thoracic Surgeons/American College of Cardiology Transcatheter Valve Therapy Registry. Circulation 2017;136(22):2132–40.

85. Reardon MJ, Van Mieghem NM, Popma JJ, et al. Surgical or transcatheter aortic-valve replacement in intermediate-risk patients. N Engl J Med 2017;376(14):1321–31.

86. Tay EL, Gurvitch R, Wijesinghe N, et al. A high-risk period for cerebrovascular events exists after transcatheter aortic valve implantation. JACC Cardiovasc Interv 2011;4(12):1290–7.

87. Miller DC, Blackstone EH, Mack MJ, et al. Transcatheter (TAVR) versus surgical (AVR) aortic valve replacement: occurrence, hazard, risk factors, and consequences of neurologic events in the PARTNER trial. J Thorac Cardiovasc Surg 2012;143(4):832–43.e13.

88. Alassar A, Soppa G, Edsell M, et al. Incidence and mechanisms of cerebral ischemia after transcatheter aortic valve implantation compared with surgical aortic valve replacement. Ann Thorac Surg 2015;99(3):802–8.

89. Van Mieghem NM, Chieffo A, Dumonteil N, et al. Trends in outcome after transfemoral transcatheter aortic valve implantation. Am Heart J 2013;165(2):183–92.

90. Carroll JD, Vemulapalli S, Dai D, et al. Procedural experience for transcatheter aortic valve replacement and relation to outcomes: the STS/ACC TVT registry. J Am Coll Cardiol 2017;70(1):29–41.

91. Ndunda PM, Vindhyal MR, Muutu TM, et al. Clinical outcomes of sentinel cerebral protection system use during transcatheter aortic valve replacement: a systematic review and meta-analysis. Cardiovasc Revasc Med 2019. https://doi.org/10.1016/j.carrev.2019.04.023. [Epub ahead of print].

92. Kotronias RA, Kwok CS, George S, et al. Transcatheter aortic valve implantation with or without percutaneous coronary artery revascularization strategy: a systematic review and meta-analysis. J Am Heart Assoc 2017;6(6) [pii:e005960].

93. Chieffo A, Giustino G, Spagnolo P, et al. Routine screening of coronary artery disease with computed tomographic coronary angiography in place of invasive coronary angiography in patients

undergoing transcatheter aortic valve replacement. Circ Cardiovasc Interv 2015;8(7):e002025.

94. Vahanian A, Alfieri O, Al-Attar N, et al. Transcatheter valve implantation for patients with aortic stenosis: a position statement from the European association of cardio-thoracic surgery (EACTS) and the European Society of Cardiology (ESC), in collaboration with the European Association of Percutaneous Cardiovascular Interventions (EAPCI). EuroIntervention 2008;4(2):193–9.

95. Goel SS, Ige M, Tuzcu EM, et al. Severe aortic stenosis and coronary artery disease—implications for management in the transcatheter aortic valve replacement era: a comprehensive review. J Am Coll Cardiol 2013;62(1):1–10.

96. Abdel-Wahab M, Mostafa AE, Geist V, et al. Comparison of outcomes in patients having isolated transcatheter aortic valve implantation versus combined with preprocedural percutaneous coronary intervention. Am J Cardiol 2012;109(4):581–6.

97. Griese DP, Reents W, Toth A, et al. Concomitant coronary intervention is associated with poorer early and late clinical outcomes in selected elderly patients receiving transcatheter aortic valve implantation. Eur J Cardiothorac Surg 2014;46(1):e1–7.

98. Mostafa AE, Geist V, Abdel-Wahab M. Ad-hoc percutaneous coronary intervention and transcatheter aortic valve implantation as a combined transfemoral procedure. J Invasive Cardiol 2011;23(5):E102–5.

99. Babaliaros VC, Liff D, Chen EP, et al. Can balloon aortic valvuloplasty help determine appropriate transcatheter aortic valve size? JACC Cardiovasc Interv 2008;1(5):580–6.

100. Babaliaros VC, Junagadhwalla Z, Lerakis S, et al. Use of balloon aortic valvuloplasty to size the aortic annulus before implantation of a balloon-expandable transcatheter heart valve. JACC Cardiovasc Interv 2010;3(1):114–8.

101. Hahn RT, Nicoara A, Kapadia S, et al. Echocardiographic imaging for transcatheter aortic valve replacement. J Am Soc Echocardiogr 2018;31(4):405–33.

102. Khan JM, Dvir D, Greenbaum AB, et al. Transcatheter laceration of aortic leaflets to prevent coronary obstruction during transcatheter aortic valve replacement: concept to first-in-human. JACC Cardiovasc Interv 2018;11(7):677–89.

103. Khan JM, Greenbaum AB, Babaliaros VC, et al. The BASILICA trial: prospective multicenter investigation of intentional leaflet laceration to prevent TAVR coronary obstruction. JACC Cardiovasc Interv 2019;12(13):1240.

104. Jilaihawi H, Doctor N, Kashif M, et al. Aortic annular sizing for transcatheter aortic valve replacement using cross-sectional 3-dimensional transesophageal echocardiography. J Am Coll Cardiol 2013;61(9):908–16.

105. Smith LA, Dworakowski R, Bhan A, et al. Real-time three-dimensional transesophageal echocardiography adds value to transcatheter aortic valve implantation. J Am Soc Echocardiogr 2013;26(4):359–69.

106. Altiok E, Koos R, Schröder J, et al. Comparison of two-dimensional and three-dimensional imaging techniques for measurement of aortic annulus diameters before transcatheter aortic valve implantation. Heart 2011;97(19):1578–84.

107. Hahn R, Khalique O, Williams MR, et al. Predicting paravalvular regurgitation following transcatheter valve replacement: utility of a novel method for three-dimensional echocardiographic measurements of the aortic annulus. J Am Soc Echocardiogr 2013;26(9):1043–52.

Transcatheter Aortic Valve Replacement
Procedure and Outcomes

Erwan Salaun, MD, PhD*, Philippe Pibarot, DVM, PhD,
Josep Rodés-Cabau, MD

KEYWORDS

- Aortic stenosis • Interventional cardiology • Outcomes • Paravalvular regurgitation
- Structural valve deterioration • Transcatheter aortic valve replacement • Transcatheter heart valve

KEY POINTS

- Transcatheter aortic valve replacement (TAVR) was initially only used in patients with severe symptomatic aortic stenosis and prohibitive risk for surgical aortic valve replacement (SAVR).
- Subsequently, this procedure was extended to patients with high and intermediate surgical risk and was reported as superior to SAVR in low-risk patients.
- Procedural outcomes have been improved owing to assessments by heart teams, the development of safer devices and delivery systems, and a better knowledge in the implantation techniques and patient management.
- Long-term durability of transcatheter heart valves remains to be confirmed to allow generalization of TAVR to low-risk patients.

INTRODUCTION

Since 2002 and the first-in-human transcatheter aortic valve replacement (TAVR) in Rouen (France),[1] this procedure has expanded rapidly worldwide. Initially, this procedure was only used in patients with severe symptomatic aortic stenosis (AS) with prohibitive risk for surgical aortic valve replacement (SAVR). Subsequently, TAVR was extended to patients with high and intermediate surgical risk.[2,3] Recently, the results of randomized trials in patients at low surgical risk showed superiority or noninferiority of TAVR versus SAVR in this population, which represents most patients with severe AS.[4,5] Thus, the number of TAVR procedures, estimated in 2019 at 144,000, is expected to double by 2025.[6] This article presents the evolution and current status of TAVR, with respect to the different types of devices and procedures as well as its outcomes.

RANDOMIZED TRIALS OF TRANSCATHETER AORTIC VALVE REPLACEMENT VERSUS SURGICAL AORTIC VALVE REPLACEMENT

After years of ex vivo testing and animal implantation of transcatheter heart valves (THVs), the first-in-human TAVR was performed by Cribier and colleagues[1] in Rouen, France, in 2002. This first THV consisted of 3 bovine pericardial leaflets mounted within a tubular, slotted, stainless steel, balloon-expandable stent,[1] and was implanted in a 57-year-old man with severe bicuspid AS, severely

Disclosure: Dr E. Salaun has nothing to disclose. Dr P. Pibarot received research grants from Edwards Lifesciences and Medtronic for echo corelab analyses in transcatheter aortic valve replacement. Dr J. Rodés-Cabau has received institutional research grants from Edwards Lifesciences.
Institut Universitaire de Cardiologie et de Pneumologie de Québec, Québec Heart & Lung Institute, Laval University, 2725 Chemin Sainte-Foy, Québec, Québec G1V-4G5, Canada
* Corresponding author.
E-mail address: erwan.salaun@criucpq.ulaval.ca

depressed left ventricle ejection fraction, and cardiogenic shock who was inoperable.[1]

After this first human experience, several human cases and series were reported in the following years. In 2010, the first randomized trial (PARTNER [Placement of AoRTic TraNscathetER Valve Trial] 1B) was published and showed a superiority of TAVR performed with the first generation of balloon-expandable THVs (Edwards SAPIEN) compared with conservative treatment in patients with symptomatic severe AS and prohibitive risk for SAVR.[7,8] The use of the first generation of self-expanding THVs (CoreValve) during TAVR was also reported to be safe and effective in patients with symptomatic severe AS at prohibitive surgical risk.[9,10]

Subsequently, randomized trials comparing TAVR with SAVR in high-surgical-risk patients with severe symptomatic AS showed (1) a noninferiority of TAVR performed with balloon-expandable THVs (Edwards SAPIEN) (PARTNER 1A trial)[11]; and (2) a superiority of TAVR versus SAVR performed with the first generation of self-expanding THVs (CoreValve) (CoreValve US High-Risk Pivotal Trial).[12]

A few years later, randomized trials (PARTNER 2A and SURTAVI [Surgical Replacement and Transcatheter Aortic Valve Implantation]) showed that TAVR, with both self-expanding and balloon-expandable THVs, was a noninferior alternative to SAVR in patients with severe symptomatic AS with intermediate surgical risk.[13,14] Moreover, outcomes of TAVR seem to be better than SAVR when TAVR was performed via the transfemoral access compared with transapical or transaortic routes and with the third generation compared with first and second generations of THVs.[11,15]

In 2019, the randomized EVOLUT Low Risk and PARTNER 3 trials reported a noninferiority of TAVR with self-expanding THV compared with SAVR in low-risk patients with severe AS,[4] whereas the PARTNER 3 trials showed a superiority of TAVR with the SAPIEN 3 THV implanted via the transfemoral approach.[5]

GUIDELINES FOR THE SELECTION OF TRANSCATHETER AORTIC VALVE REPLACEMENT VERSUS SURGICAL AORTIC VALVE REPLACEMENT

The strong body of evidence established by the randomized trials presented earlier have formed the basis of the current guidelines recommendations for the selection of TAVR versus SAVR (**Fig. 1**). In patients considered to have symptomatic severe AS and to be potential candidates for TAVR, the guidelines strongly recommend (class I) an evaluation of these patients by the heart team to confirm the indication of aortic valve replacement (AVR) and determine the optimal type of AVR: SAVR or TAVR (see **Fig. 1**).[2] This heart team generally includes cardiologists; cardiac surgeons; imaging specialists; anesthetists; and, if needed, general practitioners, geriatricians, or intensive care specialists. The guidelines also support the concept of heart valve centers to deliver optimal care to patients with complex heart disease, including

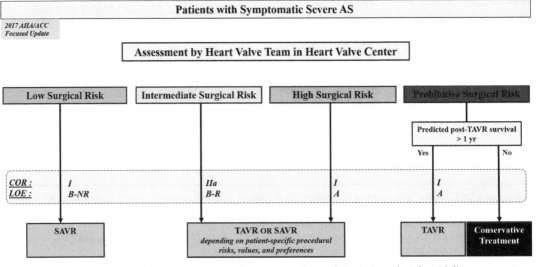

Fig. 1. Current American Heart Association (AHA)/American College of Cardiology (ACC) guidelines on management of symptomatic patients with severe AS. COR, class of recommendations; LOE, level of evidence; NR, nonrandomized trial; R, randomized trial.

diagnosis, follow-up, therapeutic decision making, and performance of valve interventions.[2,3] TAVR has evolved as the treatment of choice for elderly patients with symptomatic severe AS who are at high or extreme risk for surgery (see **Fig. 1**).[2,16] TAVR is recommended (class I) for symptomatic patients with severe AS, prohibitive risk for SAVR, and predicted post-TAVR survival longer than 1 year (see **Fig. 1**). TAVR or SAVR is recommended (class I) for symptomatic patients with severe AS and high risk for SAVR, depending on patient-specific procedural risks and patient's preferences (see **Fig. 1**). TAVR is a reasonable alternative to SAVR (class IIa) for symptomatic patients with severe AS and intermediate surgical risk. In light of the recently published trial in low-risk patients,[4,5] it is likely that the next edition of the guidelines will conclude that TAVR is also a reasonable alternative to SAVR in patients with low surgical risk. Valve-in-valve TAVR is reasonable (class IIa) for symptomatic patients with bioprosthetic valve stenosis or regurgitation at high or prohibitive risk for reoperation, and in whom improvement in hemodynamics is anticipated.[2]

PROCEDURES
Type of Transcatheter Heart Valve

Historically, 2 main types of THV systems have been used: balloon-expandable (SAPIEN, SAPIEN XT, SAPIEN 3, Edwards Lifesciences; Irvine, CA) and self-expanding (CoreValve, EVOLUT R, EVOLUT PRO; Medtronic, Inc., Minneapolis, MN, USA) THVs (see **Fig. 2**; **Fig. 3**). Other catheter-based delivery systems have also been recently developed: inflatable rings (Direct Flow THV; Direct Flow Medical), and mechanically expandable THV (Lotus THV, Boston Scientific). During the TAVR evolution, the design and properties of THVs have been improved, and delivery catheter profile have been reduced (see **Figs. 2** and **3**). These evolutions have facilitated the THV implantation (ability to recapture, reposition, or retrieve) and decreased the rate of procedural complications. The SAPIEN XT/SAPIEN 3 and CoreValve/EVOLUT have the most robust evidence and are thus the most frequently used in clinical practice.[4,5,13–15]

The SAPIEN family THVs (Edwards Lifesciences; Irvine, CA) consists of bovine pericardial leaflets sewn within a balloon-expandable

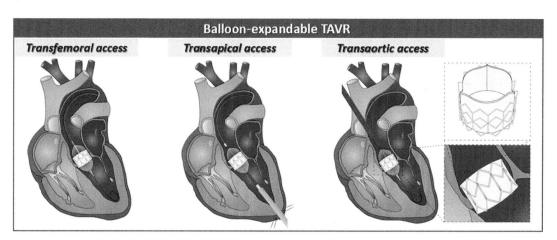

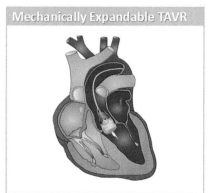

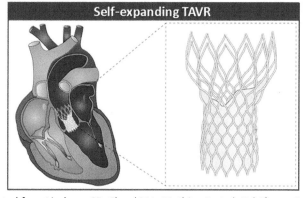

Fig. 2. Different types of TAVR procedures. (*Adapted from* Lindman BR, Clavel MA, Mathieu P, et al. Calcific aortic stenosis. Nat Rev Dis Primers 2016;2:16006; with permission.)

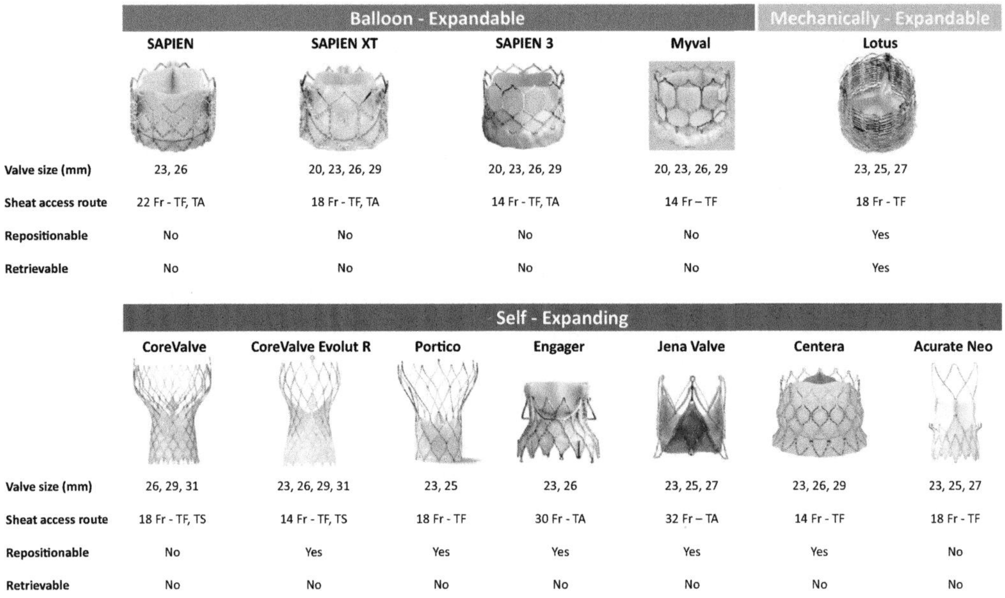

Fig. 3. Different models of THVs. TA, transapical; TF, transfemoral; TS, tanssubclavian.

	Balloon - Expandable				Mechanically - Expandable
	SAPIEN	SAPIEN XT	SAPIEN 3	Myval	Lotus
Valve size (mm)	23, 26	20, 23, 26, 29	20, 23, 26, 29	20, 23, 26, 29	23, 25, 27
Sheat access route	22 Fr - TF, TA	18 Fr - TF, TA	14 Fr - TF, TA	14 Fr – TF	18 Fr - TF
Repositionable	No	No	No	No	Yes
Retrievable	No	No	No	No	Yes

	Self - Expanding						
	CoreValve	CoreValve Evolut R	Portico	Engager	Jena Valve	Centera	Acurate Neo
Valve size (mm)	26, 29, 31	23, 26, 29, 31	23, 25	23, 26	23, 25, 27	23, 26, 29	23, 25, 27
Sheat access route	18 Fr - TF, TS	14 Fr - TF, TS	18 Fr - TF	30 Fr - TA	32 Fr – TA	14 Fr - TF	18 Fr - TF
Repositionable	No	Yes	Yes	Yes	Yes	Yes	No
Retrievable	No	No	No	No	No	No	No

cobalt-chromium stent and represent the most frequently implanted balloon-expandable THVs. The last iteration of this THV, named SAPIEN 3 THV, has an additional feature: a polyethylene terephthalate outer skirt that functions as a blood-soaked sponge to reduce paravalvular regurgitation (PVR) (see **Fig. 3**). The CoreValve family THVs are the most frequently implanted self-expanding THVs and consist of a porcine pericardial leaflet sutured in a self-expanding nitinol support frame (see **Figs. 2** and **3**). The characteristic feature of CoreValve devices is the supraannular positioning and functioning of the 3 leaflets. The last iteration of this type of devices, named EVOLUT PRO, has a pericardial wrap around the lower part of the stent to reduce PVR (see **Fig. 3**).

Access

Although the first human case was performed by an anterograde transseptal approach from the right femoral vein,[1] an arterial retrograde implantation strategy was then quickly adopted. The arterial transfemoral access is safer than other arterial accesses,[17] and is nowadays used in more than 90% of TAVR procedures.[14] The assessment of femoral accessibility is generally performed by multislice computed tomography (CT) with contrast injection and should be used to examine the presence of arterial tortuosity, significant atherosclerotic calcification, and femoral and iliofemoral diameters ($\geq$5 mm for a 14-Fr delivery system).[18,19] Three-dimensional

transesophageal echocardiography (TEE) or MRI are reliable alternatives to CT when it cannot be performed.[20,21] In the initial clinical TAVR experience, transfemoral access was performed via surgical cut-down and a large proportion of patients underwent alternative nontransfemoral access.[22] However, in recent years, with the improvements in technology, the increased experience of the clinicians, and the use of specific vascular closure devices, the fully percutaneous approach has become the preferred strategy.[23] Alternate vascular access routes can be performed, but require a systematic surgical approach: transapical,[24] transaxillary,[25] direct aortic,[26] transcaval,[27] and transcarotid.[28] The transcarotid vascular access seems to be associated with clinical benefit compared with the more invasive transapical or transaortic strategies.[29]

Heart Valve Center and Implantation Room

TAVR should be performed in experienced heart valve centers, with cardiothoracic surgery on site, after careful assessment of the patients and their clinical, hemodynamic, and anatomic conditions by the heart team.[30,31] Procedures may be performed in surgical operating room, hybrid room, or catheter laboratory, depending on the selected TAVR access and the local resources and practices.

At present, the TAVR procedure via transfemoral access and no anticipated complication is preferably performed in a catheter laboratory with a minimalist strategy (ie, local anesthesia, minimal conscious sedation, fully percutaneous access site entry and closure, and monitoring by transthoracic echocardiography).[32,33] This minimalist strategy can be performed with minimal morbidity and mortality, equivalent effectiveness, and shorter length of stay, and decreases resource use and hospitals costs.[34] However, when surgical access or general anesthesia are required, or in TAVR with specific issues, a hybrid room is preferred.

Prosthesis Implantation

Technique of implantation is related to the access route and the THV selected for the TAVR procedure. However, all THV implantations are performed with the aid of aortography and under fluoroscopy guidance. In some cases, TEE guidance is also required. Rapid ventricular pacing (180–220 beat/min) by a temporary pacing wire introduced into the right ventricle (jugular or femoral vein access) is required during balloon aortic valvuloplasty (predilatation), balloon-expandable THV deployment, and postdilatation. Self-expanding THVs may not routinely require ventricular pacing during deployment. Although predilatation was systematically performed before THV implantation with the first generations of THVs, this procedural step is not performed systematically with new-generation devices. Postdilatation is performed when significant PVR is present after the THV implantation.

Procedural Complications

Potential adverse events associated with the TAVR procedure may occur and should be avoided, recognized, and managed adequately.[35] Access and delivery complications are related to the approach selected and include (1) arterial peripheral injury (arterial dissection and perforation) and (2) apical access issues (lung injury, pneumothorax, pleural bleeding, pseudoaneurysm).[35] The TAVR procedure may also be complicated by improper THV positioning, THV embolization, need for a second valve, coronary obstruction, mitral valve injury, aortic annulus rupture, aortic dissection, cardiac tamponade, and cardiac perforation.[35] The valve academic research consortium-2 criteria provide standardized definitions of each complication and a universal classification.[36]

Diagnostic strategy is based on clinical symptoms, systematic fluoroscopic and angiographic monitoring, and echocardiographic assessment when needed.[35,37]

Although these procedural complications are associated with high morbidity and mortality,[37] the incidence of these complications is low and continuously decreased with (1) the learning curve and the increasing experience of heart teams,[38] (2) the high procedural volume of the heart valve centers,[39] and (3) the use of new generations of catheter delivery systems and devices.[40] Recent trials showed that procedural complications are rare in patients with low surgical risk (**Table 1**).

ECHOCARDIOGRAPHIC OUTCOMES

Transvalvular pressure gradients and aortic valve areas are generally better with TAVR versus SAVR and within SAVR with self-expanding THVs compared with balloon-expandable THVs (**Table 2**).[4,5,11,14] The superiority of self-expanding THVs seems to be related to the supra-annular position of the valve leaflets. This advantage is not present with the last iteration of the Edwards devices (SAPIEN 3), which have shown higher aortic mean gradient and less aortic valve area compared with surgical bioprosthesis.

Table 1
Procedural complications of transcatheter aortic valve replacement in low-risk patients

Procedural Complications	PARTNER 3[5]	EVOLUT Low Risk[4]	LRT[52,75]	NOTION[51]
≥2 THVs implanted (%)	0.2	1.2	2.0	2.8
Valve embolization (%)	0.0	—	—	—
Annulus rupture (%)	0.2	—	—	—
Aortic dissection (%)	0.0	—	—	—
Coronary obstruction (%)	0.2	0.9	0.5	0.0
Cardiac perforation (%)	0.2	—	—	1.4
Concomitant or staged PCI (%)	6.5	6.9	—	0.0
Conversion to surgery (%)	0.2	0.6	0.5	2.1

Abbreviation: LRT, Low Risk TAVR; NOTION, Nordic Aortic Valve Intervention; PCI, percutaneous coronary intervention; THVs, transcatheter heart valves.

Table 2
Echocardiographic data at 30 days after transcatheter aortic valve replacement in low-risk patients

Echocardiographic Outcomes	PARTNER 3[5]	EVOLUT Low Risk[4]	LRT[a,52,75]	NOTION[a,51]
Aortic valve area (cm²)	1.7	2.2	1.83	1.7
Mean gradient (mm Hg)	12.8	8.4	13.8	12.2
PPM moderate (%)	53.8	9.9	—	—
PPM severe (%)	8.3	1.1	—	—
Total AR mild (%)	—	36.1	23.7	61.3
Total AR ≥ moderate (%)	—	3.5	2.0	15.3
Paravalvular AR mild (%)	28.7	36.0	—	—
Paravalvular AR ≥ moderate (%)	0.8	3.4	1.0	—

Abbreviations: AR, aortic regurgitation; PPM, patient prosthesis mismatch.
 [a] Echocardiographic parameters at discharge for the LRT Trial and at 3 months for the NOTION trial.

Paravalvular Regurgitation

In the early TAVR experience, PVR was a common complication after TAVR, ranging from 20% to 80% for mild PVR,[41,42] and from 5% to 22% for moderate and severe PVR.[24,43] With new-generation devices, the incidence of PVR has markedly decreased, with a rate of greater than or equal to moderate PVR between 0% and 5% (see **Table 2**).[44] The association of PVR with worse outcomes depends on its degree of severity.[45] Moderate or greater PVR is consistently associated with an increased risk of all-cause mortality, with hazard ratios between 1.09 and 4.72.[46] The association between mild PVR and worse outcomes is inconsistent depending on the studies, and, if present, is weaker than for moderate/severe PVR. Doppler echocardiography is the primary imaging modality to assess the severity of PVR.[47] However, aortography, measurement of blood closure time adenosine diphosphate (representing the loss of high-molecular-weight multimers of von Willebrand factor when PVR is significant), and the assessment of the hemodynamic aortic regurgitation index may be useful to assess the presence and severity of PVR immediately after THV implantation.[45,48] Corrective procedures (balloon postdilatation, valve-in-valve procedures) should be performed when significant PVR is present.[44] Cardiac MRI using phase velocity imaging is also a reliable alternative to echocardiography when the assessment of PVR severity remains doubtful after a TAVR procedure and/or when there is a discordance between the transthoracic echocardiogram (TTE) assessment of PVR severity and the patient's symptomatic status.[49] A regurgitant fraction of 30% defines a moderate or greater PVR and is associated with a 2-fold increase in mortality and rehospitalization,[50] and

thus should lead to delayed corrective procedures (balloon postdilatation, valve-in-valve procedure, percutaneous closure).[44]

CLINICAL OUTCOMES
All-Cause and Cardiovascular Mortality

A recent meta-analysis by Barbanti and colleagues[40] of 37 studies and including 10,822 patients with high or intermediate risk undergoing transfemoral TAVR with new THV generations reported a 30-day all-cause and cardiovascular death rate of 2.2% (95% confidence interval [CI], 1.6%–2.8%) and 1.6% (95% CI, 0.9%–2.3%), respectively. These rates were even lower in low-risk patients,[51,52] and were less than or equal to 0.5% in the recent randomized trials (**Table 3**).[4,5] In high-risk patients and in patients contraindicated to SAVR, freedom from all-cause mortality at 5 years ranges from 20% to 55% (**Table 4**). In intermediate-risk patients, the 2-year all-cause and cardiovascular mortalities range from 11.4% to 16.7% and 7.7% and 10.1%, respectively.[13,14] In low-risk patients, the 1-year all-cause and cardiovascular death rates are low, ranging respectively from 1% to 3% and 0.8% to 1.7% (see **Table 3**).[4,5,52]

Stroke

In the meta-analysis of Barbanti and colleagues,[40] the pooled estimate rates of any stroke and major/disabling stroke were 2.6% (95% CI, 2.0%–3.3%) and 0.9% (95% CI, 0.2%–1.6%) at 30 days after TAVR, respectively. In patients with prohibitive risk or at high risk, the 1-year rate of any stroke is from 7% to 11%,[7,9,12] and major stroke occurs in close to 5% of patients after TAVR. Despite a higher rate of any stroke, no significant difference

Table 3
Clinical outcomes of transcatheter aortic valve replacement in low-risk patients

Clinical Outcomes	30-d Outcomes				1-y Outcomes			
	PARTNER 3[5]	EVOLUT Low Risk[4]	LRT[52,75]	NOTION[51]	PARTNER 3[5]	EVOLUT Low Risk[4]	LRT[52,75]	NOTION[51]
Death from any cause (%)	0.4	0.5	0.0	2.1	1.0	2.4	3.0	4.9
Cardiovascular death (%)	0.4	0.5	0.0	2.1	0.8	1.7	1.0	4.3
All stroke (%)	0.6	3.4	0.5	1.4	1.2	4.1	2.1	2.9
Disabling stroke (%)	0.0	0.5	0.0	—	0.2	0.8	0.0	—
Nondisabling stroke (%)	0.6	3.0	0.5	—	1.0	3.4	2.1	—
Transient ischemic attack	0.0	0.6	—	1.4	1.0	1.7	—	2.1
Major vascular complication (%)	2.2	3.8	3.0	5.6	2.6	3.8	—	—
Life-threatening or disabling bleeding (%)	1.2	2.4	3.0	11.3	2.8	3.2	—	—
Myocardial infarction	1.0	0.9	0.0	2.8	1.2	1.7	1.0	3.5
Acute kidney injury stage II or III (%)	0.4	0.9	0.0[b]	0.7	—	—	—	—
New permanent pacemaker (%)	6.5	17.4	6.5	34.1	7.3	19.4	7.3	38.0
New LBBB (%)	22.0	—	—	—	23.7	—	—	—
New-onset atrial fibrillation (%)	5.0	7.7	4.5	16.9	7.0	9.8	6.3	21.2
Aortic valve reintervention (%)	0.0	0.4	0.0	—	0.6	0.7	1.0	—
Endocarditis (%)	0.0	0.1	0.0	0.7	0.2	0.2	1.0	2.9
Valve thrombosis (%)	0.2	0.1	7.4[c]	—	1.0	0.2	—	—
Valve-related or procedure-related hospitalization including heart failure (%)	3.4	1.2[a]	0.0	—	7.3	3.2[a]	6.8	—

Abbreviation: LBBB, left bundle branch block.
[a] Rehospitalization for heart failure for the EVOLUT Low Risk trial.
[b] Acute kidney injury stage 3 for the LRT trial.
[c] Valve thrombosis is defined by hypoattenuation affecting motion assessed by systematic computed tomography at 30 days after transcatheter valve replacement in the LRT trial.

in terms of major stroke is observed compared with a randomized cohort of patients who underwent SAVR.[11,12] However, any stroke and major stroke occur more frequently after TAVR when alternative access was used.[10] In patients at intermediate risk, the 2-year rates of any stroke (9.5% vs 6.2%) and disabling stroke (6.2% vs 2.6%) are higher in patients implanted with a

Table 4
Structural valve deterioration following transcatheter aortic valve replacement

Study	Patients n	Valves	Median Follow-up Years	Freedom from All-Cause Mortality at 5 y (%)	Structural Valve Deterioration
Eltchaninoff et al,[76] 2018	378	Cribier-Edwards n = 79 SAPIEN n = 83 SAPIEN XT n = 216	3.1	31.7	$\geq$ Stage 2 or moderate: 3.2% at 8 y
Holy et al,[77] 2018	152	CoreValve	5.0	50.0	$\geq$ Stage 3 or severe: 7.9% (actuarial) and 4.5% (actual) at 8 y
Deutsch et al,[78] 2018	300	CoreValve n = 214 SAPIEN n = 86	7.1	40.2	$\geq$ Stage 2 or moderate: 14.9% at 7 y
Barbanti et al,[79] 2018	288	CoreValve n = 238 SAPIEN XT n = 48	6.7	54.7	Stage 2 or moderate: 5.9% at 8 y Stage 3 or severe: 6.9% at 8 y
Kumar et al,[80] 2018	276	Cribier-Edwards n = 7 SAPIEN n = 244 SAPIEN XT n = 25	3.8	44.6	$\geq$ Stage 2 or moderate: 8.3% at 5 y
Didier et al,[81] 2018	4201	SAPIEN or SAPIEN XT n = 2774 CoreValve n = 1413	—	39.2	Stage 2 or moderate: 13.3% at 5 y Stage 3 or severe: 2.5% at 5 y
Gleason et al,[82] 2018	391	CoreValve	4.2	44.7	Stage 2 or moderate: 9.2% at 5 y Stage 3 or severe: 0.8% at 5 y
Durand et al,[83] 2019	1403	Cribier-Edwards n = 77 SAPIEN n = 475 SAPIEN XT n = 512 CoreValve n = 199 Jena Valve n = 7	3.9	18.6 at 7 y	Stage 2 or moderate: 7.0% at 7 y Stage 3 or severe: 4.2% at 7 y

balloon-expandable THV compared with those implanted with a self-expanding THV.[13,14] However, the occurrence of any stroke and disabling stroke is lower using the new generations of balloon-expandable THV (SAPIEN 3) compared with the previous iteration (SAPIEN XT).[15] This finding is confirmed in patients at low risk implanted with the SAPIEN 3, in whom any stroke and disabling stroke occur in only 1.2% and 0.2% of the patients at 1 year post-TAVR (see **Table 3**).[5] The incidence of stroke post-TAVR is lower in low-surgical-risk populations, whatever the type of THV.[4,5]

A transcatheter cerebral embolic protection strategy using transcatheter filters or deflection devices was tested during TAVR. Although the use of neuroprotection devices is safe and captures embolic debris in 99% of patients, this procedure did not reduce the occurrence of new lesions on MRI, and did not improve neurocognitive function post-TAVR.[53]

Conduction Disturbance and Pacemaker Implantation

Conduction disturbances that can lead to permanent pacemaker implantation remain a common complication after TAVR.[54] New onset of left bundle branch block (LBBB) has been reported in about one-fourth (4%–65%) of patients after first-generation THV implantation, with a higher incidence after self-expanding CoreValve THV implantation.[54] LBBB rates of 12% to 22% have been reported with the new generation of Edwards SAPIEN 3 (see **Table 3**).[54] The type (CoreValve vs Edwards SAPIEN) and size (large vs small) of THV, deep implantation, and valve overexpansion are the main predictors of LBBB.[54]

Patients with baseline right bundle block branch (RBBB) may be at high risk for high-degree atrioventricular block and/or sudden cardiac death.[55] Baseline RBBB and the increase in PR length after TAVR are independent predictors of late

(≥48 hours) advanced conduction disturbances requiring permanent pacemaker implantation after TAVR.[56] New-onset LBBB is associated with worse outcomes following TAVR. Permanent pacemaker implantation after TAVR is also associated with deleterious effects on left ventricular ejection fraction and increase in the risk of heart failure at midterm or long-term follow-up.

Functional Improvement

A review including 20 studies and 2775 high-risk patients showed that functional capacity and health-related quality of life improved substantially post-TAVR irrespective of the measure used.[57] Functional status is also improved in intermediate-risk patients, with 94% of patients in New York Heart Association (NYHA) function class I or II at 1 year after TAVR.[15] Compared with SAVR, intermediate-risk patients who underwent TAVR had fewer cardiac symptoms and better improvement in quality of life at 30 days postintervention.[13,14] However, the frequency of cardiac symptoms and the quality of life did not differ significantly at later time points.[13,14]

In low-risk patients, from 68% to 80% were in NYHA function class I at 30 days after TAVR, and from 97% to 99% were NYHA function class I or II at 1 year after TAVR (**Fig. 4**). There was also an improvement in quality of life as shown by a significant increase in mean Kansas City Cardiomyopathy Questionnaire (KCCQ) from baseline to 1 year post-TAVR (see **Fig. 4**). The improvement in markers of functional status and quality of life

(NYHA class, 6-minute walk-test distance, KCCQ score) was also more rapid in low-risk patients who underwent TAVR compared with those undergoing SAVR.[4,5]

Transcatheter Aortic Valve Replacement Endocarditis

In high-risk patients, infective endocarditis is a rare complication after TAVR (incidence at 1 year, 0.50%),[58] and the incidence is similar to that reported for surgical prosthetic valve endocarditis.[59] However, infective endocarditis is associated with high rates of morbidity and mortality, and only 15% of the patients benefited from surgery to treat the endocarditic lesions.[59] The reported in-hospital and 2-year mortalities are 36% and 67%.[59] Endocarditis in TAVR is characterized by some specific issues: (1) staphylococci (45%) and enterococci (21%) are the most frequent pathogens[58]; (ii) conventional modified Duke criteria have a low diagnostic value[60]; (3) valve leaflet thickening and increased transvalvular gradient (obstructive pattern) are frequent, whereas vegetations and leaflet destruction with associated aortic regurgitation are less frequent than following SAVR.[60] In low-risk patients, the incidence of infective endocarditis at 1 year post-TAVR is low (0.2%) in the randomized trials, but is higher in LRT (Low Risk TAVR) and NOTION (Nordic Aortic Valve Intervention) trials, respectively 1% and 3% (see **Table 3**). Antibiotic prophylaxis is recommended following TAVR for dental procedures involving manipulation of gingival tissue, periapical

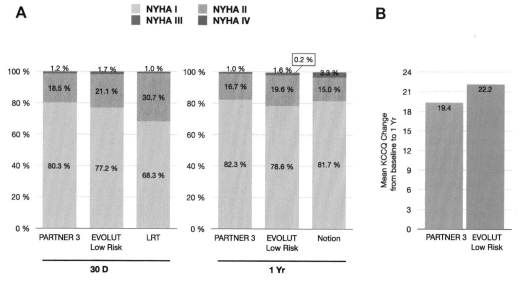

Fig. 4. Functional status and quality of life in low-risk patients who underwent TAVR. (*A*) NYHA class at 30 days and 1 year after TAVR. (*B*) Improvement in Kansas City Cardiomyopathy Questionnaire (KCCQ) score from baseline to 1 year after TAVR. (*Data from* refs.[4,5,51,52,75])

region of teeth, or perforation of oral mucosa. However, it is not recommended for TEE, esophagogastroduodenoscopy, colonoscopy, or cystoscopy (unless there is active infection).

Subclinical Valve Thrombosis

Presence of reduced aortic valve leaflet motion was noted on contrast CT in patients who had a stroke after TAVR.[61] This finding encouraged investigators to perform systematic CT examination after TAVR,[62,63] which revealed signs of possible leaflet thrombosis in 3% to 40% of the patients during the first 3 months after TAVR.[64] This rate was systematically higher after TAVR compared with SAVR in the studies including both THVs and surgical bioprostheses.[61,65] However, in most patients this CT imaging finding was not associated with clinical symptoms or abnormal transthoracic examination,[62,66] and totally resolved after a few weeks of oral anticoagulation therapy.[61,62,65]

There is a need to standardize the CT imaging protocol and definitions for subclinical valve thrombosis.[67] The association of both hypoattenuated leaflet thickening (HALT) and reduced leaflet motion (RELM) lesions on the same leaflet defines a hypoattenuation affecting leaflet motion (HAM) lesion.

This new entity of subclinical leaflet thrombosis is assessed in subsets of patients included in the ongoing low-risk trials. Such data will eventually allow assessment of the incidence of subclinical thrombosis in TAVR and SAVR, as well as its impact on clinical outcomes and valve durability. The antithrombotic therapy that is recommended in current guidelines following TAVR is (1) aspirin and clopidogrel for first 6 months; (2) aspirin after the first 6 months.

Structural Valve Deterioration

Durability of THV is determined by the occurrence of structural valve deterioration (SVD).[68] Recently, 2 standardized definitions of SVD were published and defined SVD by the onset of abnormalities in leaflet morphology and mobility (fibrocalcific remodeling and/or tear) and by the occurrence of hemodynamic valve deterioration assessed by transthoracic echocardiography.[69,70] Guidelines and consensus statements recommend systematic baseline TTE examination post-TAVR (at 1–3 months) and annually thereafter in order to allow early detection of change in valve morphology and/or hemodynamic performance.[3,69,70] At present, short-term and midterm durability of THV are encouraging, but long-term durability remains unknown. Moreover, several cases of THV failure secondary to SVD are reported,[71] and specificities related to THV (valve oversizing, manipulation, delivery, positioning, and deployment) may lead to high mechanical stress on leaflets and impair valve durability in the long term.[72]

Since 2018, several series of patients reported a satisfactory long-term durability of THV, with moderate and severe SVD occurring between 5 and 8 years post-TAVR estimated from 3% to 15% and from 1% to 8%, respectively (see **Table 4**). However, less than half of patients were alive at 5 years post-TAVR, introducing a survival bias in the estimation of the SVD rate. Thus, publication of robust data on long-term durability is needed, especially in low-risk patients with long life expectancy.

FUTURE PERSPECTIVES

The indications for TAVR are rapidly expanding. Recent registries of TAVR in patients with a bicuspid aortic valve have reported excellent results, which are as good as TAVR in patients with a tricuspid valve.[73] However, TAVR is still contraindicated in patients with a bicuspid aortic valve and large aortic annulus and/or with concomitant aortopathy requiring surgical intervention.

The ongoing EARLY-TAVR (Evaluation of Transcatheter Aortic Valve Replacement Compared to SurveiLance for Patients With AsYmptomatic Severe Aortic Stenosis) trial assess the efficacy and safety of early TAVR versus clinical surveillance strategy in asymptomatic patients with severe AS (ClinicalTrials.gov identifier: NCT03042104). In contrast, the TAVR-UNLOAD (Transcatheter Aortic Valve Replacement to UNload the Left Ventricle in Patients With ADvanced Heart Failure) trial is currently testing the efficacy and safety of TAVR versus medical therapy in patients with moderate AS and systolic heart failure (ClinicalTrials.gov identifier: NCT02661451).

The transcatheter aortic valve-in-valve procedure has been shown to be a valuable alternative to redo surgery for the treatment of failed surgical bioprostheses in patients with high or extreme surgical risk.[2] However, a large proportion of patients have severe prosthesis-patient mismatch and high residual gradients following this procedure.[74] Further studies are needed to determine whether fracturing of the stent of the surgical bioprosthesis results in significant reduction in high residual gradients following valve-in-valve procedure.

The main limitation of this future TAVI generalization remains the durability of the THVs and the risk of SVD occurrence.[68] Future studies should seek to confirm long-term durability of the specific transcatheter devices and to analyze competing risk between SVD and death. Decision making between TAVR versus SAVR should be performed by experienced heart teams after assessment of expected valve durability and life expectancy ratio.[72]

SUMMARY

TAVR has expanded rapidly since the first-in-human aortic THV implantation in 2002. In the near future, TAVR may become the treatment of choice for all patients with symptomatic severe AS who require intervention. Procedural outcomes have been improved owing to assessment by the heart teams, the development of safer devices and delivery systems, and better knowledge of the implantation techniques and patient management after the TAVR. However, long-term durability of THV remains to be confirmed to allow generalization of TAVR to low-risk patients. Further studies are also needed to establish the safety and efficacy of TAVR in some specific conditions, such as asymptomatic patients with severe AS, moderate AS with heart failure symptoms, bicuspid aortic valve, and native aortic regurgitation.

REFERENCES

1. Cribier A, Eltchaninoff H, Bash A, et al. Percutaneous transcatheter implantation of an aortic valve prosthesis for calcific aortic stenosis: first human case description. Circulation 2002;106: 3006–8.
2. Nishimura RA, Otto CM, Bonow RO, et al. 2017 AHA/ACC focused update of the 2014 AHA/ACC guideline for the management of patients with valvular heart disease: a report of the American College of Cardiology/American heart association task force on clinical practice guidelines. J Am Coll Cardiol 2017;70:252–89.
3. Baumgartner H, Falk V, Bax JJ, et al, ESC Scientific Document Group. 2017 ESC/EACTS Guidelines for the management of valvular heart disease. Eur Heart J 2017;38:2739–91.
4. Popma JJ, Deeb GM, Yakubov SJ, et al, Evolut Low Risk Trial Investigator. Transcatheter aortic-valve replacement with a self-expanding valve in low-risk patients. N Engl J Med 2019;380(18):1706–15.
5. Mack MJ, Leon MB, Thourani VH, et al, PARTNER 3 Investigators. Transcatheter aortic-valve replacement with a balloon-expandable valve in low-risk patients. N Engl J Med 2019;380(18):1695–705.
6. Cesna S, De Backer O, Sondergaard L. Rapid adoption of transcatheter aortic valve replacement in intermediate- and high-risk patients to treat severe aortic valve stenosis. J Thorac Dis 2017;9:1432–6.
7. Makkar RR, Fontana GP, Jilaihawi H, et al. Transcatheter aortic-valve replacement for inoperable severe aortic stenosis. N Engl J Med 2012;366: 1696–704.
8. Leon MB, Smith CR, Mack M, et al. Transcatheter aortic-valve implantation for aortic stenosis in patients who cannot undergo surgery. N Engl J Med 2010;363:1597–607.
9. Popma JJ, Adams DH, Reardon MJ, et al. Transcatheter aortic valve replacement using a self-expanding bioprosthesis in patients with severe aortic stenosis at extreme risk for surgery. J Am Coll Cardiol 2014;63:1972–81.
10. Reardon MJ, Adams DH, Coselli JS, et al. Self-expanding transcatheter aortic valve replacement using alternative access sites in symptomatic patients with severe aortic stenosis deemed extreme risk of surgery. J Thorac Cardiovasc Surg 2014;148:2869–76.e1-7.
11. Smith CR, Leon MB, Mack MJ, et al. Transcatheter versus surgical aortic-valve replacement in high-risk patients. N Engl J Med 2011;364:2187–98.
12. Adams DH, Popma JJ, Reardon MJ, et al, U.S. CoreValve Clinical Investigators. Transcatheter aortic-valve replacement with a self-expanding prosthesis. N Engl J Med 2014;370:1790–8.
13. Reardon MJ, Van Mieghem NM, Popma JJ, et al. Surgical or transcatheter aortic-valve replacement in intermediate-risk patients. N Engl J Med 2017; 376:1321–31.
14. Leon MB, Smith CR, Mack MJ, et al, PARTNER 2 Investigators. Transcatheter or surgical aortic-valve replacement in intermediate-risk patients. N Engl J Med 2016;374:1609–20.
15. Thourani VH, Kodali S, Makkar RR, et al. Transcatheter aortic valve replacement versus surgical valve replacement in intermediate-risk patients: a propensity score analysis. Lancet 2016;387:2218–25.
16. Baumgartner H, Falk V, Bax JJ, et al. 2017 ESC/EACTS guidelines for the management of valvular heart disease: the Task Force for the management of valvular heart disease of the European Society of Cardiology (ESC) and the European Association for Cardio-Thoracic Surgery (EACTS). Eur Heart J 2017;38:2739–91.
17. McCarthy FH, Spragan DD, Savino D, et al. Outcomes, readmissions, and costs in transfemoral and alterative access transcatheter aortic valve replacement in the US Medicare population. J Thorac Cardiovasc Surg 2017;154:1224–1232 e1.
18. Leipsic J, Gurvitch R, Labounty TM, et al. Multidetector computed tomography in transcatheter aortic valve implantation. JACC Cardiovasc Imaging 2011;4:416–29.
19. Blanke P, Weir-McCall JR, Achenbach S, et al. Computed tomography imaging in the context of transcatheter aortic valve implantation (TAVI)/transcatheter aortic valve replacement (TAVR): an expert consensus document of the Society of Cardiovascular Computed Tomography. J Cardiovasc Comput Tomogr 2019;13: 1–20.

20. Mayr A, Klug G, Reinstadler SJ, et al. Is MRI equivalent to CT in the guidance of TAVR? A pilot study. Eur Radiol 2018;28:4625–34.

21. Wang J, Jagasia DH, Kondapally YR, et al. Comparison of non-contrast cardiovascular magnetic resonance imaging to computed tomography angiography for aortic annular sizing before transcatheter aortic valve replacement. J Invasive Cardiol 2017;29:239–45.

22. Vora AN, Rao SV. Percutaneous or surgical access for transfemoral transcatheter aortic valve implantation. J Thorac Dis 2018;10:S3595–8.

23. Nakamura M, Chakravarty T, Jilaihawi H, et al. Complete percutaneous approach for arterial access in transfemoral transcatheter aortic valve replacement: a comparison with surgical cut-down and closure. Catheter Cardiovasc Interv 2014;84:293–300.

24. Walther T, Simon P, Dewey T, et al. Transapical minimally invasive aortic valve implantation: multicenter experience. Circulation 2007;116:I240–5.

25. Petronio AS, De Carlo M, Bedogni F, et al. Safety and efficacy of the subclavian approach for transcatheter aortic valve implantation with the CoreValve revalving system. Circ Cardiovasc Interv 2010;3:359–66.

26. Bauernschmitt R, Schreiber C, Bleiziffer S, et al. Transcatheter aortic valve implantation through the ascending aorta: an alternative option for no-access patients. Heart Surg Forum 2009;12:E63–4.

27. Greenbaum AB, O'Neill WW, Paone G, et al. Caval-aortic access to allow transcatheter aortic valve replacement in otherwise ineligible patients: initial human experience. J Am Coll Cardiol 2014;63: 2795–804.

28. Mylotte D, Sudre A, Teiger E, et al. Transcarotid transcatheter aortic valve replacement: feasibility and safety. JACC Cardiovasc Interv 2016;9:472–80.

29. Chamandi C, Abi-Akar R, Rodes-Cabau J, et al. Transcarotid compared with other alternative access routes for transcatheter aortic valve replacement. Circ Cardiovasc Interv 2018;11:e006388.

30. Nishimura RA, Otto CM, Bonow RO, et al. 2014 AHA/ACC guideline for the management of patients with valvular heart disease: executive summary. A report of the American College of Cardiology/American heart association task force on practice guidelines. J Am Coll Cardiol 2014;63:2438–88.

31. Vahanian A, Alfieri O, Andreotti F, et al. Guidelines on the management of valvular heart disease (version 2012). Eur Heart J 2012;33:2451–96.

32. Motloch LJ, Rottlaender D, Reda S, et al. Local versus general anesthesia for transfemoral aortic valve implantation. Clin Res Cardiol 2012;101: 45–53.

33. Durand E, Borz B, Godin M, et al. Transfemoral aortic valve replacement with the Edwards SAPIEN and Edwards SAPIEN XT prosthesis using exclusively local anesthesia and fluoroscopic guidance: feasibility and 30-day outcomes. JACC Cardiovasc Interv 2012;5:461–7.

34. Babaliaros V, Devireddy C, Lerakis S, et al. Comparison of transfemoral transcatheter aortic valve replacement performed in the catheterization laboratory (minimalist approach) versus hybrid operating room (standard approach): outcomes and cost analysis. JACC Cardiovasc Interv 2014;7:898–904.

35. Masson JB, Kovac J, Schuler G, et al. Transcatheter aortic valve implantation: review of the nature, management, and avoidance of procedural complications. JACC Cardiovasc Interv 2009;2:811–20.

36. Kappetein AP, Head SJ, Genereux P, et al. Updated standardized endpoint definitions for transcatheter aortic valve implantation: the Valve Academic Research Consortium-2 consensus document. J Am Coll Cardiol 2012;60:1438–54.

37. Pasic M, Unbehaun A, Buz S, et al. Annular rupture during transcatheter aortic valve replacement: classification, pathophysiology, diagnostics, treatment approaches, and prevention. JACC Cardiovasc Interv 2015;8:1–9.

38. Auffret V, Lefevre T, Van Belle E, et al, FRANCE TAVI Investigators. Temporal trends in transcatheter aortic valve replacement in France: FRANCE 2 to FRANCE TAVI. J Am Coll Cardiol 2017;70:42–55.

39. Cormican D, Jayaraman A, Villablanca P, et al. TAVR procedural volumes and patient outcomes: analysis of recent data. J Cardiothorac Vasc Anesth 2019. [Epub ahead of print].

40. Barbanti M, Buccheri S, Rodes-Cabau J, et al. Transcatheter aortic valve replacement with new-generation devices: a systematic review and meta-analysis. Int J Cardiol 2017;245:83–9.

41. Jerez-Valero M, Urena M, Webb JG, et al. Clinical impact of aortic regurgitation after transcatheter aortic valve replacement: insights into the degree and acuteness of presentation. JACC Cardiovasc Interv 2014;7:1022–32.

42. Lerakis S, Hayek SS, Douglas PS. Paravalvular aortic leak after transcatheter aortic valve replacement: current knowledge. Circulation 2013;127: 397–407.

43. Grube E, Schuler G, Buellesfeld L, et al. Percutaneous aortic valve replacement for severe aortic stenosis in high-risk patients using the second- and current third-generation self-expanding CoreValve prosthesis: device success and 30-day clinical outcome. J Am Coll Cardiol 2007;50:69–76.

44. Ong G, Annabi MS, Clavel MA, et al. Paravalvular regurgitation after transcatheter aortic valve replacement: is the problem solved? Interv Cardiol Clin 2018;7:445–58.

45. Sinning JM, Vasa-Nicotera M, Chin D, et al. Evaluation and management of paravalvular aortic regurgitation after transcatheter aortic valve replacement. J Am Coll Cardiol 2013;62:11–20.

46. Takagi H, Umemoto T, Group A. Impact of paravalvular aortic regurgitation after transcatheter aortic valve implantation on survival. Int J Cardiol 2016; 221:46–51.

47. Pibarot P, Hahn RT, Weissman NJ, et al. Assessment of paravalvular regurgitation following TAVR: a proposal of unifying grading scheme. JACC Cardiovasc Imaging 2015;8:340–60.

48. Van Belle E, Rauch A, Vincent F, et al. Von Willebrand factor multimers during transcatheter aortic-valve replacement. N Engl J Med 2016;375:335–44.

49. Salaun E, Jacquier A, Theron A, et al. Value of CMR in quantification of paravalvular aortic regurgitation after TAVI. Eur Heart J Cardiovasc Imaging 2016; 17:41–50.

50. Ribeiro HB, Orwat S, Hayek SS, et al. Cardiovascular magnetic resonance to evaluate aortic regurgitation after transcatheter aortic valve replacement. J Am Coll Cardiol 2016;68:577–85.

51. Thyregod HG, Steinbruchel DA, Ihlemann N, et al. Transcatheter versus surgical aortic valve replacement in patients with severe aortic valve stenosis: 1-year results from the all-comers NOTION randomized clinical trial. J Am Coll Cardiol 2015;65: 2184–94.

52. Waksman R, Corso PJ, Torguson R, et al. Transcatheter aortic valve replacement in low-risk patients: one-year results from the LRT trial. JACC Cardiovasc Interv 2019;12(10):901–7.

53. Kapadia SR, Kodali S, Makkar R, et al, SENTINEL Trial Investigators. Protection against cerebral embolism during transcatheter aortic valve replacement. J Am Coll Cardiol 2017;69:367–77.

54. Auffret V, Puri R, Urena M, et al. Conduction disturbances after transcatheter aortic valve replacement: current status and future perspectives. Circulation 2017;136:1049–69.

55. Auffret V, Webb JG, Eltchaninoff H, et al. Clinical impact of baseline right bundle branch block in patients undergoing transcatheter aortic valve replacement. JACC Cardiovasc Interv 2017;10:1564–74.

56. Mangieri A, Lanzillo G, Bertoldi L, et al. Predictors of advanced conduction disturbances requiring a late (>/=48 H) permanent pacemaker following transcatheter aortic valve replacement. JACC Cardiovasc Interv 2018;11:1519–26.

57. Straiton N, Jin K, Bhindi R, et al. Functional capacity and health-related quality of life outcomes post transcatheter aortic valve replacement: a systematic review and meta-analysis. Age Ageing 2018;47: 478–82.

58. Amat-Santos IJ, Messika-Zeitoun D, Eltchaninoff H, et al. Infective endocarditis after transcatheter aortic valve implantation: results from a large multicenter registry. Circulation 2015;131:1566–74.

59. Regueiro A, Linke A, Latib A, et al. Association between transcatheter aortic valve replacement and subsequent infective endocarditis and in-hospital death. JAMA 2016;316:1083–92.

60. Salaun E, Sportouch L, Barral PA, et al. Diagnosis of infective endocarditis after TAVR: value of a multimodality imaging approach. JACC Cardiovasc Imaging 2018;11:143–6.

61. Makkar RR, Fontana G, Jilaihawi H, et al. Possible subclinical leaflet thrombosis in bioprosthetic aortic valves. N Engl J Med 2015;373:2015–24.

62. Pache G, Schoechlin S, Blanke P, et al. Early hypoattenuated leaflet thickening in balloon-expandable transcatheter aortic heart valves. Eur Heart J 2016; 37:2263–71.

63. Hansson NC, Grove EL, Andersen HR, et al. Transcatheter aortic valve thrombosis: incidence, predisposing factors, and clinical implications. J Am Coll Cardiol 2016;68:2059–69.

64. Puri R, Auffret V, Rodes-Cabau J. Bioprosthetic valve thrombosis. J Am Coll Cardiol 2017;69:2193–211.

65. Chakravarty T, Sondergaard L, Friedman J, et al, RESOLVE, SAVORY Investigators. Subclinical leaflet thrombosis in surgical and transcatheter bioprosthetic aortic valves: an observational study. Lancet 2017;389:2383–92.

66. Leetmaa T, Hansson NC, Leipsic J, et al. Early aortic transcatheter heart valve thrombosis: diagnostic value of contrast-enhanced multidetector computed tomography. Circ Cardiovasc Interv 2015;8 [pii: e001596].

67. Jilaihawi H, Asch FM, Manasse E, et al. Systematic CT methodology for the evaluation of subclinical leaflet thrombosis. JACC Cardiovasc Imaging 2017;10:461–70.

68. Foroutan F, Guyatt GH, Otto CM, et al. Structural valve deterioration after transcatheter aortic valve implantation. Heart 2017;103:1899–905.

69. Capodanno D, Petronio AS, Prendergast B, et al. Standardized definitions of structural deterioration and valve failure in assessing long-term durability of transcatheter and surgical aortic bioprosthetic valves: a consensus statement from the European Association of Percutaneous Cardiovascular Interventions (EAPCI) endorsed by the European Society of Cardiology (ESC) and the European Association for Cardio-Thoracic Surgery (EACTS). Eur Heart J 2017;38:3382–90.

70. Dvir D, Bourguignon T, Otto CM, et al, VIVID (Valve in Valve International Data) Investigators. Standardized definition of structural valve degeneration for surgical and transcatheter bioprosthetic aortic valves. Circulation 2018;137:388–99.

71. Salaun E, Zenses AS, Clavel MA, et al. Valve-in-valve procedure in failed transcatheter aortic valves. JACC Cardiovasc Imaging 2019;12: 198–202.

72. Salaun E, Clavel MA, Rodes-Cabau J, et al. Bioprosthetic aortic valve durability in the era of

transcatheter aortic valve implantation. Heart 2018; 104:1323–32.

73. Makkar RR, Yoon SH, Leon MB, et al. Association between transcatheter aortic valve replacement for bicuspid vs tricuspid aortic stenosis and mortality or stroke. JAMA 2019;321:2193–202.

74. Zenses AS, Dahou A, Salaun E, et al. Haemodynamic outcomes following aortic valve-in-valve procedure. Open Heart 2018;5:e000854.

75. Waksman R, Rogers T, Torguson R, et al. Transcatheter aortic valve replacement in low-risk patients with symptomatic severe aortic stenosis. J Am Coll Cardiol 2018;72:2095–105.

76. Eltchaninoff H, Durand E, Avinée G, et al. Assessment of structural valve deterioration of transcatheter aortic bioprosthetic balloon-expandable valves using the new European consensus definition. EuroIntervention 2018;14:e264–71.

77. Holy EW, Kebernik J, Abdelghani M, et al. Long-term durability and haemodynamic performance of a self-expanding transcatheter heart valve beyond five years after implantation: a prospective observational study applying the standardised definitions of structural deterioration and valve failure. EuroIntervention 2018;14:e390–6.

78. Deutsch MA, Erlebach M, Burri M, et al. Beyond the five-year horizon: long-term outcome of high-risk and inoperable patients undergoing TAVR with first-generation devices. EuroIntervention 2018;14: 41–9.

79. Barbanti M, Costa G, Zappulla P, et al. Incidence of long-term structural valve dysfunction and bioprosthetic valve failure after transcatheter aortic valve replacement. J Am Heart Assoc 2018;7: e008440.

80. Kumar A, Sato K, Banerjee K, et al. Hemodynamic durability of transcatheter aortic valves using the updated Valve Academic Research Consortium-2 criteria. Catheter Cardiovasc Interv 2018;93(4): 729–38.

81. Didier R, Eltchaninoff H, Donzeau-Gouge P, et al. Five-year clinical outcome and valve durability after transcatheter aortic valve replacement in high-risk patients. Circulation 2018;138:2597–607.

82. Gleason TG, Reardon MJ, Popma JJ, et al, CoreValve U.S. Pivotal High Risk Trial Clinical Investigators. 5-Year outcomes of self-expanding transcatheter versus surgical aortic valve replacement in high-risk patients. J Am Coll Cardiol 2018;72: 2687–96.

83. Durand E, Sokoloff A, Urena-Alcazar M, et al. Assessment of long-term structural deterioration of transcatheter aortic bioprosthetic valves using the new European definition. Circ Cardiovasc Interv 2019;12:e007597.

Sex Differences in the Pathophysiology, Diagnosis, and Management of Aortic Stenosis

Nancy Côté, PhD, Marie-Annick Clavel, DVM, PhD*

KEYWORDS

- Calcific aortic stenosis • Sex differences • Pathophysiology • Diagnosis • Outcome
- Transcatheter aortic valve implantation • Surgical aortic valve replacement

KEY POINTS

- Women have higher left ventricular ejection fraction; with more concentric hypertrophy, in response to increased pressure overload; smaller cavities; and have a higher proportion of paradoxic low-flow low-gradient aortic stenosis (AS).
- Women reach similar hemodynamic severity of AS with a lower amount of aortic valve calcification compared with men.
- Sex-specific thresholds in aortic valve calcification, measured by computed tomography, to identify severe AS are 1200 AU in women and 2000 AU in men.
- Women are generally referred to surgery at a more advanced stage of the disease and have worse or comparable outcomes after surgical aortic valve replacement, but better outcomes after transcatheter valve replacement.
- Sex differences in gene expression have been found in porcine aortic valvular interstitial cells and in postmenopausal women.

INTRODUCTION

In young patients, the incidence of calcific aortic stenosis (AS) is more important in men. Indeed, congenital bicuspid aortic valve has a 3 to 1 men:-women ratio and AS is the most frequent complication in the bicuspid valve. However, recent population-based studies showed that in older patients (after 75 years of age), AS is most often encountered in women.[1] Interestingly, the valvular lesions appear to be different in men and women for the same hemodynamic impact.[2] The increased hemodynamic afterload increases left ventricular (LV) wall thickness, cardiomyocyte hypertrophy, and impairs LV function in both men

and women. However, sex-specific patterns have been described.[3] After replacement of the aortic valve, either by surgery or percutaneous procedure, outcomes appear also to be sex-related. This article thus reviews the sex differences in epidemiology, pathophysiology, clinical presentation, diagnosis and treatment in AS.

EPIDEMIOLOGY AND PATHOPHYSIOLOGY OF AORTIC STENOSIS

Sex Differences in Epidemiology and Progression of Aortic Stenosis

Historical echocardiographic data showed that the risk of developing AS was twofold higher in men

Conflict of Interest: Dr M-.A. Clavel has Core Lab contracts with Edwards Lifesciences, for which she receives no direct compensation; and research grant with Medtronic. The other author has no disclosure.
Institut Universitaire de Cardiologie et de Pneumologie de Québec (IUCPQ) - Université Laval, Québec Heart & Lung Institute, 2725 Chemin Sainte-Foy, Québec City, Québec G1V-4G5, Canada
* Corresponding author.
E-mail address: marie-annick.clavel@criucpq.ulaval.ca

Cardiol Clin 38 (2020) 129–138
https://doi.org/10.1016/j.ccl.2019.09.008

than in women.[4] However, nationwide claim-based studies in hospitalized patients showed a less pronounced disparity, with 55.1% of patients hospitalized with AS being men in United States,[5] whereas 52% are women in Sweeden,[6] and 53% in Scotland.[7] Interestingly, 60% of the young patients ($\leq$75 years old) were men and more than 50% of the elderly were women.[1] This could be explained by the rate of congenital bicuspid valve that is twofold or threefold more common in men as compared with women.

For a long time, male sex has been thought to be a predictor of faster hemodynamic progression of AS, although a large number of retrospective and prospective studies disproved this belief.[8–10] In the SEAS study, women and men had similar rates of AS progression and AS-related events[9] (**Fig. 1**).

Aortic Valve Calcification According to Sex

Aortic valve calcification (AVC) is the main culprit lesion in AS. AVC is a strong determinant of AS severity and powerful risk factor for mortality.[11,12] Interestingly, women reach a similar hemodynamic degree of AS severity with a lower amount of AVC and consequently, sex-specific thresholds have been proposed (women: 1200 Agatston units [AU] and men: 2000 AU) to identify severe AS, as well as predicting disease progression, and adverse clinical events.[10,11,13,14]

Apart from having obvious implications for AS severity evaluation, these data raised the question of the sex-specific impact and amount of noncalcified tissue in aortic valve lesions. Indeed, in patients matched for AS hemodynamic severity, age, body mass index, and comorbidities, women have relatively more valvular fibrosis compared with men.[2] Besides AVC, fibrosis contributes largely to the development of valvular stenosis and these different patterns in valve damage highlight potential differences in the pathophysiology of AS between men and women.

Sex Differences in Aortic Stenosis Pathobiology

AS pathobiology has been traditionally studied in cohorts or animal models with a vast majority of male patients and with an evident underrepresentation of women. Nevertheless, striking evidences start to build up and to demonstrate that for the same hemodynamic severity, women tend to have less calcification and more fibrosis deposits on their aortic valve[2] (see **Fig. 1**). Thus, sex seems to have a major impact on AS pathobiology, but a scarce number of studies investigated the sex-specific signaling pathways leading to these observations. The existence of intrinsic,

cellular-scale differences between male and female valvular interstitial cells (VICs) that contribute to sex discrepancies have been investigated by a global gene expression profiling between healthy male and female porcine VICs.[15] A total of 183 genes were identified as different in male and female VICs. In particular, cellular proliferation, apoptosis, migration, ossification, angiogenesis, lipid management, inflammation, and extracellular matrix reorganization were some of the pathways and processes identified as being different between male and female porcine valves. These gene expression findings also translated into functional differences behavior *in vitro*. Indeed, sex-related differences in proliferation and apoptosis were also established in cultured VICs and confirmed the microarray results that suggested greater expression of disease-related behaviors in male VICs. Polymorphism in estrogen receptor α has also been identified as a potential risk factor of AS in postmenopausal women.[16] In the postmenopausal patients and age-matched controls, the PvuII polymorphism was independently associated with an increased risk of AS. A genotype defined by at least 1 restriction site in the PvuII polymorphism and 2 restriction sites in the transforming growth factor (TGF)-b1 polymorphism was related to a highly significant increased risk of AS.

A recent study demonstrated that interferon-α alone and in combination with lipopolysaccharide trigger higher inflammation and calcification in male human VICs.[17] Dissimilarities on interleukin-6/bone morphogenetic protein-2/matrix metalloproteinase-1 secretion, which are respectively proinflammatory, pro-osteoblastic, and profibrotic molecules, might account for the lower calcification observed in female VICs of these experiments. In addition, sex differences in osteoblast markers at 24 hours suggested different kinetics in calcification progression, which seemed to be delayed in female VICs. Moreover, the mineralization inhibitor Matrix Gla Protein was also upregulated in female VICs. Altogether, these results suggest that both genetic sex differences and hormonal status may play key roles in AS pathophysiology.

PATTERNS OF LEFT VENTRICULAR REMODELING AND HYPERTROPHY ACCORDING TO SEX

Numerous studies have emphasized on understanding sex differences in the ventricular response to pressure overload imposed by AS. The geometric pattern of LV adaptive response to pressure overload in AS is heterogeneous and includes concentric remodeling, concentric

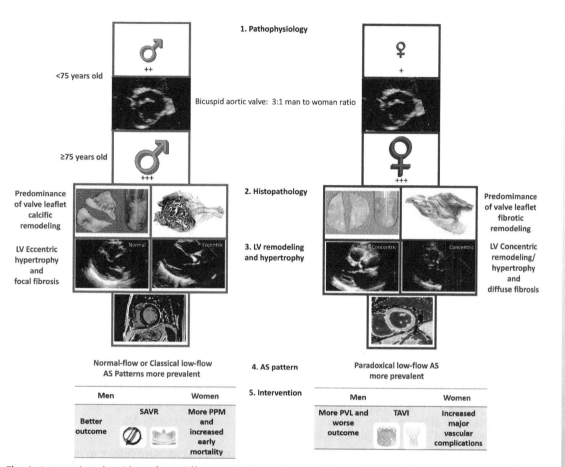

Fig. 1. Integrative algorithm of sex differences in the pathophysiology of AS. This figure represents 5 different observation areas between men and women developing AS. (1) A slightly higher rate of men (younger than 75 years) tend to develop AS when compared with women. However, in population older than 75 years, the overall percentage of the population having AS increase and is similar between both sexes. (2) Histologic observation of explanted aortic valve specimens and Trichrome Masson staining (fibrosis/collagen staining) show a more calcific AS in men and a fibrotic AS in women, for the same hemodynamic severity. (3) LV adaptive response to pressure overload in AS is sex-specific. Men have more eccentric hypertrophy, as demonstrated by echocardiographic parasternal long-axis view, and late-gadolinium enhancement measured by cardiac magnetic resonance, is increased with the presence of focal fibrosis. In women, echocardiographic findings point toward a more concentric remodeling/hypertrophy and diffuse fibrosis (increased extracellular volume) have been described using T1 mapping techniques by cardiac magnetic resonance. (4) These LV patterns lead to classical low-flow AS in men and a higher rate of paradoxic low-flow AS in women. (5) Men benefit more from a surgical aortic valve replacement whereas women have increased early mortality, but better long-term survival. Surgical aortic valve replacement leads to more PPM in women. Following a TAVI, men have higher rates of PAR and seem to have a worse 30-day outcome. Women are having more major vascular complications than men after a TAVI.

hypertrophy, and eccentric hypertrophy.[18,19] These patterns and the magnitude of LV hypertrophy remodeling are influenced by AS severity but also by several other factors including sex. Indeed, over the entire spectrum of AS severity, women have more concentric remodeling and men have more prevalence of LV hypertrophy (concentric and eccentric).[20,21] In a recent study including the whole range of AS severity, concentric LV hypertrophy was characteristic in women in association with smaller cavities and higher relative wall thickness, and this pattern of hypertrophy was a predictor of worse outcome (60% increased risk) in women but not in men.[22] Women are more likely to develop LV restrictive physiology pattern and heart failure in pressure overload cardiopathies when compared with men.[23,24] Indeed, in a recent cardiovascular magnetic resonance study, despite presenting with lower LV mass, women had similar replacement myocardial fibrosis (as assessed by late-gadolinium enhancement) and higher LV extracellular volume fraction (as assessed by T1 mapping), indicating a more pronounced diffuse fibrosis independent of the degree of AS severity.[25] A previous analysis of the Multi-Ethnic Study of Atherosclerosis also reported higher LV extracellular volume fraction in women compared with men.[26] Nevertheless, these findings are controversial, and some studies suggested a greater propensity of men to develop myocardial fibrosis than women. A recent study found higher late-gadolinium enhancement fraction and increased extracellular volume fraction indexed to LV end-diastolic volume in men.[21] However, this previous study was conducted on patients with severe AS planned for surgery in which men presented a high proportion (>70%) of LV hypertrophy and higher proportion of coronary artery disease. In the AS population, coronary artery disease is highly prevalent and this is a major confounding factor when analyzing both focal and diffuse fibrosis.

The molecular mechanisms underlying the sexually dimorphic response of the heart to the AS pressure overload–dependent myocardial fibrosis are incompletely understood. In surgical biopsies, men express a higher quantity of collagen I and III and matrix metalloproteinase-2 gene than women.[27] These data suggest that men and women differ in their matrix-related gene expression and underlying pathophysiological mechanisms related to cardiac fibrosis. A lot of effort has been devoted to analyze the cardioprotective effect of estrogen in myocardial remodeling under pressure stress in young rodents.[28,29] However, the AS population is predominantly composed of postmenopausal women who have therefore lost, at least in part, the protective effect of estrogen. Clinical studies on patients with AS showed that LV remodeling also occurs differently in postmenopausal women than in older men, many of whom have circulating testosterone levels within normal range equivalent to young men.[30,31] This observation suggests that circulating androgens may be responsible of a more detrimental remodeling in men with AS. There are controversial data on the impact of estrogen and testosterone on fibrosis. Testosterone has been demonstrated to exert antifibrotic properties through the modulation of TGF-β1 and angiotensin II signaling pathways. On the other hand, estrogens have been shown to induce fibrotic processes and histologic studies on myocardial tissues showed an overexpression of both estrogen receptors in pathologic situations.[32] Mechanistic studies demonstrated that estrogens can downregulate matrix metalloproteinase-2, causing extracellular matrix disruption via collagen degradation and consequently LV remodeling.[33]

However, estrogens have a potential protective effect against cardiac detrimental fibroblast proliferation.[27,29]

Moreover, chronic activation of the renin-angiotensin-aldosterone system is thought to play a key role in cardiac remodeling as well as profibrotic process.[34] Some evidence suggests that these processes may predominantly affect female hearts. In premenopausal and postmenopausal women, plasma level of aldosterone is associated with LV concentric remodeling.[35] Moreover, women commonly present a distinctive pattern of LV function with supernormal ejection fraction.[36,37] In a mouse model of genetically produced hypertrophic cardiomyopathy, estrogens prevented diastolic dysfunction by stimulating the energy metabolism via mitochondrial activation in the cardiac myocytes, and by reducing the myocardial oxidative stress. These results are in agreement with data showing improvement in diastolic functions in other conditions, including animal models of spontaneous hypertension and pressure overload and could partially explain the greater LV function observed in women with AS compared with men.[38] Further studies are needed to determine the underlying mechanisms for the sex differences in the magnitude of myocardial fibrosis in patients with AS.

LOW-FLOW LOW-GRADIENT AORTIC STENOSIS

Albeit having a higher LV ejection fraction at any degree of AS severity, women have a lower stroke volume index and a reduced flow rate across the valve compared with men. This entity called paradoxical low-flow AS is thus largely observed in women.[39–47] Paradoxical low-flow, low-gradient (aortic valve area <1.0 cm^2, indexed aortic valve area <0.6 cm^2/m^2, mean gradient <40 mm Hg, LV ejection fraction ≥50%, and presence of low-flow: stroke volume index <35 mL/m^2) may be a reason for underdiagnosis and underestimation of AS severity in women. Moreover, it has been associated with later referral to surgery.[40,48–50] Patients with paradoxic low-flow AS have worse outcomes under medical treatment, and higher operative mortality and/or long-term postoperative mortality.[39,48,51]

On the other hand, men will present more often with coronary artery disease and reduced ejection fraction, that is, classical low-flow, low-gradient AS.[52] This entity is probably the one with the worst outcome in AS; however, being well-known, low ejection fraction is a class I indication for aortic valve replacement (AVR) in severe AS.[53]

TREATMENT OPTIONS AND OUTCOMES IN WOMEN COMPARED WITH MEN
Surgical Aortic Valve Replacement

Surgical AVR (SAVR) is the primary intervention to treat patients with severe and symptomatic AS that has been proven to improve quality of life and life expectancy.[54–56] Studies assessing the differential impact of sex on outcomes of SAVR yielded conflicting results. Some investigations established that female sex has as a positive influential effect that contributes to a better recovery of ventricular geometry and function following SAVR that may ultimately favorably affects subsequent survival.[27,57] However, in 2009, the Society of Thoracic Surgeons National Database was queried for all isolated surgical aortic valve replacements, leading to a study including 108,791 patients and it was found that women present worse outcomes for mortality, stroke, and postoperative stay than men.[58] Other studies emphasized on a lower LV mass regression, increased 30-day mortality, higher rate of postoperative stroke, longer postoperative stay, and higher long-term mortality with or without concomitant procedures in women.[58–61] A recent study presented nuanced results. Indeed, they found that although women undergoing AVR have relatively more risk factors than do men, early mortality and overall survival were worse in women than in men; however, after adjustment for preoperative risk factors, there was no difference in overall survival between women and men.[62] These discrepancies may be related to preoperative and operative comorbidities as well as a higher rate of patient-prothesis mismatch in women, which has been associated with impaired outcomes after SAVR[63–70] (see **Fig. 1**).

Transcatheter Aortic Valve Implantation

In a recent meta-analysis, which analyzed 11,310 patients (51% female) in 5 registries, including the PARTNER trial, the preprocedural Logistic EuroSCORE has been found to be lower in women although sex is a score component by which female sex adds to overall risk. Importantly, women presenting for transcatheter aortic valve implantation (TAVI) generally have fewer cardiovascular risk factors and atherosclerotic burden, with lower rates of prior myocardial infarction, revascularization, previous stroke, and peripheral vascular disease, as well as better LV systolic function at presentation. Of note, many studies have shown a positive effect of TAVI on LV function and reduction of remodeling after decreased afterload pressure and volume. This positive effect seems to be more important in women than in men[71,72] (see **Fig. 1**).

Paravalvular regurgitations

Paravalvular leaks (PVL) that were present in approximately 70% to 80% of patients after the TAVI procedure[73–75] have decreased to 30% in new-generation devices.[76] Nevertheless, these PVLs have been demonstrated to be predictors of a fatal outcome after TAVI.[77,78] Interestingly, women have smaller annular size, which may be associated with lower rates of PVLs[79,80] (see **Fig. 1**). In 2011, the results from a German TAVI registry showed that postprocedural paravalvular regurgitation (PAR) was more common in men (57%) and that male gender was an independent predictor of PVL.[79] In a different study including a series of 358 patients undergoing TAVI procedure, 48% of the patients developed post-TAVI leakage (32% of PARs, 13% of transvalvular regurgitation, and 3% both) and still, male sex was a predictor of postprocedural leakages.[80]

Patient-prosthesis mismatch

Following TAVI, patient-prosthesis mismatch (PPM) appears to be lower than in SAVR and the difference increased in patients with smaller aortic annulus.[63,81] Many studies have investigated the possible PPM differences post-TAVI. Only one study found a trend for higher rates of PPM among women,[82] whereas most TAVI studies have shown that women do not have increased PPM despite the frequent need for smaller valves,[83,84] as opposed to SAVR studies. Future studies are needed to compare face-to-face SAVR and TAVI in terms of PPM rates according to sex. However, these data underline the possible benefit of TAVI in women who are surgical candidates, but who have smaller aortic annulus (see **Fig. 1**).

Outcomes

A recent meta-analysis including 7973 patients (14 observational studies) compared outcome after TAVI in men and women. At 30 days and during the follow-up, women had a lower mortality rate.[85] However, female gender was associated with a 1.72-fold greater risk rate of major vascular complications defined by the Valve Academic Research Consortium consensus document (VARC) criteria.[72,86–89] Major bleeding and stroke rate were not different according to sex and permanent pacemaker rate was slightly elevated in men compared with women. Nevertheless, all these observations need to be evaluated in prospective studies designed to evaluate sex differences (see **Fig. 1**).

Valve-in-valve

Bioprostheses have a limited durability and over time degenerate and eventually fail, requiring the need for replacement. Valve-in-valve (ViV) procedure emerged as an alternative to the gold standard redo-SAVR. Data from the VIVID (Valve-in-Valve International Data) registry showed that structural bioprosthesis degeneration due to stenosis is more frequent in women and especially in large body-size women who received small surgical valves.[90] The reason for this difference may be attributable to a possible PPM of the original implanted surgical valve, given that PPM has been shown to accelerate bioprosthesis degeneration.[91] However, in patients with prior PPM, strategies other than ViV may be more suitable (ie, redo cardiac surgery using a larger valve) due to the high residual gradient linked to PPM.[92]

Other complications

The risk of aortic root and annular rupture is higher in women compared with men,[93] which could be linked to smaller annular size and perhaps more friable tissue that is subject to rupture at lower level than men. Moreover, the balloon inflation and deployment of the valve may occur with higher force in women with smaller annular dimensions and consequently, result in an increased rate of rupture. Another complication associated with TAVI procedure is coronary obstruction, which is more common in women (80%) due to lower coronary heights and smaller sinus of Valsalva.[94–96] Major peripheral vascular complications and major bleeding are also more frequent in women compared with men. Reduced femoral diameters were associated with more frequent iliac complications.[86,97]

SEX-SPECIFIC MANAGEMENT AND TREATMENT

Sex-specific thresholds in AVC measured by multidetector computed tomography (MDCT) to identify severe AS (ie, 1200 AU in women and 2000 AU in men) have recently been added to the latest European Society of Cardiology guidelines.[11,98,99] The preference for transcatheter over SAVR in women should be considered in the future guidelines and practice. Because fibrosis has been found to be more abundant in aortic valve of women with AS and calcification seems to be the main culprit in men with AS, specific treatment platforms should be sex-adapted.[22] Treatment targeting fibrotic pathways should be develop and preferred in women whereas anti-calcifying drugs may be more effective to prevent the development of AS in men. However, sex-specific management and therapy in AS is still at an early stage. Clinical research studies should systematically assess the impact of sex and report results according to the sex of the patients. Sex-specific

studies on AS management should be performed such as the assessment of risk/benefit in TAVI versus SAVR and also, sex discrepancies in the management of patients with low-flow, low-gradient AS and especially in paradoxical low-flow, low-gradient AS. Critically, it is now evident that appropriate AS animal models should help understand the biological outcomes of hormone repletion or supplementation in male and female individuals. More basic science studies should be performed to evaluate sex hormone levels and chromosomal complements in both sexes and/or according to the specific sex of culture material and animal models. Another major area of doubt that should be investigated is the influence of sex (both hormonal and chromosomal) on the ventricular responses to LV overload in cohorts and appropriate animal models and should aim at developing therapies to prevent/restore LV function in patients with advanced AS.

SUMMARY

The pathophysiology and presentation of AS regarding valvular disease as well as LV function and remodeling, surgical risk, and outcomes are sex-specific. Women present with more concentric LV remodeling, smaller LV cavities, and more diffuse fibrosis. Female sex may be a risk factor for adverse outcome following SAVR and oppositely confers a survival advantage when undergoing TAVI. Despite their increased age and frailty, the lower mortality seen following TAVI in women compared with men may reflect their longer life expectancy, smaller annular size, less postprocedure PVLs, and more favorable LV reverse remodeling. Moreover, women will present with symptomatic severe AS with less aortic valve calcium but more fibrosis than men. Further studies examining molecular mechanisms underlying sex-related differences in the development and progression of AS are needed because a better understanding of these mechanisms could ultimately lead to individualized medical therapy that could prevent or reverse AS.

REFERENCES

1. Andell P, Li X, Martinsson A, et al. Epidemiology of valvular heart disease in a Swedish nationwide hospital-based register study. Heart 2017;103(21): 1696–703.
2. Simard L, Côté N, Dagenais F, et al. Sex-related discordance between aortic valve calcification and hemodynamic severity of aortic stenosis: is valvular fibrosis the explanation? Circ Res 2017;120(4): 681–91.

3. Kararigas G, Dworatzek E, Petrov G, et al. Sex-dependent regulation of fibrosis and inflammation in human left ventricular remodelling under pressure overload. Eur J Heart Fail 2014;16(11):1160–7.

4. Stewart BF, Siscovick D, Lind BK, et al. Clinical factors associated with calcific aortic valve disease. Cardiovascular Health Study. J Am Coll Cardiol 1997;29(3):630–4.

5. Badheka AO, Singh V, Patel NJ, et al. Trends of hospitalizations in the United States from 2000 to 2012 of patients >60 years with aortic valve disease. Am J Cardiol 2015;116(1):132–41.

6. Martinsson A, Li X, Andersson C, et al. Temporal trends in the incidence and prognosis of aortic stenosis: a nationwide study of the Swedish population. Circulation 2015;131(11):988–94.

7. Berry C, Lloyd SM, Wang Y, et al. The changing course of aortic valve disease in Scotland: temporal trends in hospitalizations and mortality and prognostic importance of aortic stenosis. Eur Heart J 2013;34(21):1538–47.

8. Kamath AR, Pai RG. Risk factors for progression of calcific aortic stenosis and potential therapeutic targets. Int J Angiol 2008;17(2):63–70.

9. Cramariuc D, Rogge BP, Lønnebakken MT, et al. Sex differences in cardiovascular outcome during progression of aortic valve stenosis. Heart 2015; 101(3):209–14.

10. Tastet L, Enriquez-Sarano M, Capoulade R, et al. Impact of aortic valve calcification and sex on hemodynamic progression and clinical outcomes in AS. J Am Coll Cardiol 2017;69(16):2096–8.

11. Clavel MA, Pibarot P, Messika-Zeitoun D, et al. Impact of aortic valve calcification, as measured by MDCT, on survival in patients with aortic stenosis: results of an international registry study. J Am Coll Cardiol 2014;64(12):1202–13.

12. Pawade T, Clavel MA, Tribouilloy C, et al. Computed tomography aortic valve calcium scoring in patients with aortic stenosis. Circ Cardiovasc Imaging 2018; 11(3):e007146.

13. Aggarwal SR, Clavel MA, Messika-Zeitoun D, et al. Sex differences in aortic valve calcification measured by multidetector computed tomography in aortic stenosis. Circ Cardiovasc Imaging 2013;6(1):40–7.

14. Clavel MA, Messika-Zeitoun D, Pibarot P, et al. The complex nature of discordant severe calcified aortic valve disease grading: new insights from combined Doppler-echocardiographic and computed tomographic study. J Am Coll Cardiol 2013;62(24): 2329–38.

15. McCoy CM, Nicholas DQ, Masters KS. Sex-related differences in gene expression by porcine aortic valvular interstitial cells. PLoS One 2012;7(7): e39980.

16. Nordstrom P, Glader CA, Dahlen G, et al. Oestrogen receptor alpha gene polymorphism is related to aortic valve sclerosis in postmenopausal women. J Intern Med 2003;254(2):140–6.

17. Parra-Izquierdo I, Castanos-Mollor I, Lopez J, et al. Calcification induced by type i interferon in human aortic valve interstitial cells is larger in males and blunted by a Janus Kinase inhibitor. Arterioscler Thromb Vasc Biol 2018;38(9):2148–59.

18. Grossman W, Jones D, McLaurin LP. Wall stress and patterns of hypertrophy in the human left ventricle. J Clin Invest 1975;56:56–64.

19. Gerdts E. Left ventricular structure in different types of chronic pressure overload. Eur Heart J 2008; 10(Supplement E):E23–30.

20. Cramariuc D, Rieck AE, Staal EM, et al. Factors influencing left ventricular structure and stress-corrected systolic function in men and women with asymptomatic aortic valve stenosis (a SEAS Substudy). Am J Cardiol 2008;101(4):510–5.

21. Treibel TA, Kozor R, Fontana M, et al. Sex dimorphism in the myocardial response to aortic stenosis. JACC Cardiovasc Imaging 2018;11(7):962–73.

22. Capoulade R, Clavel MA, Le Ven F, et al. Impact of left ventricular remodelling patterns on outcomes in patients with aortic stenosis. Eur Heart J Cardiovasc Imaging 2017;18(12):1378–87.

23. Douglas PS, Katz SE, Weinberg EO, et al. Hypertrophy remodeling: gender differences in the early response to left ventrcular pressure overload. J Am Coll Cardiol 1998;32(4):1118–25.

24. Gjesdal O, Bluemke DA, Lima JA. Cardiac remodeling at the population level–risk factors, screening, and outcomes. Nat Rev Cardiol 2011;8(12):673–85.

25. Everett RJ, Tastet L, Clavel MA, et al. Progression of hypertrophy and myocardial fibrosis in aortic stenosis: a multicenter cardiac magnetic resonance study. Circ Cardiovasc Imaging 2018;11(6): e007451.

26. Liu CY, Liu YC, Wu C, et al. Evaluation of age-related interstitial myocardial fibrosis with cardiac magnetic resonance contrast-enhanced T1 mapping: MESA (Multi-Ethnic Study of Atherosclerosis). J Am Coll Cardiol 2013;62(14):1280–7.

27. Petrov G, Regitz-Zagrosek V, Lehmkuhl E, et al. Regression of myocardial hypertrophy after aortic valve replacement: faster in women? Circulation 2010;122(11 Suppl):S23–8.

28. Piro M, Della Bona R, Abbate A, et al. Sex-related differences in myocardial remodeling. J Am Coll Cardiol 2010;55(11):1057–65.

29. Weinberg EO, Thienelt CD, Katz SE, et al. Gender differences in molecular remodeling in pressure overload hypertrophy. J Am Coll Cardiol 1999; 34(1):264–73.

30. Villar AV, Llano M, Cobo M, et al. Gender differences of echocardiographic and gene expression patterns in human pressure overload left ventricular hypertrophy. J Mol Cell Cardiol 2009;46(4):526–35.

31. Villari B, Campbell SE, Schneider J, et al. Sex-dependent differences in left ventricular function and structure in chronic pressure overload. Eur Heart J 1995;16(10):1410–9.

32. Nordmeyer J, Eder S, Mahmoodzadeh S, et al. Up-regulation of myocardial estrogen receptors in human aortic stenosis. Circulation 2004;110(20): 3270–5.

33. Regitz-Zagrosek V, Seeland U. Sex and gender differences in myocardial hypertrophy and heart failure. Wien Med Wochenschr 2011;161(5–6):109–16.

34. Pacurari M, Kafoury R, Tchounwou PB, et al. The Renin-Angiotensin-aldosterone system in vascular inflammation and remodeling. Int J Inflam 2014; 2014:689360.

35. Vasan RS, Evans JC, Benjamin EJ, et al. Relations of serum aldosterone to cardiac structure: gender-related differences in the Framingham Heart Study. Hypertension 2004;43(5):957–62.

36. Aurigemma GP, Silver KH, McLaughlin M, et al. Impact of chamber geometry and gender on left ventricular systolic function in patients over 60 years of age with aortic stenosis. Am J Cardiol 1994;74: 794–8.

37. Cramariuc D, Gerdts E, Davidsen ES, et al. Myocardial deformation in aortic valve stenosis - relation to left ventricular geometry. Heart 2010;96(2):106–12.

38. Chen Y, Zhang Z, Hu F, et al. 17beta-estradiol prevents cardiac diastolic dysfunction by stimulating mitochondrial function: a preclinical study in a mouse model of a human hypertrophic cardiomyopathy mutation. J Steroid Biochem Mol Biol 2015;147: 92–102.

39. Clavel MA, Berthelot-Richer M, LV F, et al. Impact of classic and paradoxical low flow on survival after aortic valve replacement for severe aortic stenosis. J Am Coll Cardiol 2015;65(7):645–53.

40. Hachicha Z, Dumesnil JG, Bogaty P, et al. Paradoxical low flow, low gradient severe aortic stenosis despite preserved ejection fraction is associated with higher afterload and reduced survival. Circulation 2007;115(22):2856–64.

41. Lancellotti P, Donal E, Magne J, et al. Impact of global left ventricular afterload on left ventricular function in asymptomatic severe aortic stenosis: a two-dimensional speckle-tracking study. Eur J Echocardiogr 2010;11(6):537–43.

42. Adda J, Mielot C, Giorgi R, et al. Low-flow, low-gradient severe aortic stenosis despite normal ejection fraction is associated with severe left ventricular dysfunction as assessed by speckle tracking echocardiography: a multicenter study. Circ Cardiovasc Imaging 2012;5(1):27–35.

43. Le Ven F, Freeman M, Webb J, et al. Impact of low flow on the outcome of high risk patients undergoing transcatheter aortic valve replacement. J Am Coll Cardiol 2013;62(9):782–8.

44. Mehrotra P, Jansen K, Flynn AW, et al. Differential left ventricular remodelling and longitudinal function distinguishes low flow from normal-flow preserved ejection fraction low-gradient severe aortic stenosis. Eur Heart J 2013;34(25):1906–14.

45. Melis G, Frontera G, Caldentey G, et al. Systolic volume index by Doppler echocardiography is an useful marker for stratification and prognostic evaluation in patients with severe aortic stenosis and preserved ejection fraction. Rev Esp Cardiol 2013;66(4):261–8.

46. Mohty D, Magne J, Deltreuil M, et al. Outcome and impact of surgery in paradoxical low-flow, low-gradient severe aortic stenosis and preserved left ventricular ejection fraction: a cardiac catheterization study. Circulation 2013;128(26 Suppl 1): S235–42.

47. Eleid MF, Michelena HI, Nkomo VT, et al. Causes of death and predictors of survival after aortic valve replacement in low flow vs. normal flow severe aortic stenosis with preserved ejection fraction. Eur Heart J Cardiovasc Imaging 2015;16(11):1270–5.

48. Clavel MA, Dumesnil JG, Capoulade R, et al. Outcome of patients with aortic stenosis, small valve area and low-flow, low-gradient despite preserved left ventricular ejection fraction. J Am Coll Cardiol 2012;60(14):1259–67.

49. Dayan V, Vignolo G, Magne J, et al. Outcome and impact of aortic valve replacement in patients with preserved LV ejection fraction and low gradient aortic stenosis: a meta-analysis. J Am Coll Cardiol 2015;66(23):2594–603.

50. Girard SE, Miller FAJ, Edwards WD, et al. Subvalvular stenosis at repeat aortic valve replacement for patient-prosthesis mismatch. J Am Coll Cardiol 2000;35:534A, 2 (Suppl.A).

51. Eleid MF, Sorajja P, Michelena HI, et al. Survival by stroke volume index in patients with low-gradient normal EF severe aortic stenosis. Heart 2015; 101(1):23–9.

52. Clavel MA, Fuchs C, Burwash IG, et al. Predictors of outcomes in low-flow, low-gradient aortic stenosis: results of the multicenter TOPAS Study. Circulation 2008;118(14 Suppl):S234–42.

53. Nishimura RA, Otto CM, Bonow RO, et al. 2014 AHA/ACC guideline for the management of patients with valvular heart disease: executive summary. A report of the American College of Cardiology/American heart association task force on practice guidelines. J Am Coll Cardiol 2014;63(22):2438–88.

54. Pai RG, Varadarajan P, Razzouk A. Survival benefit of aortic valve replacement in patients with severe aortic stenosis with low ejection fraction and low gradient with normal ejection fraction. Ann Thorac Surg 2008;86(6):1781–9.

55. Shan L, Saxena A, McMahon R, et al. A systematic review on the quality of life benefits after aortic valve

replacement in the elderly. J Thorac Cardiovasc Surg 2013;145(5):1173–89.

56. Speir A, Henry LL, Hunt SL, et al. Health-related quality of life following isolated aortic valve surgery: is earlier intervention better? J Heart Valve Dis 2013; 22(3):270–5.

57. Morris JJ, Schaff HV, Mullany CJ, et al. Determinants of survival and recovery of left ventricular function after aortic valve replacement. Ann Thorac Surg 1993;56:22–30.

58. Brown JM, O'Brien SM, Wu C, et al. Isolated aortic valve replacement in North America comprising 108,687 patients in 10 years: changes in risks, valve types, and outcomes in the Society of Thoracic Surgeons National Database. J Thorac Cardiovasc Surg 2009;137(1):82–90.

59. Vaturi M, Shapira Y, Rotstein M, et al. The effect of aortic valve replacement on left ventricular mass assessed by echocardiography. Eur J Echocardiogr 2000;1:116–21.

60. Onorati F, D'Errigo P, Barbanti M, et al. Different impact of sex on baseline characteristics and major periprocedural outcomes of transcatheter and surgical aortic valve interventions: results of the multicenter Italian OBSERVANT Registry. J Thorac Cardiovasc Surg 2014;147(5):1529–39.

61. Stamou SC, Robich M, Wolf RE, et al. Effects of gender and ethnicity on outcomes after aortic valve replacement. J Thorac Cardiovasc Surg 2012; 144(2):486–92.

62. Ter Woorst JF, Hoff AHT, van Straten AHM, et al. Impact of sex on the outcome of isolated aortic valve replacement and the role of different preoperative profiles. J Cardiothorac Vasc Anesth 2019;33(5): 1237–43.

63. Popma JJ, Khabbaz K. Prosthesis-patient mismatch after "high-risk" aortic valve replacement. J Am Coll Cardiol 2014;64(13):1335–8.

64. Urso S, Sadaba R, Vives M, et al. Patient-prosthesis mismatch in elderly patients undergoing aortic valve replacement: impact on quality of life and survival. J Heart Valve Dis 2009;18(3):248–55.

65. Tasca G, Brunelli F, Cirillo M, et al. Impact of the improvement of valve area achieved with aortic valve replacement on the regression of left ventricular hypertrophy in patients with pure aortic stenosis. Ann Thorac Surg 2005;79(4):1291–6.

66. Fuster RG, Montero Argudo JA, Albarova OG, et al. Patient-prosthesis mismatch in aortic valve replacement: really tolerable? Eur J Cardiothorac Surg 2005;27(3):441–9.

67. Nozohoor S, Nilsson J, Luhrs C, et al. The influence of patient-prosthesis mismatch on in-hospital complications and early mortality after aortic valve replacement. J Heart Valve Dis 2007;16(5):475–82.

68. Astudillo LM, Santana O, Urbandt PA, et al. Clinical predictors of prosthesis-patient mismatch after aortic valve replacement for aortic stenosis. Clinics (Sao Paulo) 2012;67(1):55–60.

69. Hernandez-Vaquero D, Garcia JM, Diaz R, et al. Moderate patient-prosthesis mismatch predicts cardiac events and advanced functional class in young and middle-aged patients undergoing surgery due to severe aortic stenosis. J Card Surg 2014;29(2): 127–33.

70. Kandler K, Moller CH, Hassager C, et al. Patient-prosthesis mismatch and reduction in left ventricular mass after aortic valve replacement. Ann Thorac Surg 2013;96(1):66–71.

71. Connolly HM, Oh JK, Orszulak TA, et al. Aortic valve replacement for aortic stenosis with severe left ventricular dysfunction: prognostic indicators. Circulation 1997;95(10):2395–400.

72. Williams M, Kodali SK, Hahn RT, et al. Sex-related differences in outcomes following transcatheter or surgical aortic valve replacement in patients with severe aortic stenosis: insights from the PARTNER Trial. J Am Coll Cardiol 2014;63(15):1522–8.

73. Hahn RT, Pibarot P, Stewart WJ, et al. Comparison of transcatheter and surgical aortic valve replacement in severe aortic stenosis: a longitudinal study of echocardiography parameters in cohort A of the PARTNER Trial (placement of aortic transcatheter valves). J Am Coll Cardiol 2013;61(25): 2514–21.

74. Sinning JM, Vasa-Nicotera M, Chin D, et al. Evaluation and management of paravalvular aortic regurgitation after transcatheter aortic valve replacement. J Am Coll Cardiol 2013;62(1):11–20.

75. Rodés-Cabau J, Webb JG, Cheung A, et al. Long-term outcomes after transcatheter aortic valve implantation: insights on prognostic factors and valve durability from the canadian multicenter experience. J Am Coll Cardiol 2012;60(19):1864–75.

76. Mack MJ, Leon MB, Thourani VH, et al. Transcatheter aortic-valve replacement with a balloon-expandable valve in low-risk patients. N Engl J Med 2019;380(18):1695–705.

77. Kodali SK, Williams MR, Smith CR, et al. Two-year outcomes after transcatheter or surgical aortic-valve replacement. N Engl J Med 2012;366(18): 1686–95.

78. Adams DH, Popma JJ, Reardon MJ, et al. Transcatheter aortic-valve replacement with a self-expanding prosthesis. N Engl J Med 2014;370(19): 1790–8.

79. Abdel-Wahab M, Zahn R, Horack M, et al. Aortic regurgitation after transcatheter aortic valve implantation: incidence and early outcome. Results from the German transcatheter aortic valve interventions registry. Heart 2011;97(11):899–906.

80. Unbehaun A, Pasic M, Dreysse S, et al. Transapical aortic valve implantation: incidence and predictors of paravalvular leakage and transvalvular

regurgitation in a series of 358 patients. J Am Coll Cardiol 2012;59(3):211–21.

81. Pibarot P, Weissman NJ, Stewart WJ, et al. Incidence and sequelae of prosthesis-patient mismatch in transcatheter versus surgical valve replacement in high-risk patients with severe aortic stenosis- A PARTNER trial cohort A analysis. J Am Coll Cardiol 2014;64(13):1323–34.

82. Kukucka M, Pasic M, Dreysse S, et al. Patient-prosthesis mismatch after transapical aortic valve implantation: incidence and impact on survival. J Thorac Cardiovasc Surg 2013;145(2):391–7.

83. Jilaihawi H, Chin D, Spyt T, et al. Prosthesis-patient mismatch after transcatheter aortic valve implantation with the Medtronic-Corevalve bioprosthesis. Eur Heart J 2010;31(7):857–64.

84. Bleiziffer S, Hettich I, Hutter A, et al. Incidence and impact of prosthesis-patient mismatch after transcatheter aortic valve implantation. J Heart Valve Dis 2013;22(3):309–16.

85. Stangl V, Baldenhofer G, Laule M, et al. Influence of sex on outcome following transcatheter aortic valve implantation (TAVI): systematic review and meta-analysis. J Interv Cardiol 2014;27(6):531–9.

86. Hayashida K, Morice MC, Chevalier B, et al. Sex-related differences in clinical presentation and outcome of transcatheter aortic valve implantation for severe aortic stenosis. J Am Coll Cardiol 2012; 59(6):566–71.

87. Humphries KH, Toggweiler S, Rodés-Cabau J, et al. Sex differences in mortality after transcatheter aortic valve replacement for severe aortic stenosis. J Am Coll Cardiol 2012;60(10):882–6.

88. Ferrante G, Pagnotta P, Petronio AS, et al. Sex differences in postprocedural aortic regurgitation and mid-term mortality after transcatheter aortic valve implantation. Catheter Cardiovasc Interv 2014; 84(2):264–71.

89. Al-Lamee R, Broyd C, Parker J, et al. Influence of gender on clinical outcomes following transcatheter aortic valve implantation from the UK transcatheter aortic valve implantation registry and the National Institute for Cardiovascular Outcomes Research. Am J Cardiol 2014;113(3):522–8.

90. Dvir D, Webb JG, Bleiziffer S, et al. Transcatheter aortic valve implantation in failed bioprosthetic surgical valves. JAMA 2014;312(2):162–70.

91. Flameng W, Herregods MC, Vercalsteren M, et al. Prosthesis-patient mismatch predicts structural valve degeneration in bioprosthetic heart valves. Circulation 2010;121(19):2123–9.

92. Zenses AS, Dahou A, Salaun E, et al. Haemodynamic outcomes following aortic valve-in-valve procedure. Open heart 2018;5(2):e000854.

93. Barbanti M, Yang TH, Rodés CJ, et al. Anatomical and procedural features associated with aortic root rupture during balloon-expandable transcatheter aortic valve replacement. Circulation 2013;128(3): 244–53.

94. Ribeiro HB, Webb JG, Makkar RR, et al. Predictive factors, management and clinical outcomes of coronary obstruction following transcatheter aortic valve implantation: insights from a large multicenter registry. J Am Coll Cardiol 2013;62(17):1552–62.

95. Ribeiro HB, Sarmento-Leite R, Siqueira DA, et al. Coronary obstruction following transcatheter aortic valve implantation. Arq Bras Cardiol 2014;102(1): 93–6.

96. Buellesfeld L, Stortecky S, Kalesan B, et al. Aortic root dimensions among patients with severe aortic stenosis undergoing transcatheter aortic valve replacement. JACC Cardiovasc Interv 2013;6(1): 72–83.

97. O'Connor SA, Morice MC, Gilard M, et al. Revisiting sex equality with transcatheter aortic valve replacement outcomes: a collaborative, patient-level meta-analysis of 11,310 patients. J Am Coll Cardiol 2015;66(3):221–8.

98. Vahanian A, Baumgartner H, Bax J, et al. Guidelines on the management of valvular heart disease: the task force on the management of valvular heart disease of the European Society of Cardiology. Eur Heart J 2007;28(2):230–68.

99. Baumgartner H, Falk V, Bax JJ, et al. 2017 ESC/ EACTS guidelines for the management of valvular heart disease: the Task Force for the management of valvular heart disease of the European Society of Cardiology (ESC) and the European Association for Cardio-Thoracic Surgery (EACTS). Eur Heart J 2017;38(36):2739–91.

Aortic Stenosis
What Risks Do the Stresses of Noncardiac Surgery or Pregnancy Pose and How Should They Be Managed?

Jordi S. Dahl, MD, PhD[a],*, Lucia Baris, MD[b], Rasmus Carter-Storch, MD, PhD[a], Roger Hall, MD[b]

KEYWORDS

- Aortic stenosis • Noncardiac surgery • Pregnancy • Risks

KEY POINTS

- Pregnancy outcomes in asymptomatic women with moderate or severe AS are generally favorable.
- Women with symptomatic severe AS, however, are at high risk of pregnancy complications, mainly heart failure, and should undergo AVR before pregnancy.
- Preconception counseling and the formulation of a pregnancy plan as far in advance as possible is essential in all women with AS.
- Non cardiac surgery may be performed with a low rate of complications in patients with asymptomatic severe AS, particularly when NCS is low risk or intermediate risk.
- In patients with symptomatic severe AS it is advisable to recommend AVR before NCS, although one has to consider if the benefit of AVR to reduce cardiovascular risk outweighs the potential delay of non cardiac surgery.

INTRODUCTION

Both noncardiac surgery (NCS) and pregnancy are situations that stress the heart by requiring increased cardiac output and may lead to sudden changes in the loading conditions of the heart. Aortic stenosis (AS) usually has different origins in these two situations but the same hemodynamic consequences. In pregnant patients who have AS it is nearly always congenital or rheumatic in origin, whereas in NCS the patients are often elderly and consequently the AS is frequently of degenerative origin.

The main consequences of AS in terms of morbidity and mortality are the result of increased resistance to left ventricular (LV) outflow caused by the narrowed valve and consequently the increased work this imposes on the LV. This pressure overload leads to LV hypertrophy and concentric remodeling, a response regarded as a physiologic adaptation preserving end-systolic wall stress, and increasing contractility to maintain cardiac output. However, these adaptive mechanisms occur at the expense of altered LV function and increased filling pressures because of increased stiffness of the hypertrophied and sometimes fibrosed LV myocardium. Combined with reduced coronary flow reserve,[1] which results from an altered coronary artery-LV pressure gradient, these abnormalities may lead to myocardial ischemia, reduced function particularly in response to increased demand, and eventually to

[a] Department of Cardiology, Odense University Hospital, Søndre boulevard 29, 5000 Odense C, Denmark;
[b] Department of Cardiology, Norwich Medical School, University of East Anglia, Norwich Research Park, Norwich NR4 7TJ, UK
* Corresponding author.
E-mail address: jordi.sanchez.dahl@rsyd.dk

Cardiol Clin 38 (2020) 139–148
https://doi.org/10.1016/j.ccl.2019.09.009

heart failure. Although the occurrence of symptoms is regarded as a class I indication for aortic valve replacement (AVR), asymptomatic patients are generally considered to be low-risk and follow-up rather than intervention is generally recommended.[2,3] However, AS-related LV remodeling, altered coronary flow reserve, and a reduced valve area may lead to sudden deterioration in asymptomatic patients with severe AS if they experience rapid changes in loading conditions as may occur during pregnancy or anesthesia. The inability to adequately increase stroke volume, because of a fixed orifice and a reduced LV chamber size, may be troublesome during arterial vasodilation or volume depletion (reduced preload) because small changes in these variables may lead to severe hypotension as the heart cannot adequately increase its output and compensate; with this comes a vicious circle of reduced coronary perfusion leading to further impairment of LV function and so on. Furthermore, vasoconstriction with reduced systemic arterial compliance (increased afterload) or hypervolemia (increased preload) may also stress the LV leading to congestion and overt heart failure. Consequently, various studies have suggested that patients with AS have increased risk in pregnancy and delivery and during anesthesia and surgery, although there are significant degrees of uncertainty as to the exact risks and consequently the best way to manage such patients. The purpose of this study is to review current literature regarding the impact of AS on pregnancy and anesthesia during NCS. It is important at the outset to understand the shortcomings of the scientific evidence. Most of the available studies are observational and they are also often retrospective and therefore there is bound to be a great deal of bias. This leads to difficulty in drawing conclusions in terms of how to apply the published information to clinical management.

AORTIC STENOSIS AND NONCARDIAC SURGERY

Since the seminal paper by Skinner and Pearce in 1964,[4] demonstrating high rates of cardiovascular complications and death among patients with aortic lesions, the risk of NCS in patients with AS has been recognized. These findings were later corroborated by Goldman and colleagues[5] in 1977, showing that patients with severe AS had a 13% risk of death before discharge. Although since then, several clinical studies[6–20] and a few meta-analysis[21,22] have studied AS a risk factor, the management of NCS in patients with AS remains a clinical conundrum. Should patients undergo AVR with the risks associated with this procedure and of delaying important NCS, or should NCS be conducted at an increased risk? The introduction of percutaneous aortic valve procedures with lower risk, but requiring additional antithrombotic therapy and with limited experience among asymptomatic patients has further increased the complexity of this topic.

NCS can, according to the procedure and risk of death, be classified as low risk (<1%), intermediate risk (1%–5%), and high risk (>5%) (**Box 1**). Current European Society of Cardiology (ESC) guidelines[2] and American College of Cardiology/American Heart Association Guidelines[3] recommend that elective NCS be postponed in symptomatic patients and in asymptomatic patients undergoing a high-risk procedure until after aortic valve surgery, particularly when the AVR is low risk. In contrast,

---

Box 1
Risk of noncardiac surgery (30-day mortality) with examples of types of surgery

Low risk (<1% risk)

    Minor orthopedic surgery (eg, knee surgery)

    Minor urologic surgery

    Eye surgery

    Dental surgery

    Mamma surgery

    Asymptomatic carotid artery surgery

Intermediate risk (1%–5% risk)

    Symptomatic carotid artery surgery

    Peripheral vascular angioplasty

    Intraperitoneal surgery

    Head and neck surgery

    Major orthopedic surgery (hip or spine)

    Minor intrathoracic surgery

    Kidney transplant

High risk (>5% risk)

    Open peripheral vascular surgery

    Aortic surgery

    Lung and liver transplant

    Duodenal, pancreas, and gallbladder surgery

    Major urologic surgery

    Intracranial surgery

    Major intrathoracic surgery

Data from Schwarze ML, Barnato AE, Rathouz PJ, et al. Development of a list of high-risk operations for patients 65 years and older. JAMA surgery. 2015;150(4):325-331.

patients in whom AVR is high-risk should undergo NCS under strict monitoring without prior AVR. However, the basis for these management decisions is controversial, because they are based primarily on studies of retrospective and observational nature, with heterogeneous populations using different AS severity definitions and events.

The potential harms of NCS in patients with severe AS are several. In a study comparing 30 patients with severe asymptomatic AS with more than 75 years of age, gender-matched patients with mild to moderate AS, undergoing predominantly intermediate risk NCS, Calleja and colleagues[15] demonstrated that the risk of hypotension or the need of catecholamines during hospitalization was nearly two-fold (30% vs 17%) compared with patients with mild and moderate AS despite nonsignificant ($P = .11$). These findings have since been reinforced by others,[6,15,18,19] and it has been speculated that patients with severe AS are more vulnerable to anesthesia-induced decrease in systemic vascular resistance. Indeed, a fixed valvular obstruction may impede the increase of stroke volume needed in this situation to maintain systemic blood pressure and consequently, leads to hypotension. However, studies examining the impact of vasodilatation with angiotensin-converting enzyme inhibitors[23,24] or nitroprusside[25–27] in patients with AS have failed to demonstrate an unfavorable impact on hemodynamics, and have even demonstrated an increase in stroke volume. Most of these studies were conducted among patients with concomitant hypertension, and support the importance of treating hypertension in patients with AS to avoid a double-loaded LV, but also probably explains why preexisting hypertension seems to protect against surgery-induced hypotension.[11] However, Eleid and colleagues[25] demonstrated an increase in stroke volume and cardiac output after nitroprusside-induced vasodilation among patients without reduced stroke volume irrespective of hypertension, supporting previous findings. This probably reflects that mild vasodilatation may be appropriate when stroke volume is reduced, although it rarely improves stroke volume when it is preserved.[26] However, when vasodilation exceeds the capacity of the LV to increase stroke volume, it may lead to hypotension. If not corrected, this may cause a progressive negative spiral of reduced coronary pressure, ischemia, reduced LV systolic function, and further exacerbation of hypotension. The risk of hypotension is especially high in patients with concomitant coronary artery disease,[11,16] indicating that other factors in addition to valvular resistance impede compensatory increases in stroke volume.

Although ischemic heart disease commonly coexists with AS, reduced coronary flow may occur in the absence of coronary artery disease because increasing LV pressures reduce the coronary artery/LV pressure gradient and coronary flow, even leading to systolic flow-reversal[28,29] limiting coronary perfusion to diastole. Patients with severe AS are particularly vulnerable to tachycardia and tachyarrhythmia, because when the heart rate rises, diastolic perfusion time falls and this is likely to lead to ischemia and consequently increased filling pressures. The latter is also the consequence of AS-associated LV remodeling in which LV hypertrophy, concentric geometry with reduced LV chamber, and myocardial fibrosis despite preserving wall-stress and increasing contractility occur at the price of reduced LV compliance, delayed LV relaxation, and increased LV filling pressures. Diastolic dysfunction and increased filling pressures may partially explain the transition from asymptomatic to symptomatic AS.[30] In a recent study, Lyhne and colleagues[31] demonstrated that even asymptomatic severe AS patients with a normal functional capacity had an inappropriate hemodynamic response during exercise with an abnormal increase in LV filling pressures. The steeper pressure-volume relationship during diastole and impaired LV relaxation may thus explain the increased risk of heart failure in patients with AS undergoing NCS because the same response is likely to occur in response to any cardiac stress. Increased systemic vascular resistance for example, because of catecholamines or hypertension, a rapid increase in preload caused by fluid shifts and/or excessive fluid/blood administration, or tachycardia reducing the contribution of the atrium of the LV filling and diastolic filling time, may altogether or separately lead to decompensation and overt heart failure in patients with AS. In a large study from the Mayo Clinic, Tashiro and colleagues[18] demonstrated that after NCS, compared with patients without AS those with severe AS were more likely to experience the combined end point of death, heart failure, myocardial infarction, ventricular arrhythmia, and stroke, although this difference was largely driven by differences in the incidence of heart failure. These findings are in agreement with other studies, demonstrating an increased risk of heart failure in patients with AS undergoing NCS.[5,9–12,15–19,22]

Although some studies have suggested that AS may increase the risk of myocardial infarction[11,16,22] and stroke, a recent Danish registry study including data from 2823 patients with AS and 2823 matched patients was not able to demonstrate any difference in myocardial infarction, stroke, or the combination of end points (n = 229 [8%] vs n = 207 [7%] in AS and control subjects, respectively).[17]

Although AS did not associate with outcome, the presence of symptoms interpreted as a history of heart failure or treatment with nitrates/diuretics, and emergency surgery did. These findings parallel previous studies identifying symptom status,[16–18,20,22] emergency surgery,[17,18,20] and mitral valve regurgitation[16] as markers of postoperative outcome. Smaller studies have also found that patients with AS had a higher incidence of perioperative gastrointestinal bleeding,[12,19] delirium,[19] and length of stay.[16]

The impact of AS on mortality in patients undergoing NCS is more controversial. It is generally accepted that the risk is lower than previously reported by Skinner and Pearce[4] and Goldman and coworkers,[5] probably reflecting improvement in anesthesia, and that patients undergoing NCS with AS have a higher long-term mortality than control subjects after NCS.[16,18,19] The latter is not unexpected, given that patients with AS despite successful AVR have a worse outcome than the general population.[32] However, it is also likely that there are now fewer symptomatic patients with AS in the population because AVR has become more widespread and also applied to the elderly who in the past were denied surgery and consequently developed conditions needing NCS while remaining untreated for their symptomatic AS.

However, although some studies find that AS in general is a significant risk factor for in-hospital or 30-day all-cause mortality after NCS,[12,16,17,19] other studies do not. A large retrospective study by Zahid and colleagues[11] did not find that AS was associated with an increased risk of postoperative mortality, although AS severity was not defined and most procedures were low-risk. Furthermore, most studies failing to demonstrate the impact of AS on mortality were limited by small sample size[15] or by the inclusion of patients undergoing surgery in regional blockade.[7,13,14] In a larger set of patients, Agarwal and colleagues[16] demonstrated an increased 30-day mortality among 634 patients with at least moderate AS compared with 2536 propensity-score-matched patients (2.1% vs 1.0%; $P = .04$). The risk was, at first sight, paradoxically higher in patients with moderate AS than in severe AS (2.3% vs 1.6%; $P = .06$). However, this probably reflects that patients with low-flow low-gradient AS with reduced LV ejection fraction were included and that patients failing to increase mean gradients greater than 30 mm Hg during a dobutamine stress test were labeled as moderate AS. This group includes patients with pseudosevere AS

and patients lacking flow-reserve on dobutamine, entities highly associated with a poor outcome.[33,34] The validity of this study is probably hampered by the inclusion of patients with reduced LV ejection fraction and patients with severe mitral regurgitation. In contrast, Tashiro and colleagues[18] reported, in a study of 256 patients with severe AS undergoing intermediate- and high-risk NCS, no differences in 30-day cardiac mortality compared with age- and gender-matched patients without AS. These findings have since been corroborated by two recent meta-analyses.[21,22]

Management of Patients with Aortic Stenosis Undergoing Noncardiac Surgery

Although the previously mentioned information emphasizes that the data regarding the risks of NCS in AS are confusing, clinical common sense demands extreme care in a situation that, based on physiologic first principles and clinical experience, is hazardous. This is particularly so because of the concerns about the degree of bias in observational and often small and retrospective studies.

Management of patients with AS undergoing NCS should include careful assessment of symptoms. In case of symptoms, American and European guidelines recommend AVR before NCS if possible.[35,36] Although we believe this is an appropriate recommendation, particularly because these patients already have a class I recommendation for valvular surgery, and AVR may reduce the risk of developing heart failure, it must be emphasized that in case of "malignant disease," valvular surgery should be performed urgently to avoid delay of potentially life-saving NCS. Furthermore the reverse remodeling process after aortic valve surgery is slow, or may not occur[37] in some patients and diastolic function may even deteriorate after AVR.[38] Irrespective of whether this reflects irreversible changes[39] or coexisting morbidities as amyloid, which are common among elderly with severe AS,[40] the increased risk of heart failure may still be prevalent after AVR.

Although the American guidelines do not present recommendations for asymptomatic severe AS,[35] the European guidelines recommend that these patients should undergo NCS without prior AVR if surgery is low or intermediate risk. In contrast, evaluation for AVR before NCS is recommended in high-risk surgery; patients with a low risk of AVR should be considered for AVR and patients with high risk for AVR should be considered for transcatheter AVR or balloon valvuloplasty, although to our knowledge there are no data to support these recommendations.[36] Alternatively, it is proposed that all patients with severe AS undergoing high-risk NCS, including patients who have declined AVR or where this is contraindicated, should preferably be operated at a tertiary cardiac center under strict hemodynamic monitoring to avoid episodes of hypotension and tachycardia.[35,36]

We recommend, based on the available and rather limited evidence and in accordance with the recommendations of Osnabrugge and colleagues,[41] that NCS should be undertaken under close hemodynamic surveillance in asymptomatic AS patients. Episodes of hypotension should be avoided and treated appropriately with fluid and catecholamines. However, there is no evidence to suggest that AVR should be undertaken before NCS in asymptomatic patients, even in the case of high-risk surgery (see **Box 1**). In symptomatic patients, AVR should be considered first, and if the risk associated with surgical or transcatheter AVR is too high, balloon aortic valvuloplasty could be considered to provide a window in which to undertake the necessary NCS.[42–44] These recommendations are summarized in **Fig. 1**.

Conclusion

NCS is performed with a low rate of complications in patients with asymptomatic severe AS, particularly when NCS is low risk or intermediate risk. In these cases NCS can be undertaken under close hemodynamic surveillance, without previous AVR. In patients with symptomatic severe AS it is advisable to recommend AVR (surgical or transcatheter) before NCS, although one has

to consider if the benefit of AVR to reduce cardiovascular risk outweighs the potential delay of NCS.

AORTIC STENOSIS AND PREGNANCY
Hemodynamic Changes During Pregnancy

During pregnancy, many profound changes take place in the mother's hemodynamics, including a 30% to 50% increase in cardiac output. The presence of LV outflow obstruction in AS reduces or in extreme circumstances prevents this increase in cardiac output depending on its severity. In women with severe AS, cardiac output depends entirely on heart rate and preload, because increases in stroke volume are limited by the low effective valve area of the stenotic aortic valve. Although often well tolerated, this can lead to congestive heart failure, cardiogenic shock, and death. Thus, during pregnancy there is an increased risk of maternal mortality and morbidity, and fetal complications brought on by the mother's impaired hemodynamics. The hemodynamic changes that occur during pregnancy are summarized in **Fig. 2**.

Aortic Stenosis in Women of Childbearing Age

In women of childbearing age, the main cause of AS is a congenital bicuspid aortic valve. Most of these women are aware of their valve condition and undergo (frequent) outpatient follow-up care, allowing ample opportunity for preconception counseling and prepregnancy optimization. Another important cause of AS in women of

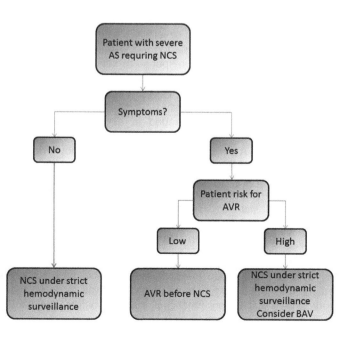

Fig. 1. Recommendations for the management of patients with severe AS undergoing NCS. BAV, balloon aortic valvulotomy.

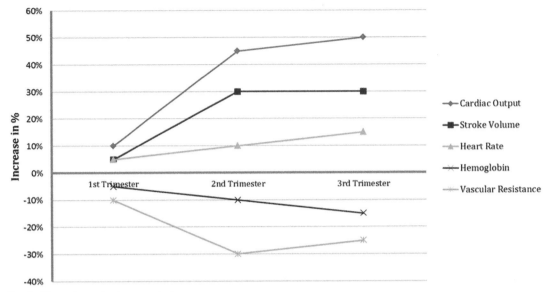

Fig. 2. Hemodynamic changes during pregnancy.

childbearing age is rheumatic heart disease. Rheumatic heart disease, although especially endemic in low-to-middle-income countries, is more frequently encountered nowadays in the Western world because of immigration. As opposed to women with congenital AS, many women with AS caused by rheumatic valve disease are often unaware of their condition before pregnancy. The hemodynamic changes of pregnancy often unmask these previously unrecognized lesions, leaving no space for preconceptional counseling and posing diagnostic and treatment-related problems.

Pregnancy Risks and Preconception Counseling

The outcome of pregnancy and the problems that are expected in women with AS are dependent on the severity of the valve stenosis, and on symptomatology, LV function, and the presence of LV hypertrophy. Women with moderate AS tolerate pregnancy well and have low rates of complications, and the same goes for women with severe AS who are asymptomatic before pregnancy.[45] Historically, pregnancy in women with AS is associated with increased maternal mortality rates but numbers vary, ranging from 0% to 17.4%.[46–50] In the current era, maternal mortality seems to be close to zero in women with AS (moderate and severe).[45,51] In contrast, however, women with severe AS who are also symptomatic before pregnancy are at substantially increased risk of maternal morbidity during pregnancy, predominantly heart failure. Thus, women with severe AS

form a high-risk group and should always be counseled accordingly prepregnancy: they should be made aware of the risks and a management plan should be set up for care during pregnancy, labor, delivery, and the postpartum period.

Otherwise healthy women with severe AS who are symptomatic require AVR (either surgical or percutaneous) before pregnancy according to the 2017 ESC guidelines for the management of valvular heart disease and the 2018 ESC guidelines on the management of pregnancy in women with heart disease.[51,52] Before valve replacement, these women should be counseled against pregnancy.[51] It is recommended that in women with asymptomatic severe AS, an exercise test before pregnancy is performed to assess exercise tolerance and the response to hemodynamic fluctuations. This test can first unmask concealed symptoms. However, with normal exercise tolerance and normal LV functions, pregnancy should not be discouraged in asymptomatic women, even those with severe AS.

A pregnancy management plan should be made in which regular clinical and echocardiographic follow-up is set up by multidisciplinary teams (cardiologist, obstetrician, and obstetric anesthesiologist) in specialized centers.

Management During Pregnancy

Although women with severe AS represent a high-risk group, most tolerate pregnancy well, especially those who are asymptomatic (New York Heart Association functional class I) before pregnancy. Symptomatic women with severe AS who despite counsel against pregnancy become pregnant, should be monitored intensively. The same goes for women who are asymptomatic before pregnancy and who become symptomatic during pregnancy. Monthly evaluations by specialized teams including regular echocardiographic imaging are advised. In addition, in symptomatic women, bed rest and limited heart failure therapy are the first choices of treatment. Heart failure therapy is mainly limited to diuretics that should be used with caution because of the risk of placental hypoperfusion and β-blockers when indicated (ie, LV dysfunction); angiotensin-converting enzyme inhibitors are contraindicated in pregnancy.

Balloon valvuloplasty for severe AS is performed in symptomatic patients in whom conventional therapy and bed rest are not sufficient.[53] Balloon valvuloplasty, however, carries the risk of causing severe aortic regurgitation, which necessitates emergency surgery. Because cardiac surgery with cardiopulmonary bypass is associated with high rates of complications, especially fetal, it should be avoided whenever possible. Therefore, in the case of fetal viability, caesarian section (CS) before balloon valvuloplasty or valvular surgery is recommended.

Management of Labor and Delivery

In nearly all cardiac patients, the preferred mode of delivery is vaginal delivery. CS should be reserved for obstetric indications only, and very few high-risk cardiac exceptions (eg, in the case of fulminant heart failure). In women with severe AS who are symptomatic despite maximum medical therapy, CS should be considered. However, CS with both general and spinal anesthesia is associated with major blood pressure fluctuations caused by blockade of the autonomic system[54] with high risks of hypotension and subsequent coronary hypoperfusion. However, in comparison with general anesthesia, a better controlled situation with greater hemodynamic stability is created when continuous spinal anesthesia is used, because this allows for personalized titration of the anesthetic.[55]

Asymptomatic women with severe AS can have a vaginal delivery. However, because their cardiac output depends largely on heart rate and preload, tachycardia but also bradycardia should be avoided during delivery and care must be taken to maintain an adequate preload during labor. Thus, a prolonged second stage of labor and active pushing is not desirable because this can reduce cardiac output. In addition, caval compression should be avoided and women should be positioned in the left lateral tilt position during labor. In nonlaboring patients, aortocaval compression by the gravid uterus is usually asymptomatic. However, during active labor, particularly in women with a (to some extent) fixed cardiac output caused by AS, aortocaval compression can lead to insufficient preload and thus hemodynamic collapse.[56] Epidural anesthesia reduces stress and pain and thus catecholamine production during labor and delivery. Its use in women with severe AS, however, is controversial, because it also causes peripheral vasodilatation leading to hypotension and thus a decreased preload. In addition, tachycardia is more often seen, as is a decrease in diastolic relaxation time. Therefore general, spinal, and epidural anesthesia should be handled by specialized anesthesiologists and preferably delivery and anesthesia plans should be made before or in the early stages of pregnancy.

Close monitoring of cardiac output and other hemodynamic parameters during labor and delivery is advised, preferably continuously. The gold standard for continuous cardiac output monitoring is Swan-Ganz thermodilution, but its use in pregnancy is controversial because of its invasive nature. Noninvasive cardiac output monitoring using impedance cardiography is a suitable option to monitor these high-risk women during labor and delivery.[57]

The use of oxytocin and ergometrine during and after delivery in women with severe AS is contraindicated because of their hemodynamic effects including induction of hypotension, coronary artery spasms, vasoconstriction, and tachycardia. However, in some situations the benefit of these drugs outweighs any potential disadvantages (eg, in such situations as severe postpartum hemorrhage or retained placenta, and then slow infusion is preferred to an intravenous bolus).[58]

In the absence of active infection, routine antibiotic endocarditis prophylaxis is not recommended during delivery in women with severe native valve AS.[59–61]

SUMMARY

Pregnancy outcomes in asymptomatic women with moderate or severe AS are generally favorable. Women with symptomatic severe AS, however, are at high risk of pregnancy complications, mainly heart failure, and should undergo AVR before pregnancy. Preconception counseling and the formulation of a pregnancy plan as far in advance as possible is essential in all women with AS. Furthermore, these women should be managed in specialized centers by multidisciplinary teams. Surgical and percutaneous valve interventions during pregnancy are available in the case of persistent heart failure despite optimal medical therapy. During delivery, either caesarean or vaginal, anesthesia poses potential hemodynamic problems and should therefore be managed by specialized obstetric anesthesiologists.

DISCLOSURE/CONFLICTS OF INTERESTS

None.

REFERENCES

1. Rajappan K, Rimoldi OE, Dutka DP, et al. Mechanisms of coronary microcirculatory dysfunction in patients with aortic stenosis and angiographically normal coronary arteries. Circulation 2002;105(4): 470–6.
2. Baumgartner H, Falk V, Bax JJ, et al. 2017 ESC/EACTS guidelines for the management of valvular heart disease: the task force for the management of valvular heart disease of the European Society of Cardiology (ESC) and the European Association for Cardio-Thoracic Surgery (EACTS). Eur Heart J 2017;38(36):2739–91.
3. Nishimura RA, Otto CM, Bonow RO, et al. 2014 AHA/ACC guideline for the management of patients with valvular heart disease: executive summary: a report of the American College of Cardiology/American Heart Association Task Force on practice guidelines. Circulation 2014;129(23):2440–92.
4. Skinner JF, Pearce ML. Surgical risk in the cardiac patient. J Chronic Dis 1964;17:57–72.
5. Goldman L, Caldera DL, Nussbaum SR, et al. Multifactorial index of cardiac risk in noncardiac surgical procedures. N Engl J Med 1977;297(16):845–50.
6. O'Keefe JH Jr, Shub C, Rettke SR. Risk of noncardiac surgical procedures in patients with aortic stenosis. Mayo Clin Proc 1989;64(4):400–5.
7. Raymer K, Yang H. Patients with aortic stenosis: cardiac complications in non-cardiac surgery. Can J Anaesth 1998;45(9):855–9.
8. Torsher LC, Shub C, Rettke SR, et al. Risk of patients with severe aortic stenosis undergoing noncardiac surgery. Am J Cardiol 1998;81(4):448–52.
9. Rohde LE, Polanczyk CA, Goldman L, et al. Usefulness of transthoracic echocardiography as a tool for risk stratification of patients undergoing major noncardiac surgery. Am J Cardiol 2001;87(5):505–9.
10. Kertai MD, Bountioukos M, Boersma E, et al. Aortic stenosis: an underestimated risk factor for perioperative complications in patients undergoing noncardiac surgery. Am J Med 2004;116(1): 8–13.
11. Zahid M, Sonel AF, Saba S, et al. Perioperative risk of noncardiac surgery associated with aortic stenosis. Am J Cardiol 2005;96(3):436–8.
12. Adunsky A, Kaplan A, Arad M, et al. Aortic stenosis in elderly hip fractured patients. Arch Gerontol Geriatr 2008;46(3):401–8.
13. Leibowitz D, Rivkin G, Schiffman J, et al. Effect of severe aortic stenosis on the outcome in elderly patients undergoing repair of hip fracture. Gerontology 2009;55(3):303–6.
14. McBrien ME, Heyburn G, Stevenson M, et al. Previously undiagnosed aortic stenosis revealed by auscultation in the hip fracture population: echocardiographic findings, management and outcome. Anaesthesia 2009;64(8):863–70.
15. Calleja AM, Dommaraju S, Gaddam R, et al. Cardiac risk in patients aged >75 years with asymptomatic, severe aortic stenosis undergoing noncardiac surgery. Am J Cardiol 2010;105(8):1159–63.
16. Agarwal S, Rajamanickam A, Bajaj NS, et al. Impact of aortic stenosis on postoperative outcomes after noncardiac surgeries. Circ Cardiovasc Qual Outcomes 2013;6(2):193–200.
17. Andersson C, Jorgensen ME, Martinsson A, et al. Noncardiac surgery in patients with aortic stenosis: a contemporary study on outcomes in a matched sample from the Danish health care system. Clin Cardiol 2014;37(11):680–6.
18. Tashiro T, Pislaru SV, Blustin JM, et al. Perioperative risk of major non-cardiac surgery in patients with severe aortic stenosis: a reappraisal in contemporary practice. Eur Heart J 2014;35(35):2372–81.
19. Keswani A, Lovy A, Khalid M, et al. The effect of aortic stenosis on elderly hip fracture outcomes: a case control study. Injury 2016;47(2):413–8.
20. MacIntyre PA, Scott M, Seigne R, et al. An observational study of perioperative risk associated with aortic stenosis in non-cardiac surgery. Anaesth Intensive Care 2018;46(2):207–14.
21. Tarantini G, Nai Fovino L, Tellaroli P, et al. Asymptomatic severe aortic stenosis and noncardiac surgery. Am J Cardiol 2016;117(3):486–8.
22. Kwok CS, Bagur R, Rashid M, et al. Aortic stenosis and non-cardiac surgery: a systematic review and meta-analysis. Int J Cardiol 2017;240:145–53.
23. Chockalingam A, Venkatesan S, Subramaniam T, et al. Safety and efficacy of angiotensin-converting enzyme inhibitors in symptomatic severe aortic stenosis: symptomatic cardiac obstruction-pilot study of enalapril in aortic stenosis (SCOPE-AS). Am Heart J 2004;147(4):E19.
24. Jimenez-Candil J, Bermejo J, Yotti R, et al. Effects of angiotensin converting enzyme inhibitors in hypertensive patients with aortic valve stenosis: a drug withdrawal study. Heart 2005;91(10): 1311–8.
25. Eleid MF, Nishimura RA, Sorajja P, et al. Systemic hypertension in low-gradient severe aortic stenosis with preserved ejection fraction. Circulation 2013; 128(12):1349–53.

26. Lloyd JW, Nishimura RA, Borlaug BA, et al. Hemodynamic response to nitroprusside in patients with low-gradient severe aortic stenosis and preserved ejection fraction. J Am Coll Cardiol 2017;70(11): 1339–48.

27. Khot UN, Novaro GM, Popovic ZB, et al. Nitroprusside in critically ill patients with left ventricular dysfunction and aortic stenosis. N Engl J Med 2003;348(18):1756–63.

28. Carroll RJ, Falsetti HL. Retrograde coronary artery flow in aortic valve disease. Circulation 1976;54(3): 494–9.

29. Fujiwara T, Nogami A, Masaki H, et al. Coronary flow velocity waveforms in aortic stenosis and the effects of valve replacement. Ann Thorac Surg 1989;48(4): 518–22.

30. Dahl JS, Christensen NL, Videbaek L, et al. Left ventricular diastolic function is associated with symptom status in severe aortic valve stenosis. Circ Cardiovasc Imaging 2014;7(1):142–8.

31. Christensen NL, Dahl JS, Carter-Storch R, et al. Association between left atrial dilatation and invasive hemodynamics at rest and during exercise in asymptomatic aortic stenosis. Circ Cardiovasc Imaging 2016;9(10) [pii:e005156].

32. Ashikhmina EA, Schaff HV, Dearani JA, et al. Aortic valve replacement in the elderly: determinants of late outcome. Circulation 2011;124(9): 1070–8.

33. van Gils L, Clavel MA, Vollema EM, et al. Prognostic implications of moderate aortic stenosis in patients with left ventricular systolic dysfunction. J Am Coll Cardiol 2017;69(19):2383–92.

34. Quere JP, Monin JL, Levy F, et al. Influence of preoperative left ventricular contractile reserve on postoperative ejection fraction in low-gradient aortic stenosis. Circulation 2006;113(14):1738–44.

35. Fleisher LA, Fleischmann KE, Auerbach AD, et al. 2014 ACC/AHA guideline on perioperative cardiovascular evaluation and management of patients undergoing noncardiac surgery: a report of the American College of Cardiology/American Heart Association Task Force on Practice Guidelines. Circulation 2014;130(24):e278–333.

36. Kristensen SD, Knuuti J, Saraste A, et al. 2014 ESC/ESA Guidelines on non-cardiac surgery: cardiovascular assessment and management: the Joint Task Force on non-cardiac surgery: cardiovascular assessment and management of the European Society of Cardiology (ESC) and the European Society of Anaesthesiology (ESA). Eur Heart J 2014;35(35): 2383–431.

37. Krayenbuehl HP, Hess OM, Monrad ES, et al. Left ventricular myocardial structure in aortic valve disease before, intermediate, and late after aortic valve replacement. Circulation 1989;79(4): 744–55.

38. Gjertsson P, Caidahl K, Bech-Hanssen O. Left ventricular diastolic dysfunction late after aortic valve replacement in patients with aortic stenosis. Am J Cardiol 2005;96(5):722–7.

39. Weidemann F, Herrmann S, Stork S, et al. Impact of myocardial fibrosis in patients with symptomatic severe aortic stenosis. Circulation 2009;120(7): 577–84.

40. Treibel TA, Fontana M, Gilbertson JA, et al. Occult transthyretin cardiac amyloid in severe calcific aortic stenosis: prevalence and prognosis in patients undergoing surgical aortic valve replacement. Circ Cardiovasc Imaging 2016;9(8) [pii:e005066].

41. Osnabrugge RL, Kappetein AP, Serruys PW. Noncardiac surgery in patients with severe aortic stenosis: time to revise the guidelines? Eur Heart J 2014; 35(35):2346–8.

42. Calicchio F, Guarracino F, Giannini C, et al. Balloon aortic valvuloplasty before noncardiac surgery in severe aortic stenosis: a single-center experience. J Cardiovasc Med (Hagerstown) 2017;18(2): 109–13.

43. Kogoj P, Devjak R, Bunc M. Balloon aortic valvuloplasty (BAV) as a bridge to aortic valve replacement in cancer patients who require urgent non-cardiac surgery. Radiol Oncol 2014;48(1):62–6.

44. Levine MJ, Berman AD, Safian RD, et al. Palliation of valvular aortic stenosis by balloon valvuloplasty as preoperative preparation for noncardiac surgery. Am J Cardiol 1988;62(17):1309–10.

45. Orwat S, Diller GP, van Hagen IM, et al. Risk of pregnancy in moderate and severe aortic stenosis: from the multinational ROPAC registry. J Am Coll Cardiol 2016;68(16):1727–37.

46. Arias F, Pineda J. Aortic stenosis and pregnancy. J Reprod Med 1978;20(4):229–32.

47. Siu SC, Sermer M, Colman JM, et al. Prospective multicenter study of pregnancy outcomes in women with heart disease. Circulation 2001; 104(5):515–21.

48. Avila WS, Rossi EG, Ramires JA, et al. Pregnancy in patients with heart disease: experience with 1,000 cases. Clin Cardiol 2003;26(3):135–42.

49. Hameed A, Karaalp IS, Tummala PP, et al. The effect of valvular heart disease on maternal and fetal outcome of pregnancy. J Am Coll Cardiol 2001; 37(3):893–9.

50. Yap SC, Drenthen W, Pieper PG, et al. Risk of complications during pregnancy in women with congenital aortic stenosis. Int J Cardiol 2008;126(2):240–6.

51. Regitz-Zagrosek V, Roos-Hesselink JW, Bauersachs J, et al. 2018 ESC Guidelines for the management of cardiovascular diseases during pregnancy. Eur Heart J 2018;39(34):3165–241.

52. Baumgartner H, Hung J, Bermejo J, et al. Recommendations on the echocardiographic assessment of aortic valve stenosis: a focused update from the

European Association of Cardiovascular Imaging and the American Society of Echocardiography. J Am Soc Echocardiogr 2017;30(4):372–92.

53. Myerson SG, Mitchell AR, Ormerod OJ, et al. What is the role of balloon dilatation for severe aortic stenosis during pregnancy? J Heart Valve Dis 2005;14(2): 147–50.

54. Xia VW, Messerlian AK, Mackley J, et al. Successful epidural anesthesia for cesarean section in a parturient with severe aortic stenosis and a recent history of pulmonary edema: a case report. J Clin Anesth 2006;18(2):142–4.

55. Lopez MM, Guasch E, Schiraldi R, et al. Continuous spinal anaesthesia with minimally invasive haemodynamic monitoring for surgical hip repair in two patients with severe aortic stenosis. Braz J Anesthesiol 2016;66(1):82–5.

56. Lee SW, Khaw KS, Ngan Kee WD, et al. Haemodynamic effects from aortocaval compression at different angles of lateral tilt in non-labouring term pregnant women. Br J Anaesth 2012;109(6):950–6.

57. Fanning N, Balki M, Sermer M, et al. Noninvasive cardiac output monitoring during general anesthesia for cesarean delivery in a patient with severe aortic stenosis. Can J Anaesth 2011;58(9):837–41.

58. Sliwa K, Johnson MR, Zilla P, et al. Management of valvular disease in pregnancy: a global perspective. Eur Heart J 2015;36(18):1078–89.

59. American College of O, Gynecologists Committee on Obstetric P. ACOG Committee Opinion No. 421, November 2008: antibiotic prophylaxis for infective endocarditis. Obstet Gynecol 2008; 112(5):1193–4.

60. Nishimura RA, Otto CM, Bonow RO, et al. 2014 AHA/ACC guideline for the management of patients with valvular heart disease: a report of the American College of Cardiology/American Heart Association Task Force on practice guidelines. Circulation 2014; 129(23):e521–643.

61. Wilson W, Taubert KA, Gewitz M, et al. Prevention of infective endocarditis: guidelines from the American Heart Association: a guideline from the American Heart Association Rheumatic Fever, Endocarditis, and Kawasaki Disease Committee, Council on Cardiovascular Disease in the Young, and the Council on Clinical Cardiology, Council on Cardiovascular Surgery and Anesthesia, and the quality of care and outcomes research interdisciplinary working group. Circulation 2007;116(15): 1736–54.

Moving?

Printed and bound by CPI Group (UK) Ltd, Croydon, CR0 4YY

12/10/2024

01773358-0001